Innovative Medical Devices

By involving China and international experts in medical devices and allied technologies, the book series covers both original research and practical approaches to device innovation and aims to be served as an important reference to researchers and developers in medical devices and related fields. The book series include 7 topics, which are strategic frontiers, medical imaging, in vitro diagnosis, advanced therapeutics, medical rehabilitation, health promotion and biomedical materials.

The book series reflects the latest developments in the fields and is suitable for senior undergraduates, postgraduates, managers, and research and development engineers in medical devices companies and regulatory bodies, as well as medical students. The book series is also suitable for training in related topics.

Jingsong Li • Yu Tian • Tianshu Zhou

Healthcare Information Systems

Progress, Challenges and Future Directions

上海交通大學出版社
Shanghai Jiao Tong University Press

Springer

Jingsong Li
College of Biomedical Engineering and Instrumental Science
Zhejiang University
Hangzhou, P.R. China

Yu Tian
College of Biomedical Engineering and Instrumental Science
Zhejiang University
Hangzhou, P.R. China

Tianshu Zhou
Research Center for Data Hub and Security
Zhejiang Laboratory
Hangzhou, China

ISSN 2731-7730 ISSN 2731-7749 (electronic)
Innovative Medical Devices
ISBN 978-981-97-9550-5 ISBN 978-981-97-9551-2 (eBook)
https://doi.org/10.1007/978-981-97-9551-2

Jointly published with Shanghai Jiao Tong University Press
The print edition is not for sale in China (Mainland). Customers from China (Mainland) please order the print book from: Shanghai Jiao Tong University Press.

This Springer imprint is published by the registered company Springer Nature Singapore Pte Ltd.
The registered company address is: 152 Beach Road, #21-01/04 Gateway East, Singapore 189721, Singapore

Preface

Since the twenty-first century, information technology has developed rapidly, especially demonstrating immense potential in its cross-disciplinary integration with other fields. The increasing demand for medical care promotes the wide application of information technology in the field of medical care. Various medical health information systems have penetrated into all aspects of people's lives, exerting profound influences on institutional construction, clinical research and development, diagnosis and treatment, as well as lifestyles. Concurrently, the rapid development of medical health information systems has led to an explosive growth in medical health data. Socioeconomic growth, improved living standards, accelerated population aging, and shifts in the disease spectrum have expanded people's needs in the medical health field beyond mere "effective and accessible healthcare" to new horizons. Driven by new technologies and changing needs, health information systems are playing an increasingly important role in promoting the high-quality development of health services.

This book is based on the author's years of research experience and original achievements in the field of medical informatics, combined with practical work cases. It comprehensively and systematically introduces the latest research progress, challenges, and future development trends of various medical and health information systems. This book is divided into three parts, comprising a total of 12 chapters. Chapter 1 serves as an introduction, briefly outlining the formation, development, and typical research achievements of medical informatics. Chapters 2–8 systematically introduce relatively mature medical health information systems, including electronic medical record systems, laboratory information systems, picture archiving and communication systems, clinical decision support systems, Internet of medical things systems, telemedicine systems and mobile health systems, and public health information systems. Chapters 9–12, starting from big data technology and the evolution of medical informatization, introduce rapidly developing Internet hospitals, proactive health systems, and intelligent systems for medical and elderly care combination in the era of big data.

The compilation of this book has been greatly assisted by numerous experts and scholars from various fields. We sincerely express our gratitude for their care and support. During the compilation process, we have cited works and research findings from some scholars, and we offer our heartfelt thanks for their contributions.

Hangzhou, P.R. China Jingsong Li
Hangzhou, P.R. China Yu Tian
Hangzhou, China Tianshu Zhou

Contents

1 Introduction ... 1
1.1 Informatics ... 2
1.1.1 Overview of Information Theory ... 2
1.1.2 The Nature of Information ... 3
1.1.3 Information Systems ... 6
1.2 Medical Informatics ... 8
1.2.1 Overview of Medical Informatics ... 8
1.2.2 The Development History of Medical Informatics ... 10
1.2.3 The Role and Significance of Medical Informatics ... 12
1.3 Medical Informatization ... 15
1.3.1 Overview of Medical Information System ... 15
1.3.2 Current Research Status of Medical Information System at Home and Abroad ... 16
1.3.3 Development History of Medical Informatization ... 17
1.3.4 Framework of Medical Informatization System ... 22
1.3.5 Frontier Research in Medical Informatization ... 24
1.4 Summary ... 26
References ... 27

2 Electronic Medical Record Systems ... 29
2.1 Overview of Electronic Medical Record Systems ... 31
2.1.1 Electronic Medical Records and Electronic Medical Record Systems ... 31
2.1.2 Components of Electronic Medical Record Systems ... 31
2.1.3 Current Research on Electronic Medical Record Systems ... 35
2.1.4 Case Studies of Electronic Medical Record Systems ... 36
2.2 Main Functions of the Electronic Medical Record System ... 41
2.2.1 Medical Order Processing ... 41
2.2.2 Medical Record Editing ... 42
2.2.3 Nursing Business Support ... 44
2.2.4 Medical Record Browsing ... 45

2.3 Frontier Research on Electronic Medical Record Entry and Quality Control 46
2.3.1 Intelligent Assisted Entry of Electronic Medical Records . . . 46
2.3.2 Voice-Enabled Electronic Medical Records 47
2.3.3 Intelligent Quality Control of Electronic Medical Records 49
2.4 Frontiers in Electronic Medical Record Data Integration and Application 51
2.4.1 Construction of Clinical Data Centers 51
2.4.2 Clinical Data Center Services for Real-World Studies 54
2.4.3 Post-Market Research on Pharmaceutical Products Using Electronic Medical Records 56
2.4.4 EMR Services for Infectious Disease Early Warning 58
2.5 Frontier Research on Information Sharing of Electronic Medical Records 59
2.5.1 Framework for Information Sharing in Electronic Medical Record Systems 59
2.5.2 Regional Medical Electronic Medical Record Transformation 63
2.5.3 Transformation of Electronic Medical Records for Internet-Based Healthcare 65
2.6 Conclusion 68
References 68

3 Laboratory Information Systems 69
3.1 Overview of Laboratory Information Systems 70
3.1.1 Introduction to Laboratory Testing and Laboratory Testing Systems 70
3.1.2 Development History of Laboratory Information Systems 72
3.1.3 Current Research Status of Laboratory Information Systems Both Domestically and Internationally 74
3.2 Main Framework and Workflow of Laboratory Information Systems 76
3.2.1 Main Framework of Laboratory Information Systems 76
3.2.2 Workflow of Clinical Laboratory System 81
3.3 Case Analysis 83
3.3.1 Neusoft Smart Laboratory Information System 83
3.3.2 Shanghai Ruimei Examination Information System 85
3.4 Frontier Research on Clinical Laboratory Systems 86
3.4.1 Clinical Biological Sample Library 86
3.4.2 Miniaturized and Portable Point-of-Care Testing Equipment and Systems 90
3.4.3 Regional Test Center 93
3.5 Summary 94
References 94

4 Picture Archiving and Communication Systems 97
4.1 Overview of Picture Archiving and Communication Systems 98
4.1.1 Introduction to Picture Archiving and Communication Systems 98
4.1.2 Development History of Picture Archiving and Communication Systems. 100
4.1.3 Current Research Status of Picture Archiving and Communication Systems at Home and Abroad 102
4.1.4 Technological Development of Picture Archiving and Communication Systems. 103
4.2 DICOM Standard. 104
4.2.1 Overview of the DICOM Standard 104
4.2.2 Development History of the DICOM Standard 105
4.2.3 Introduction to DICOM 3.0 Standard 107
4.3 Main Functions and Key Technologies of Picture Archiving and Communication Systems. 111
4.3.1 Main Functions of Picture Archiving and Communication Systems. 111
4.3.2 Key Technologies of Picture Archiving and Communication Systems. 115
4.4 Cutting-Edge Research in Picture Archiving and Communication Systems. 120
4.4.1 Miniaturized and Mobile Imaging Devices and Systems . . . 120
4.4.2 Image Reconstruction and 3D Printing 122
4.4.3 Regional Imaging Center. 123
4.5 Summary 126
Reference 127

5 Clinical Decision Support Systems 129
5.1 Overview of Clinical Decision Support Systems. 130
5.1.1 Introduction to Clinical Decision Support Systems. 130
5.1.2 Classification of Clinical Decision Support Systems 133
5.1.3 Development History of Clinical Decision Support Systems 135
5.2 Construction Methods and Inference Algorithms of Clinical Decision Support Systems 138
5.2.1 Construction Methods of Clinical Decision Support Systems 138
5.2.2 Inference Algorithms of Clinical Decision Support Systems 142
5.3 Case Studies of Clinical Decision Support Systems 150
5.3.1 MYCIN 150
5.3.2 Dxplain. 152
5.3.3 SimuConsult. 152
5.3.4 CADUCEUS 152
5.3.5 ISABEL 153

5.4 Frontier Research in Clinical Decision Support Systems 153
5.4.1 Multimodal Fusion Assisted Diagnosis 153
5.4.2 Disease Prognosis Prediction and Risk Factor Warning 156
5.4.3 Shared Decision-Making and Health Management 158
5.4.4 Assisted Precision Screening for Rare and Genetic Diseases 159
5.5 Summary 161
References 162

6 Internet of Medical Things Systems 163
6.1 Overview of Internet of Medical Things Systems 164
6.1.1 Introduction to Internet of Medical Things and Internet of Medical Things Systems 164
6.1.2 Development History of Internet of Medical Things Systems 165
6.1.3 Current Research Status of Internet of Medical Things at Home and Abroad 167
6.2 Main Functions and Applications of Internet of Medical Things Systems 170
6.2.1 Patient Management 171
6.2.2 Remote Monitoring 171
6.2.3 Medication Management 172
6.2.4 Hospital Supplies Management 173
6.2.5 Hospital Logistics Personnel Management 174
6.3 Case Studies 175
6.3.1 Application of In-Hospital Medical Supplies Management 175
6.3.2 Application in Public Health Management 177
6.4 Frontiers in Medical Internet of Things Research 179
6.4.1 5G Smart Wards 179
6.4.2 Unmanned Material Distribution 180
6.5 Summary 182

7 Telemedicine Systems and Mobile Health Systems 183
7.1 Overview of Telemedicine Systems and Mobile Health Systems 184
7.1.1 Introduction to Telemedicine Systems and Mobile Health Systems 184
7.1.2 Introduction to Mobile Health and Mobile Health Systems 185
7.1.3 Development History 186
7.1.4 Current Status of Research Domestically and Internationally 188
7.2 Components and Related Technologies of Telemedicine Systems 190
7.2.1 Composition and Functions of Telemedicine Systems 190
7.2.2 Technologies Related to Telemedicine 192

7.3 Mobile Health System Compositions and Related Technologies . . . 194
7.3.1 Composition and Functions of Mobile Health Systems 194
7.3.2 Mobile Health-Related Technologies 195
7.4 Case Studies 197
7.4.1 Case Studies of Telemedicine Systems 197
7.4.2 Mobile Healthcare System Case Study 198
7.5 Frontier Research 199
7.5.1 Advancements in Data Exchange Technology 199
7.5.2 Virtual Reality Remote Surgery 201
7.5.3 5G Pre-hospital Emergency Care 203
7.6 Summary 204
References 205

8 Public Health Information Systems 207
8.1 Overview of Public Health Information Systems 208
8.1.1 Introduction to Public Health Information Systems 208
8.1.2 Development History of Public Health Information Systems 210
8.1.3 Current State of Domestic and International Research on Public Health Information Systems 213
8.2 Data Sources and Architectural Composition of Public Health Information Systems 215
8.2.1 Data Sources of Public Health Information Systems 215
8.2.2 Architectural Composition of Public Health Information Systems 218
8.3 Public Health Information Systems and Personal Health Statistics 223
8.3.1 Comprehensive and Lifelong Personal Electronic Health Records 223
8.3.2 Population Statistics Analysis 227
8.3.3 Health Statistics Analysis 229
8.4 Case Study 231
8.4.1 CDC's INPHO System in the USA 231
8.4.2 Australia's Public Health Information System Response to the COVID-19 Transition 232
8.4.3 Infectious Disease Surveillance and Early Warning Platform Based on Big Data in Yinzhou District, Ningbo City 233
8.5 Cutting-Edge Research 236
8.5.1 Early Warning and Efficient Response to Emerging Major Infectious Diseases 236
8.5.2 Identification of Occupational Health Risk Factors 240
8.5.3 Public Health Event Early Warning Based on Social Networks 244
8.6 Summary 246
References 247

9 Big Data Technology and Healthcare Informatics 249
9.1 Overview of Big Data Technologies 250
9.1.1 Introduction to Big Data 250
9.1.2 Introduction to Big Data Technology 252
9.1.3 Medical Information Systems Require Big Data Technology 254
9.1.4 Development of Big Data Technology in Medical Information Systems 255
9.2 Fundamental Technologies of Medical Big Data 257
9.2.1 Data Storage Management 257
9.2.2 Efficient Data Processing 258
9.2.3 Data Analysis Techniques 259
9.2.4 Data Visualization 260
9.3 Construction of Medical Big Data Platform 263
9.3.1 Platform Construction Philosophy 263
9.3.2 Big Data Platform Ecosystem 264
9.3.3 Big Data Platform Implementation Standards 268
9.4 Case Analysis 270
9.4.1 Medical Information System Based on Cloud Platform . . . 270
9.4.2 Multi-Center Intelligent Medical Information Platform . . . 271
9.5 Summary 274
References 274

10 Internet Hospitals 275
10.1 Overview of Internet Hospitals 276
10.1.1 Introduction to Internet Hospitals 276
10.1.2 Development History of Internet Hospitals 276
10.1.3 Current Status of Internet Hospitals Domestically and Internationally 277
10.2 Internet Hospital Technology System 279
10.2.1 Internet Hospital Technology Framework 279
10.2.2 Internet Hospital System Framework 280
10.2.3 Main Functions and Implementation of Internet Hospitals 281
10.2.4 Interconnection with In-Hospital Systems 281
10.2.5 Security Construction of Internet Hospitals 282
10.3 Internet Hospital Service Model 283
10.3.1 Online Consultation 283
10.3.2 Online Prescription 284
10.3.3 Hierarchical Medical System 284
10.4 Issues in the Development of Internet Hospitals 285
10.4.1 Potential Security Risks 285
10.4.2 Operational Difficulties 286
10.4.3 Talent Scarcity 287
10.4.4 Relevant Laws and Policies 287

10.5 Case Studies . . . 289
10.5.1 Implementation of Physical Community Internet Hospitals . . . 289
10.5.2 Innovative Internet Hospital Combining Tertiary Hospitals and Internet Enterprises . . . 291
10.5.3 Role of Internet Hospitals During the COVID-19 Pandemic . . . 291
10.6 Summary . . . 293

11 Proactive Health Systems . . . 295
11.1 Overview of Proactive Health Technology . . . 296
11.1.1 Concept of Proactive Health . . . 296
11.1.2 Overview of Proactive Health Systems . . . 298
11.1.3 The Development History of Proactive Health . . . 300
11.2 Key Technologies for Proactive Health . . . 301
11.2.1 Proactive Health Monitoring Technology . . . 301
11.2.2 Health Status Identification and Risk Warning Technology . . . 303
11.2.3 Proactive Health Intervention and Management Techniques . . . 305
11.3 Case Analysis . . . 307
11.3.1 Intelligent Health Management Systems . . . 307
11.3.2 Digital Health Family Service Systems . . . 308
11.4 Summary . . . 310

12 Intelligent Systems for Medical and Elderly Care Combination . . . 311
12.1 Overview of Integrated Medical and Care Intelligent Systems . . 312
12.1.1 Concept of Integrated Medical and Care . . . 312
12.1.2 Concept of Integrated Medical and Care Intelligent Systems . . . 313
12.1.3 Current Status of Integrated Medical and Care Intelligent Systems . . . 314
12.1.4 Development History of Integrated Medical and Care Intelligent Systems . . . 315
12.2 Main Functions and Applications of Integrated Medical and Care Intelligent Systems . . . 316
12.2.1 Telemedicine . . . 316
12.2.2 Health Risk Assessment and Health Plan Development . 317
12.2.3 Assisted Chronic Disease Management . . . 318
12.2.4 Health Education . . . 318
12.2.5 Dietary and Medication Guidance . . . 319
12.2.6 Community Care . . . 319
12.3 Key Technologies of Integrated Medical and Nursing Care Intelligent Systems . . . 320

12.3.1 Comprehensive Assessment and Chronic Disease Risk Assessment for the Elderly 320
12.3.2 Aging-Friendly Human–Computer Interaction Technology. 323
12.4 Case Studies. 325
12.4.1 Case Study: Zhejiang Elderly Care Hospital 325
12.4.2 Elderly Health Intervention and Management Technology. 326
12.4.3 Smart Health and Care System Integrating Medical Treatment and Elderly Care 327
12.5 Summary 329
References. 329

Introduction 1

Contents

1.1 Informatics ... 2
1.1.1 Overview of Information Theory ... 2
1.1.2 The Nature of Information ... 3
1.1.2.1 Introduction to the Nature of Information ... 3
1.1.2.2 Information, Messages, Signals, Data, and Knowledge ... 5
1.1.3 Information Systems ... 6
1.1.3.1 Source ... 7
1.1.3.2 Transmitter ... 7
1.1.3.3 Receiver ... 7
1.1.3.4 Channel ... 7
1.1.3.5 Destination ... 7
1.1.3.6 Noise and Interference ... 7
1.2 Medical Informatics ... 8
1.2.1 Overview of Medical Informatics ... 8
1.2.2 The Development History of Medical Informatics ... 10
1.2.3 The Role and Significance of Medical Informatics ... 12
1.3 Medical Informatization ... 15
1.3.1 Overview of Medical Information System ... 15
1.3.2 Current Research Status of Medical Information System at Home and Abroad ... 16
1.3.3 Development History of Medical Informatization ... 17
1.3.3.1 Typical International Representatives ... 20
1.3.3.2 Domestic Representatives ... 21
1.3.4 Framework of Medical Informatization System ... 22
1.3.5 Frontier Research in Medical Informatization ... 24
1.3.5.1 Smart Hospitals ... 24
1.3.5.2 Big Data Management ... 25
1.4 Summary ... 26
References ... 27

J. Li et al., *Healthcare Information Systems*, Innovative Medical Devices,
https://doi.org/10.1007/978-981-97-9551-2_1

In the 1940s, three fundamental theories were proposed that would profoundly influence both the natural and social sciences: systems theory, information theory, and cybernetics [1]. These are collectively celebrated as the "three great theories of the twentieth century." Information theory, in particular, systematically and scientifically introduced basic theories such as information system, information entropy, and data compression, which are crucial for information processing. As we entered the twenty-first century, with rapid advancements in computer science and materials science, the avenues for information acquisition expanded, the magnitude of information grew, and the types of information became more diverse, underscoring the increasing importance of information theory to human development. Undoubtedly, the twenty-first century is the information age.

With the implementation of electronic medical record (EMR), hospital information system (HIS), laboratory information system (LIS), and picture archiving and communication system (PACS) in hospitals, the medical field has become an intensely information-rich sector. By 2013, a medium-sized Chinese city with a population of about one million had accumulated financial data, medical images, surgery recordings, videos, and health records amounting to 10 petabytes over 50 years. The information gleaned from processing this data is innumerable. Medical informatics was born against this backdrop, guided by information theory to analyze vast amounts of medical data to extract valuable medical information. This facilitates clinical decision-making, patient health management, and public health monitoring.

This chapter will provide a brief introduction to the formation, development, and significant research achievements of medical informatics from three perspectives: informatics, medical informatics, and medical informatization.

1.1 Informatics

Informatics, formerly known as information science, focuses on information as its primary subject of study. This field encompasses the analysis, collection, classification, processing, storage, retrieval, dissemination, and protection of information.

1.1.1 Overview of Information Theory

People had a vague idea of information as early as the early nineteenth century when many scientists were working on how to transmit and process waveforms. Notable contributions came from American physicist Harry Nyquist, who made significant advances in areas such as thermal noise, stability of feedback amplifiers, and facsimile transmission. Another scientist, R.V.L. Hartley, proposed using the formula NlgD for measuring information. However, a comprehensive and systematic understanding of how to convert messages into transmittable waveforms (information) had not yet been developed. A major breakthrough occurred in October 1948 when Claude Elwood Shannon published "A Mathematical Theory of

Communication" in the *Bell System Technical Journal*. Building on the theoretical work of Nyquist and others, Shannon defined information as a description of the uncertainty of the motion state or existence mode of things. He expanded Hartley's formula to account for situations with different probabilities. The publication of this paper marked the beginning of modern information theory research, earning Shannon the title "Father of Information Theory" [2].

One of the key components of information theory is the measurement of information, most famously through the concept of entropy. Originally a concept in physics, entropy measures the disorder or randomness within a thermodynamic system. The physicist Boltzmann once described entropy as a measure of the information that is lost. Shannon built upon this concept to define "information entropy" as the average amount of information contained in each message received. This concept is also known as source entropy, average self-information, or Shannon entropy. Shannon argued that the greater the randomness of the source, the higher the entropy, because more information is provided when an improbable event occurs. For example, the outcome of a coin toss (with two equally likely outcomes) conveys less information (lower entropy) than the outcome of a dice roll (with six equally likely outcomes). Entropy is typically measured in bits, which are the smallest units of information. From Shannon's foundational work, the academic and industrial communities have developed many other measures of information, including conditional entropy (the remaining entropy of a random variable Y given the known value of another random variable X), joint entropy (a measure of the uncertainty of a set of variables), and mutual information (a measure of the dependency between variables).

As communication technologies have rapidly advanced, the definition of information has expanded beyond Shannon's original scope. It now includes theories on weak signal detection, estimation theory, modulation, and signal processing. The broader view of information theory analyzes signals from both objective and subjective perspectives, covering the entire process from acquisition to utilization. Unlike Shannon's information theory, which was confined to electronic communications, the generalized theory encompasses related fields such as psychology, linguistics, semantics, and cybernetics. The relationship between information theory and these fields is depicted in Fig. 1.1. However, because it incorporates subjective elements, this broader interpretation of information theory is still evolving and has not yet achieved a comprehensive, reasonable explanation. Therefore, information theory is generally still considered in the narrow sense proposed by Shannon.

1.1.2 The Nature of Information

1.1.2.1 Introduction to the Nature of Information

Here, we primarily discuss the characteristics of information: abstraction, universality, representativeness, supportiveness, transmissibility, compressibility, transformability, and timeliness, among others.

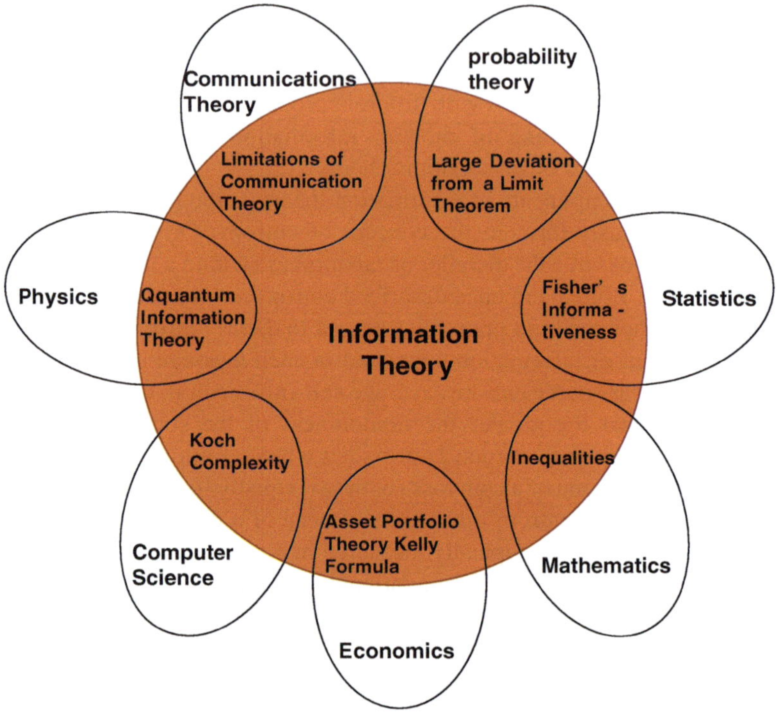

Fig. 1.1 Relationship between information theory and other fields

Abstraction

Information is abstract. Unlike tangible materials or energy, which can be considered a form of material motion, information represents a new level in the process of human understanding and transforming the world. Humans acquire information through thinking and processing material with the brain and use this information to guide production and everyday life. Information permeates all aspects of life; it can be measured, shared, held by a few, or known by many. The essence of information has long been a hot topic of research in both the philosophical and scientific communities.

Universality

Information is ubiquitous. The process of any object's motion can generate information, making it omnipresent. For example, the expressions of joy, anger, sorrow, or pleasure on a person's face convey information about their mood to others.

Representativeness

Information can be seen as a representation of the universal attributes of objective entities. Humans process the attributes of external objects through the brain, forming information that is stored in the mind. Different information is represented in various ways, such as through text, images, and audio.

Supportiveness

Information must be carried by some form of matter to be manifested. For instance, in the historical anecdote "beacons play the princes," the urgent military alert about an enemy invasion was conveyed through the lighting of beacons. Thus, matter is the foundation for the existence of information.

Transmissibility

The value of information is realized through its transmission, sharing, or dissemination. George Bernard Shaw famously illustrated this with his "apple theory": If you have an apple and I have an apple, and we exchange these apples, we each still only have one apple. But if you have an idea and I have an idea, and we exchange these ideas, each of us ends up with two ideas.

Compressibility

Information is compressible. In the real world, to ensure the efficient and rapid transmission of large amounts of information, it often needs to be compressed. Common compression formats include lossless compression (such as ZIP format) and lossy compression (such as MP3 and JPEG formats). After compression, the entropy of information increases.

Transformability

Information can be transformed. To fully utilize information, it often needs to be converted into different representational forms. For example, in a clinical decision support system for rational drug use, if there is an irrational combination of two drugs in a patient's current prescription, this information can be alerted to doctors or nurses in various forms such as interface warning pop-ups or alarm sounds.

Timeliness

Information has timeliness. The timeliness of information refers to the interval and efficiency from when information is sent from the source to when it is received, processed, transmitted, and utilized. The shorter the time interval, the more timely the use of the information, the higher the degree of usage, and the stronger the timeliness.

1.1.2.2 Information, Messages, Signals, Data, and Knowledge

In discussions about information, there is often confusion among the concepts of information, messages, signals, data, and knowledge. These concepts are fundamentally distinct, and their relationships are illustrated in Fig. 1.2.

Information is an abstract entity that is implicit within messages and can change the knowledge state of the receiver or their uncertainty about something.

Messages consist of independent units of communication conveyed from a sender to one or more recipients. Messages can be transmitted in various ways,

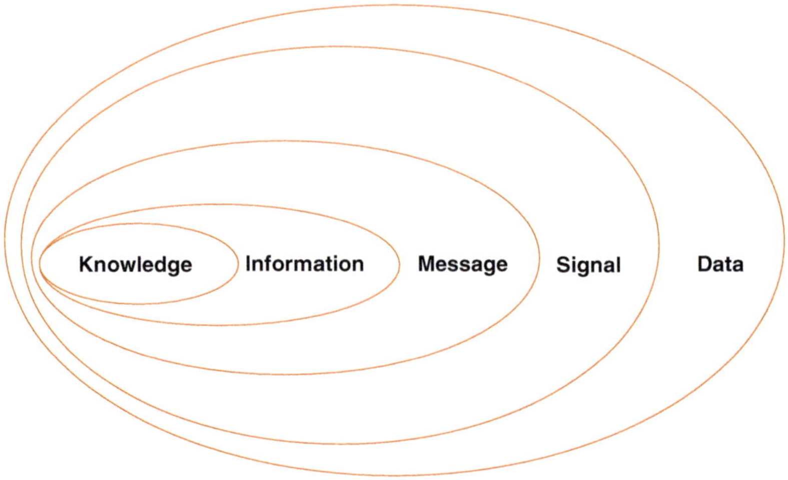

Fig. 1.2 Information, messages, signals, data, and knowledge

including via couriers, newspapers, and data cables. By transmitting messages, uncertainty is reduced, and information is obtained. It can be said that messages are carriers of information, but they lack physical properties, making them challenging to transmit.

Signals are the physical manifestations of messages. In the process of message transmission, engineers often need to digitize and modulate messages through a series of processing steps, converting them into discrete physical quantities for transmission. Signals serve as the physical carriers of information.

Data is obtained through observation as numerical characteristics or information, containing information useful to people. However, a considerable portion of data content is redundant, which can be expressed as: Data = Information + Redundant Data. The focus and challenge for data scientists today is how to extract information from data.

Knowledge is an understanding of the regularities of things, derived from further processing of information. Typically, knowledge lacks timeliness. It is verified, correct, and widely believed information.

1.1.3 Information Systems

An information system is a fundamental model and the primary subject of study in information theory. Information systems process and transmit information to ensure the reliability and accuracy of information transmission. The structure of an information system is illustrated in Fig. 1.3.

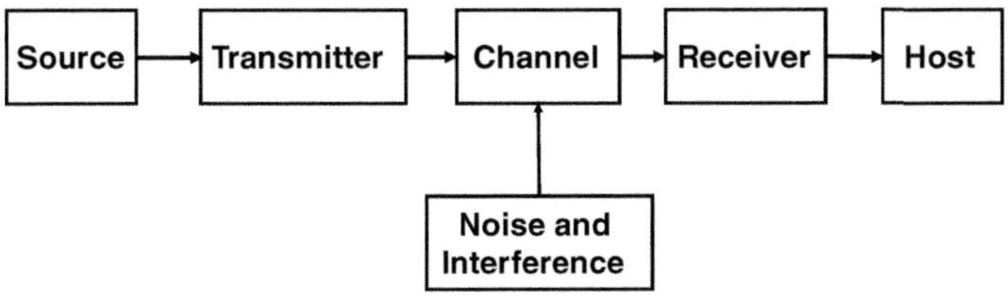

Fig. 1.3 Structure of an information system

1.1.3.1 Source

The source is the originator of messages, which can be either a person or an object. It generates messages that are transmitted to the destination. There are various types of messages, such as letter sequences in telegrams, telephone calls, or functions.

1.1.3.2 Transmitter

The transmitter converts messages into a suitable form for transmission and sends them through the channel.

1.1.3.3 Receiver

The receiver has the opposite function to the transmitter; it primarily aims to restore the signals transmitted through the channel back to their original message form as accurately as possible.

1.1.3.4 Channel

The channel is the medium through which signals are transmitted. It could be electrical wires, coaxial cables, radio frequencies, optical fibers, etc.

1.1.3.5 Destination

The destination (receiver) is the recipient of the message and the target of the information transmission, which can be either a person or an object.

1.1.3.6 Noise and Interference

Information systems often operate in noisy environments. Common sources of noise and interference include white noise and Gaussian noise. White noise is a random signal or process with a constant power spectral density, while Gaussian noise has a probability density function that follows a normal distribution (also known as Gaussian distribution).

Building on this basic structure, the engineering field has developed models for analog and digital information systems based on whether the source outputs analog or digital signals, primarily involving adjustments to the transmitters and receivers. In analog information systems, the transmitter is composed of a signal converter and a modulator, while the receiver consists of a demodulator and a signal converter. Analog information systems mainly process analog signals directly in the time or frequency domain (such as amplification, filtering, and modulation) before transmission and perform band processing and demodulation at the receiving end to restore the signal to its original form. The digital information system model, which involves converting analog signals into digital signals, requires that the messages output by the source undergo compression and encryption encoding, converting the messages into digital sequences to enhance communication efficiency and transmission security. Additionally, this system applies channel coding to the digital sequences, employing error control coding and code conversion to resist noise interference from the channel, thereby providing some error detection capabilities. Similarly, at the receiving end, the system includes channel and source decoders to decode the signals, essentially reversing the encoding process to restore the signals back to their original state.

1.2 Medical Informatics

1.2.1 Overview of Medical Informatics

Medical informatics is an interdisciplinary field that primarily uses information technology to study medical information. The sources and types of medical information are incredibly diverse, with common sources including in-hospital electronic medical records, clinical notes, medical imaging, and medical trials, as well as external sources like health insurance claims and medical research literature. The diverse origins of medical information also result in various forms, including textual information from medical journals, medical reports, prescriptions, and medical orders; structured data from medical trials and public health surveys; image information from electrocardiograms, magnetic resonance imaging (MRI), and computer tomography (CT) scans; and audio data from cardiac or respiratory sound examinations [1].

The definition of medical informatics has been articulated in various ways within the academic community. At the Third World Conference on Medical Informatics (Medinfo 80) held in Tokyo in 1980, medical informatics was defined as "the discipline that applies computer technology to all fields of medicine—healthcare, medical education, and medical research." Both Jan H. van Bemmel, a former president of the American Medical Informatics Association, and Edward H. Shortliffe have offered definitions of medical informatics. Bemmel views medical informatics as consisting of two aspects: information processing and communication theory and applications, with the subject matter being the knowledge and experience obtained through the healthcare process. Shortliffe sees medical informatics as an emerging, rapidly developing interdisciplinary field that studies the information, data, and knowledge in biomedicine, collecting, storing, presenting, and retrieving its patterns, which can be used for decision-making and problem-solving in health management, clinical diagnosis and treatment, and knowledge analysis [3–4].

Although definitions of medical informatics vary, it is evident that the field has evolved in response to advances in medicine and has increasingly intersected and integrated with computer science, healthcare, and data science. It primarily explores how information technology can be optimally applied in environments such as patient care, clinical diagnosis and treatment, and clinical research.

The application areas of medical informatics are extremely broad, ranging from cellular-level studies such as the processing of biological signals, to organ-level studies like MRI and CT image analysis, to individual-level studies including electronic medical records, institutional-level research like digital hospitals, and societal-level studies such as public health information systems. Common information technologies used include signal processing analysis, medical imaging technology, networking, communications technology, and artificial intelligence.

In the information field, concepts such as medical informatics, bioinformatics, biomedical informatics, and health informatics are often confused. In reality, these concepts have different focuses, as shown in Table 1.1.

Table 1.1 Distinctions between concepts related to medical informatics

Concepts	Research subjects	Research purposes	Research directions
Medical informatics	Mainly focuses on the information generated during medical research, clinical diagnosis and treatment, and medical management	To study the nature, acquisition, conversion, coding, transmission, control, and application of medical information to solve problems in the medical field	Medical information systems, medical big data, medical artificial intelligence, etc.
Bioinformatics	Mainly focuses on the transmission of biological information, such as genetic information, gene group information, and protein group information	To study the storage, transmission, and expression of information in biological systems and processes, especially in terms of biological data, to explore the mysteries of life inheritance	Sequence comparison, biochips, biological computing, etc.
Biomedical informatics	The scope is relatively broad, covering both biological and medical information	To study how to translate the results of basic research, such as gene and protein expression processes, into clinical applications	Precision medicine, translational medicine, integrated biomedical research information systems, etc.
Health informatics	Mainly involves all information produced and applied by healthcare providers	To study the acquisition, storage, retrieval, and use of healthcare information to ensure optimal collaboration between patients and healthcare providers	Wearable health technology, mobile health, medical education, etc.

1.2.2 The Development History of Medical Informatics

Medical informatics is a "young" discipline that originated in the 1950s. In 1946, the University of Pennsylvania in the United States invented the world's first general-purpose computer, "ENIAC." With the advent of computers, people began to apply them to the medical field. In 1950, Professor Robert Steven Ledley in the United States applied computers to dentistry to help dentists determine the chewing angle of teeth, marking the earliest application of computer technology in medicine. As the cross-application of computer science and medicine became increasingly common, many medical literature at the time used terms such as "medical computer science," "biomedical computing," and "medical information science" to refer to the application of information technology in medicine. At that time, medical informatics had not yet fully developed into an independent discipline. During this period, significant achievements in medical informatics included the development of the MYCIN system at Stanford University (a decision support system for the treatment of bacteremia, which was the first rule-based reasoning decision support system), the INTERNIST I system developed at the University of Pittsburgh (a system used to guide internists in prescribing medication), and the Massachusetts General Hospital Utility Multi-Programming System (MUMPS) developed by the Octo Barnett Laboratory in the United States.

Due to the increasingly rich research results and the continuous proposal of related theories, Western countries formally proposed in the 1970s to designate "medical informatics" as an independent discipline and began teaching this discipline in universities. In 1967, the International Medical Informatics Association (IMIA) was established. In 1974, the first volume of the IFIP Transactions on Medical Informatics, titled "Education of Health Care Personnel in Informatics," was published, marking the first use of "medical informatics" as a professional term. In 1976, the journal *Medical Informatics* was founded. Bleich and Slack established the first clinical informatics department at Harvard Medical School. In 1982, Shortliffe began a graduate program in medical informatics at Stanford University. Since then, the education of medical informatics has developed rapidly. Universities in many European and American countries have set up medical informatics programs, cultivating a large number of professionals in the field and producing many significant research results and theories. For example, van Bemmel proposed the structural framework of medical informatics, providing a foundation for understanding the methodological and technical knowledge required for this discipline. Reichertz discussed the functions and architectural perspectives of hospital information systems. The Institute of Medicine proposed methods for converting paper medical records to electronic records and first demonstrated the clinical application value of electronic health records (EHRs). In addition, the standardization of medical informatics research began, with the formulation of standards such as Health Level Seven (HL7), Logical Observation Identifiers Names and Codes (LOINC), and Systematized Nomenclature of Medicine-Clinical Terms (SNOMED CT), which standardized medical information practices and improved the interoperability and data usability of information systems [5].

The development of medical informatics in China started relatively late, initially focusing mainly on medical intelligence research and related fields. In 1980, the China Medical Informatics Association (CMIA) was established. In 1994, the Medical Informatics Branch of the Chinese Medical Association was founded. In 1995, the Ministry of Health proposed the "Golden Health Project," initiating the construction of a national medical information backbone and a local area network for medical and health information management.

Regarding talent education, from 1985 to 1987, China approved the establishment of medical library and information science programs at Tongji Medical University (now Tongji Medical College of Huazhong University of Science and Technology), Bethune Medical University (now Bethune Medical College of Jilin University), China Medical University, and Hunan Medical University (now Xiangya School of Medicine, Central South University). This marked the beginning of medical informatics education in China. In 2003, "Medical Informatics" officially became a discipline outside the higher education professional directory. By 2009, more than 40 colleges and universities had been filed or approved by the Ministry of Education to offer information management and information system programs or medical informatics programs aimed at the medical and health fields.

In recent years, with the continuous advancement of medical informatization in China, the gap between China and Western countries has been steadily narrowing. In 2019, the sudden outbreak of the novel coronavirus pneumonia (COVID-19) saw China quickly utilize informatization methods to conduct high-risk population screening, develop information collection systems for hospital visitors, and pre-examination and triage screening systems, effectively streamlining outpatient services in emergency departments and respiratory clinics. Some hospitals also launched online free consultation clinics, convenient online outpatient services, and online drug delivery services, providing comprehensive and intelligent medical services through multiple channels. Hangzhou was the first to introduce the "health code" for screening the movement and health status of the city's population. This code was gradually promoted nationwide, helping the country to scientifically and orderly resume work and production activities. This series of rapid and efficient information utilization methods was based on the accumulation of China's medical informatization achievements over the years, and the success of China's anti-epidemic efforts received high praise from both domestic and international communities. World Health Organization (WHO) Director-General Tedros Adhanom Ghebreyesus commented that "China's actions in response to the epidemic are admirable."

Currently, with the continuous development of information technology and medicine, medical informatization has entered a new stage. New technologies such as artificial intelligence algorithms, knowledge graphs, and mobile Internet of Things are continuously being applied in the medical field, with more and more medical information products being approved for clinical use to improve clinical practice. It is believed that in the future, medical informatics will further promote the development of human health.

1.2.3 The Role and Significance of Medical Informatics

The main roles of medical informatics can be summarized as follows:

1. Providing theoretical guidance for clinical applications, education, and research in medicine. As an interdisciplinary field, medical informatics cannot directly apply the theories of computer science or other disciplines due to the unique characteristics of the healthcare industry. Instead, it requires modification and organic integration to guide relevant practitioners in developing and using tools. For example, Shortliffe developed the world's first rule-based clinical decision support system (CDSS). He separated the patient information database from the knowledge base, creating a CDSS that utilized taxonomy to construct the knowledge base, which accelerated searches and improved efficiency. This CDSS construction model has become a reference for many experts in building their own CDSS. Additionally, facing the heterogeneity of medical data and processes, HL7 FHIR (Fast Healthcare Interoperability Resources) was proposed. It integrates web standards from the computing field and the advantages of previous HL7 V2, V3, and Clinical Document Architecture (CDA). It uses tags, metadata, basic languages, and inherent rules to describe and define various concepts involved in medical processes, such as diagnoses, treatments, examinations, and roles like patients, doctors, and nurses. This helps different systems recognize and understand the true meanings of these medical concepts and data, and its modular assembly method efficiently handles interoperability issues among complex and diverse information systems in healthcare institutions.
2. Modernizing medical science through the application of standardized, intelligent, automated, and digitized information methods. In today's information society, the development of information technology has brought solutions to many problems that have troubled medical experts. For instance, issues such as uneven regional development of healthcare, grassroots medical institutions unable to meet the needs of local populations, and difficulty in quickly mobilizing medical resources during public health emergencies can be addressed through telemedicine, which leverages communication technology, audio and video technology, and virtual reality (VR) technology. This can improve the diagnostic and treatment capabilities of grassroots medical institutions and help alleviate the imbalance in the distribution of medical resources between urban and rural areas. At the same time, the development of sensor technology enables patients to monitor certain health indicators anytime and anywhere, assisting doctors in follow-up work. Information technology has turned many previous "impossibilities" in medicine into "possibilities," driving the rapid development of the medical field.
3. Utilizing accumulated medical data for data mining to promote the generation and discovery of new medical knowledge. The development of medical devices and software has expanded the scope of human perception, enabling healthcare professionals to observe more changes in the structure and tissues of the human body, make accurate decisions and diagnoses, and provide data assurance for

medical informatics experts to discover new knowledge through data-driven methods. Especially in the field of drug repurposing, since the development of new drugs is an extremely time-consuming, labor-intensive, and high-risk process, requiring an average of 10–15 years and $800 million to $1.5 billion from concept to market approval, the accumulation of large drug databases provides a foundation for discovering new uses for existing drugs. Therefore, many pharmaceutical companies are researching how to use computer-assisted drug repurposing. For example, Liu et al. used causal inference and machine learning algorithms to simulate randomized clinical trials in large-scale medical claims databases, successfully identifying drugs and drug combinations that significantly improve coronary artery disease but are not yet used for treatment. During the COVID-19 pandemic, many researchers used artificial intelligence methods to study drug repurposing of existing antiviral drugs for severe acute respiratory syndrome (SARS), Middle East respiratory syndrome (MERS), AIDS, and malaria, quickly identifying candidate drugs such as favipiravir and tocilizumab and conducting clinical trials on them. Information technology allows doctors to discover new patterns from large amounts of data, accelerating the progress of medical research [6, 7].

The significance of medical informatics mainly includes the following aspects:

1. Improving the Quality of Patient Care and Healthcare: With the explosive growth of medical theories and the increasing number of patient visits, doctors face problems such as high information load and repetitive labor intensity, which makes them prone to errors in actual diagnosis and treatment. Clinical decision support systems (CDSS) can help doctors solve these problems. Based on vast knowledge bases, CDSS can alert doctors and patients to potential adverse reactions to medications and surgeries, provide key points for differential diagnoses and treatment plans, and predict future disease risks for patients. The development of mobile health also promotes patient participation in the diagnostic and treatment process, enhancing their understanding of their diseases and health management. For example, CloudMedX, a well-known healthcare data collection and analysis service provider, conducted an experiment in hospitals to predict patient readmission risks. The results showed that their algorithm could help hospitals reduce the readmission rate by 30%, significantly improving healthcare quality.
2. Reducing Hospital Operating Costs: One of the earliest applications of medical informatics in hospitals was in billing and charge management. Medical information systems can assist hospitals in refined management, providing an automated, comprehensive management system that covers all business processes, addressing common issues in hospital operations such as slow information transmission and unclear process relationships and service entities. They help standardize the management of medical supplies and equipment and regularly calculate and analyze hospital financial costs, thereby reducing hospital maintenance costs. Additionally, by helping doctors reduce diagnostic errors and

improve healthcare quality, medical informatics can shorten patient hospital stays and lower service costs. Researchers have found that DXplain can help medical centers save more than $two million annually.

3. Accelerating the Discovery of New Medical Knowledge: There are many undiscovered patterns in vast amounts of medical data. Finding these hidden patterns using information technology is a hot topic in current research. Literature-based discovery involves using computer data to find new relationships between existing knowledge based on literature and other data. This has led to extensive research in drug discovery, drug repurposing, and adverse drug reactions. Statistics show that about 30% of new uses for drugs and vaccines developed through drug repurposing are approved by the US FDA (Food and Drug Administration). Furthermore, traditional Chinese medicine (TCM) differs from modern medicine, as TCM includes philosophical concepts such as yin-yang theory and the five elements theory. Many researchers use TCM knowledge to find relationships between diseases and genes. For example, Shen et al. identified genes related to kidney yang deficiency syndrome and successfully determined one of the genes, c1q-related factors.
4. Assisting in the Training of Medical Professionals: Some medical information systems have large-scale knowledge bases and medical rule databases. These databases are built based on a large amount of medical literature, medical guidelines, expert consensus, and authoritative textbooks, often possessing reliable differential diagnostic capabilities. They can be used as educational tools for medical students for simulation and learning. For instance, the well-known clinical decision support system DXplain is a common educational tool in American medical schools, widely used in clinical physician training. Many studies have shown that diagnostic decision support tools have a significant beneficial impact on the quality of differential diagnosis and management plans for first-year residents [8, 9].
5. Assisting Hospitals and Government Agencies in Scientific Decision-Making: The popularization of information technology in medicine has changed the traditional mode of manual data reporting in the medical field, achieving rapid and automatic data uploading. The statistical tools integrated into medical information systems also provide reliable evidence for managers and leaders in formulating and implementing decisions. Since the SARS epidemic in 2003, China has strengthened the construction of public health information systems centered on infectious disease and public health emergency surveillance and reporting. This system provides a guarantee for public health service management and emergency command in China. During the COVID-19 pandemic, Beijing, based on its public health information system, achieved a time of only 42 minutes from diagnosis in medical institutions to online reporting. The rapid collection of case data also provided a basis for the timely allocation and optimization of medical emergency resources in China.

1.3 Medical Informatization

1.3.1 Overview of Medical Information System

Medical information system (MIS) refers to information systems that combine biomedical and health science theories and methods with information technology to solve medical and health problems and provide support for clinical and management decisions. These systems are a generalized term for a variety of systems, with common examples including hospital information system (HIS), public health information system (PHIS), clinical decision support system (CDSS), and telemedicine system.

Hospital information system (HIS), also known as hospital management software (HMS) or hospital management system, refers to the use of modern technologies such as computer hardware and software, network communication technologies, and other advanced tools to comprehensively manage the flow of people, logistics, and financial resources within hospitals and their departments. These systems collect, store, process, extract, transmit, summarize, and generate various information from the data produced at each stage of medical activities, thereby providing comprehensive and automated management and service information for the overall operation of the hospital. Depending on the application area, HIS can be further divided into outpatient information system, inpatient information system, pharmaceutical information system, and medical management information system.

Public health information system (PHIS) utilizes computer technology, network technology, and communication technology to digitally collect, exchange, process, store, and retrieve information according to the application goals of various levels of public health departments, such as health administration, disease prevention and control, health supervision centers, and maternal and child health centers. PHIS can be classified into emergency command information system, community health service information system, disease prevention and control information system, among others, based on their purposes.

Clinical decision support system (CDSS) primarily assists in improving decision-making processes within clinical workflows, linking actual observations with medical knowledge to influence clinical doctors' decisions and subsequently improve healthcare. CDSS can be divided into knowledge-based and non-knowledge-based types.

Telemedicine system utilizes remote communication technology, audio and video technology, and presence technology to provide medical information services. Depending on their functions, telemedicine systems can be further classified into teleconsultation system, remote consultation system, remote monitoring system, and remote education system.

1.3.2 Current Research Status of Medical Information System at Home and Abroad

The early development of medical information systems (MIS) is closely related to the development of database technology. It originated in the 1960s when mainframe-based hospital information systems were developed to integrate patient data into a single database, such as the COSTAR system developed by Massachusetts General Hospital. At that time, the storage capacity of computers and the high cost of storage greatly limited database capacity. For example, clinical laboratory systems were mainly offline, batch-oriented systems that used punched cards to transfer data to the hospital mainframe. In the 1970s, with the advent of real-time access disk storage, integrated database management systems emerged. Many researchers attempted to design more efficient databases that were independent of their applications and subsystems to handle almost all types of data and meet the functionalities required for patient records. During this period, many medical information systems were proposed. In 1972, the Regenstrief Institute developed the first electronic medical record (EMR) system; in 1974, NASA and Houston's SCI System conducted telemedicine consultation experiments; and in 1976, the Shortliffe team at Stanford University developed the first expert system, MYCIN. As storage technology efficiency continued to improve, the medical data warehouse emerged in the 1980s, integrating vast amounts of medical data from various sources to support MIS in quickly and efficiently accessing and analyzing large volumes of data. At that time, some state health departments in the United States developed computer-based systems to monitor infectious diseases [3]. With the maturity and development of mobile terminal devices, sensors, and multimedia, mobile health system was subsequently born, helping patients monitor their health at home and providing more convenient healthcare services. Based on this foundation, China proposed the concept of proactive health in 2015. Proactive health system combines the characteristics of telemedicine and mobile health, integrating online health management and offline health monitoring to help patients actively participate in their health management process.

Currently, with the development of information technology, MIS is also advancing rapidly. More and more new technologies are being applied to MIS. In addition to conventional hospital management and decision support, medical informatics is penetrating broader application fields, especially in the health management of patients outside the hospital. For example, Jiang et al. used mobile health technology to monitor lung transplant patients, providing decision support for their health management [10]. According to a 2015 survey in the United States, 58% of smartphone users had downloaded health-related applications for self-management of lifestyle. Vergara et al. used Internet of Things (IoT) technology to detect and monitor focal myoclonic epilepsy seizures. Santos et al. built an intelligent personal assistant based on IoT, using body sensor networks to automatically collect information about users' locations, heart rates, and potential falls, sending this information to smart terminal devices to help caregivers monitor the health status of those they care for at all times. To address data processing issues in IoT, cloud computing and fog computing have been proposed. Cloud computing provides an ubiquitous, distributed way to process medical data. Rao et al. reported on a project called "Dhathri," which used cloud computing and wireless technology to help doctors access patients' medical information at any time [11]. Fog computing, derived from cloud computing, was proposed to address severe latency issues in cloud computing input and response. Unlike cloud computing, which processes all data on cloud-based servers, fog computing processes data and applications on edge devices, helping real-time applications achieve ultra-low latency and improving data privacy and security through distributed data. Fog computing is gradually replacing cloud computing in MIS.

Although the accumulation of large amounts of data facilitates researchers in uncovering hidden patterns, the issue of medical information security is becoming increasingly prominent. Data breaches can be devastating to MIS. Therefore, data security research is also a major focus of MIS. In recent years, secure multi-party computation, random perturbation techniques, anonymization techniques, and homomorphic encryption have been widely used in MIS. Ovunc Kocabas et al. used fully homomorphic encryption to compute private health information without actually observing the data.

Additionally, VR is another hot research topic. Tashjian et al. used VR technology for a cohort study on pain management in hospitalized patients, finding that VR can significantly reduce patients' pain responses [12]. Furthermore, VR can help children mitigate the potential psychological impacts of cancer treatment and hospitalization.

Besides widespread application, how to thoroughly utilize MIS to apply medical information is a current development focus. In 2010, the Centers for Medicare & Medicaid Services and the Office of the National Coordinator for Health Information Technology in the United States issued the final rules for the Electronic Health Records (EHR) Incentive Program, proposing Meaningful Use Criteria. These criteria set five priority health outcome policy areas and ten care goals, providing application quality assessments for EHR systems to promote the improvement of healthcare quality. In 2015, China proposed the Hospital Information Interconnection Standards and Maturity Assessment, and in 2020, a new assessment plan was proposed. This plan evaluates the degree of hospital information sharing from quantitative and qualitative perspectives and divides it into seven levels (Table 1.2).

Despite the profound changes brought about by information technology in the medical field, many challenges still exist. These include the interpretability of machine learning applications in medicine, alert fatigue in decision support systems, and insufficient monitoring sensitivity in public health information systems. It is hoped that future technological advancements will address these issues.

1.3.3 Development History of Medical Informatization

The development of medical informatization has gone through a journey from scratch, evolving from small-to large-scale applications. The American College of

Table 1.2 Hospital information interconnection standardization maturity grading scheme

Grade	Grading requirements
Level I	Deployment of a hospital information management system and compliance of electronic medical record data for the inpatient component with national standards
Level II	Deployment of a hospital information management system, with some electronic medical record data for outpatient (emergency) clinics meeting national standards
Level III	Realize the integration of electronic medical record data Build an independent electronic medical record shared document library, and the shared document of the inpatient part of the electronic medical record meets the national standard Realize the document registration and query service that meets the standard requirements The number of public service application functions is not less than 3 The number of connected external institutions is not less than 3
Level IVB	Outpatient (emergency) clinic part of the electronic medical record sharing documents in line with national standards Realize the registration and query services for individuals, healthcare personnel and healthcare institutions in line with the standard requirements On the basis of the integration of hospital information, realize the number of public service application functions of not less than 11, the number of healthcare application functions of not less than 5, and the number of health management application functions of not less than 10 The number of connected business systems of not less than 15 The number of connected external institutions of not less than 3

(continued)

Table 1.2 (continued)

Grade	Grading requirements
Level IVA	To build a more complete hospital information platform based on electronic medical records To build an independent clinical information database based on the platform To realize interactive services based on the platform in accordance with the standard requirements and to increase the support for interactive services for consultation, doctor's orders, application forms, and part of the status information Based on the hospital information platform, the number of public service application functions is not less than one, the number of medical service application functions is not less than 14, and the number of health management application functions is not less than 17 Provide internet diagnosis and treatment services, start the construction of the clinical knowledge base, and provide richer auxiliary decision-making support in health management The number of connected business systems is not less than 31 The number of external organizations connected is not less than 5
Level VB	Statutory medical reports and health checkups partly share documents in line with national standards Increase support for appointment, terminology, status information interaction services Platform to realize the unification of hospital terminology and dictionaries and realize interaction with higher-level platforms based on the form of shared documents Realize the number of public service application functions to be no less than 27, and the number of medical service application functions to be no less than 30 Provide more complete internet diagnosis and treatment services. Initially realize clinical decision support, closed-loop management and big data application based on the platform The platform initially realizes interconnection and interoperability with higher-level information platforms The number of external organizations connected to the platform is not less than 7
Level VA	The hospital information platform enables rich interaction with the superior platform, realizing the unification of the hospital with the superior terminology and dictionary Based on the platform, it provides more complete clinical decision support, closed-loop management, and realizes rich artificial intelligence and big data applications The platform realizes rich cross-agency business collaboration and interconnection applications The number of connected external organizations is not less than 9

Surgeons began contemplating and seeking ways to improve record creation standards in clinical environments as early as 1928. However, due to the immature state of information technology at the time, hospitals continued to use paper medical records. With the invention of computers and the maturation of database technology, American universities started exploring the integration of computers and medical records, marking the beginning of the informatization phase in the medical industry.

Today, the medical informatization industry is one of the most dynamic sectors, with numerous companies emerging rapidly.

1.3.3.1 Typical International Representatives

Cerner Corporation

Cerner Corporation is a renowned American provider of health information technology services, solutions, equipment, and hardware. Cerner designs, installs, supports, and develops applications centered around health network architecture, allowing clinics, hospitals, doctors, and integrated health organizations to share clinical and management data across multiple disciplines and facilities. Notable products from Cerner include Millennium, Cerner RadNet Radiology Information System (RadNet RIS), and Cerner Learning Framework. Millennium is a cloud-based electronic medical record (EMR) system suitable for small-to medium-sized medical practices. RadNet RIS provides radiologists with rapid access to patient data and personalized care services. The Cerner Learning Framework is an online education platform designed for webinars and courses. In 2021, Cerner collaborated with Apple to help iOS 15 users track metrics like heart rate, sleep, and steps, allowing users to share personal health data with healthcare providers or family members.

McKesson Corporation

McKesson Corporation is the oldest and largest healthcare company in the United States, serving over 75% of American hospitals, more than 20% of home care agencies, and over 30% of doctors. McKesson was a pioneer in using barcode scanning, pharmacy robots, and radio-frequency identification (RFID) technology in drug distribution. Currently, McKesson offers over 80 products and services covering clinical audits, pharmaceutical retail, home medical equipment, medical claims, oncology management, and more.

IBM Corporation

IBM is a well-known American technology company that invented numerous important technologies such as the automated teller machine (ATM), floppy disk drive, magnetic stripe card, relational database, SQL programming language, UPC barcode, and dynamic random-access memory (DRAM). IBM's most famous product in the medical information field is Watson. Originally developed to answer questions on the quiz show "Jeopardy!" Watson was later adapted by IBM for clinical decision support. Based on a powerful knowledge base and its ability to process large amounts of data, Watson can identify critical information in the patient's treatment process, find diagnostic evidence related to the patient's medical history, and provide personalized treatment plans. Watson's emergence sparked a wave of medical artificial intelligence interest, leading IBM to partner with renowned American hospitals and clinics like the Cleveland Clinic, Mayo Clinic, and MD Anderson Cancer Center. However, Watson has encountered setbacks in recent years, highlighting the complexity and uniqueness of the healthcare field and the long road ahead for the widespread application of medical AI.

GE Healthcare

GE Healthcare is part of the well-known American enterprise GE. It primarily develops information technology for medical imaging, medical diagnostics, patient monitoring, and drug discovery and manufactures medical diagnostic equipment such as CT scanners, X-ray machines, and MRI machines. GE Healthcare has conducted extensive research in medical imaging technology. For example, they have studied hyperpolarized gas MRI technology for lung imaging, which provides information on alveoli, capillaries, and pulmonary ventilation for lung diagnosis. They have also developed diffusion-weighted imaging technology that allows patients to breathe freely during MRI scans, addressing the issue of breath-holding in patients with biliary diseases during MRI examinations. GE Healthcare has formed a comprehensive precision medical ecosystem from disease diagnosis to treatment and monitoring.

Epic System Corporation

Epic System is one of the largest providers of electronic medical records (EMRs) in the United States. It is reported that hospitals using its software service 54% of American patients and 2.5% of global patients. Epic develops, manufactures, licenses, supports, and sells proprietary EMR software applications. Epic not only provides standalone application software but also offers cloud storage services to reduce the cost of using and storing EMRs. The core of Epic's EMR system is the EpicCare software, which is used for clinical care. Epic collaborates with health tracking manufacturers to integrate data collected from wearable devices into its electronic health record (EHR) applications. One major criticism of Epic is its data sharing capabilities. Unlike Cerner and McKesson, Epic has refused to join the CommonWell Health Alliance, an organization that aims to facilitate patient data flow and interoperability, making it unable to share data with systems developed by other EMR providers.

1.3.3.2 Domestic Representatives

Neusoft Group

Neusoft Group, founded in 1991, is an IT solutions and services provider and the first listed software company in China. In the healthcare sector, Neusoft is a leader and enabler of medical and health technology and business innovation. Neusoft and its invested companies in the healthcare field promote the deep integration of information technology with healthcare, covering areas such as smart healthcare informatization, medical insurance, medical big data and intelligent technology research, medical IoT and 5G, medical equipment manufacturing, and cloud hospital platforms.

B-Soft co., Ltd.

B-Soft Co., Ltd., founded in 1997, focuses on providing informatization services and innovation for the healthcare sector. With the development of technologies such as 5G, the Internet, IoT, and big data, B-Soft's products cover various service scenarios, including medical care, health, medical insurance, elderly care, and more.

Hangzhou Century co., Ltd.
Hangzhou Century Co., Ltd., founded in 2003, relies on core technologies such as IoT, big data, artificial intelligence, and blockchain. Its products cover the entire field of digital health and smart healthcare informatization, providing accessible and coherent smart healthcare information services from residents to healthcare professionals.

HAITAI Medical Information Systems co., Ltd.
Nanjing HAITAI Medical Information Systems Co., Ltd., known as HAITAI Medical, is a professional medical informatization solutions provider in China, mainly offering electronic medical record (EMR) systems and hospital information systems (HIS). HAITAI Medical has developed solutions centered around "EMR-centered hospital informatization," "clinical drug trial management," "telemedicine," and "cloud EMR," which have been applied in over 400 large-and medium-sized hospitals.

1.3.4 Framework of Medical Informatization System

After years of development, medical informatization has achieved many accomplishments, particularly in the development of the system architecture for medical information systems. As the largest source of medical data acquisition and the most commonly used tool by healthcare personnel, designing an efficient and interoperable medical information system architecture has always been a challenge for medical informatics experts and system providers.

The basic architecture of a hospital information system is shown in Fig. 1.4. It mainly includes the hospital management information system, service information system, clinical information system, and the corresponding supporting infrastructure and external interfaces. Specifically, hospital management information system mainly supports administrative and transaction management within the hospital. Clinical information system primarily assists and supports clinical activities of healthcare personnel. Service information system provides transactional services for patients and all staff and offers collaborative services between society and industry. Infrastructure ensures the normal operation of the system. External interfaces provide connection points between subsystems and cooperate with other systems, such as public health information systems, to achieve real-time data transmission [13].

Medical information systems mainly adopt a distributed service framework. Compared to traditional centralized architectures, distributed architectures connect hospital computers, printers, and medical instruments through a large-scale computer network. Although these systems are physically separated, resources within the same network can be shared, ensuring the secure management of large volumes

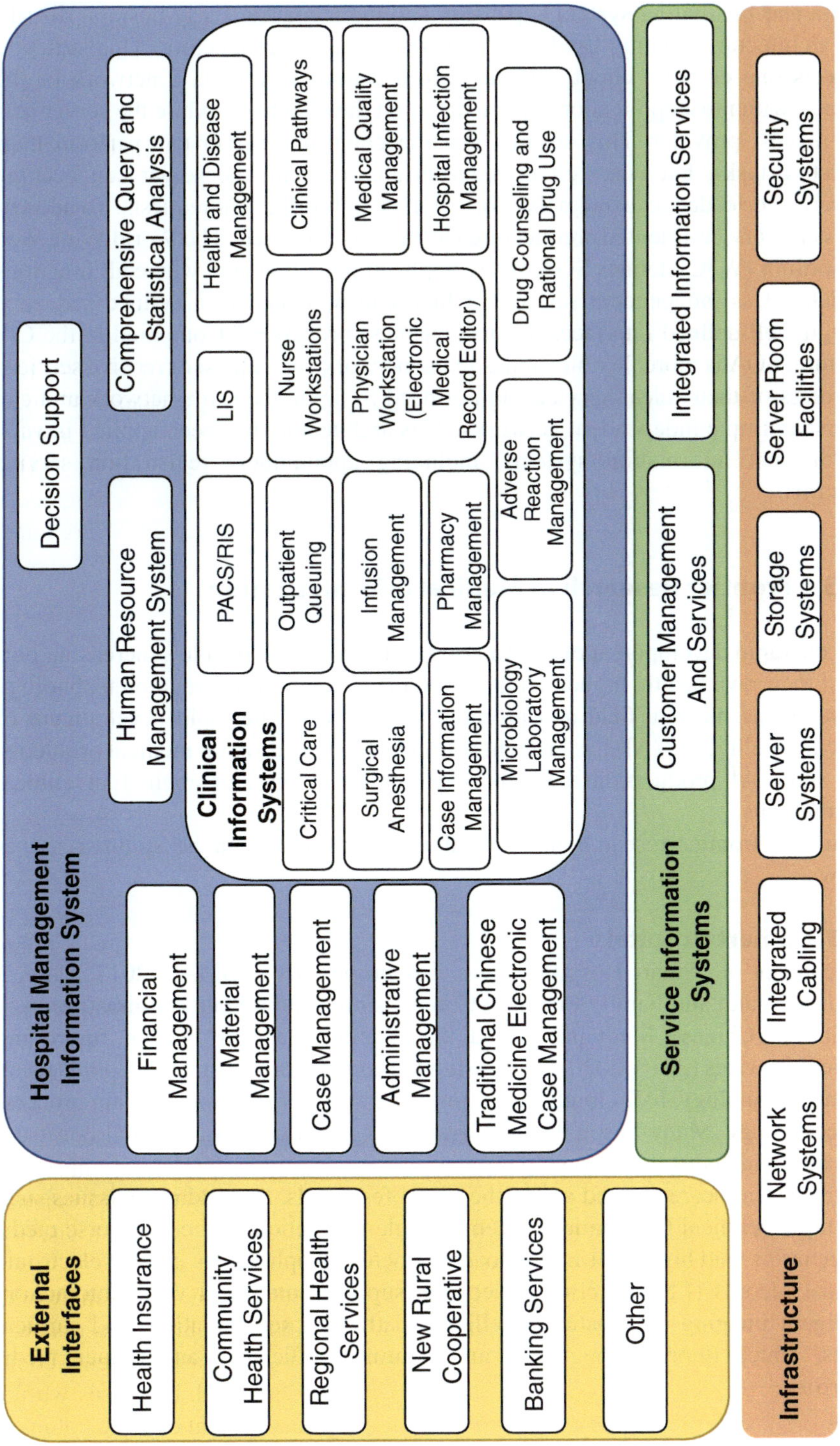

Fig. 1.4 Framework of medical informatization systems

of data and facilitating system expansion and maintenance. Early hospital distributed architectures mainly used the client/server (C/S) architecture. This structure connects one or more client computers to a central server via a network or the Internet, with most application logic located on the client side while the server acts as a request provider. This ensures that the client and server can perform their respective tasks, but when client requests are frequent, the server can become severely overloaded, causing delays or inability to fulfill client requests. To address this issue, service-oriented architecture (SOA) was proposed. The World Wide Web Consortium (W3C) defines SOA as "an application architecture where all functions are defined as independent services, which can be called in a defined sequence through well-defined interfaces to form business processes." Compared to the C/S structure, SOA is more flexible; nodes in the network can request or receive services regardless of their roles. Services do not need to be on the same network and can traverse multiple independent networks. This architecture has been applied in various medical information systems, including appointment registration service platforms.

1.3.5 Frontier Research in Medical Informatization

With the rapid development of information technology and people's increasing pursuit of their own health, higher demands are placed on how information technology can serve the medical field and promote its progress. The rapid development of artificial intelligence (AI) has brought solutions to many difficult medical problems, with some AI products already approved by the FDA and applied in clinical environments.

Current frontier research in medical informatization can be summarized as follows:

1.3.5.1 Smart Hospitals

The concept of "Smart Hospitals" was first proposed by IBM. In 2017, China's National Health and Family Planning Commission and the State Administration of Traditional Chinese Medicine issued the "Action Plan for Further Improving Medical Services (2018–2020)," proposing the construction of smart hospitals using Internet technology, IoT, cloud computing, wearable devices, and big data processing technology. Many hospitals are currently engaged in smart hospital construction, which includes the following aspects:

Smart Healthcare: Aimed at healthcare professionals, this addresses issues such as complex clinical information systems, single interaction methods, diverse medical scenarios, and high information load on doctors. Applications include electronic medical records (EMRs), clinical decision support, intelligent voice interaction, intelligent imaging diagnostics, intelligent pathology segmentation, and surgical robots, which improve diagnostic and treatment efficiency and reduce medical errors.

Smart Services: Targeted at patients, this addresses issues such as low adherence to medical advice, complex and variable disease conditions, and high heterogeneity in education and economic levels. Applications include online consultations, intelligent guidance, smart bed interaction, intelligent follow-up, and smart billing, aimed at improving the patient experience.

Smart Management: Aimed at hospitals, which are large and complex organizations with intricate diagnostic and treatment processes. To ensure efficient operation, hospitals must adopt standardized, refined, and scientific management. Research areas include logistics robots, intelligent security, smart management of medical waste and equipment, smart logistics, and smart lighting.

1.3.5.2 Big Data Management

With the rapid advancement of medical informatization and the widespread adoption of wearable medical devices, medical data is growing explosively. By 2020, the global volume of medical data was estimated to be 44 times that of 2009. Medical data is characterized by diverse structures, rich types, rapid growth, and high value. This vast amount of data provides a foundation for medical information experts to explore hidden patterns and for medical researchers to conduct scientific research. Current research in medical big data management includes:

1. Data Integration: This involves integrating multi-center medical data and multimodal data. Different medical institutions have varied data coding and database structures, and there are differences in patient privacy protection and data sharing strategies between institutions. Even within the same institution, medical data can be textual, numerical, image-based, audio, and video. Ensuring safe and effective integration of multi-institution, multimodal data and achieving standardized data representation is a hot research topic. Research areas include blockchain and homomorphic encryption for security and privacy protection, Hadoop and graph databases for big data storage, data virtualization for data management, OMOP/I2B2 for medical data standardization, and multimodal data fusion technologies.
2. Data Processing: The massive integration of medical data means that conventional software cannot process it within a reasonable time frame, necessitating new processing algorithms to quickly and efficiently utilize the data for medical value. Research areas include efficient computing techniques based on distributed computing, distributed model training based on federated learning, medical data annotation using unsupervised and semi-supervised machine learning algorithms, model compression techniques using pruning/weight decomposition/shared weights/precision reduction, pathological image segmentation based on convolutional networks, and image/disease recognition technologies based on AI.
3. Ubiquitous Services: Modern diagnostic and treatment models are increasingly focusing on out-of-hospital health management for patients and healthy individuals, leveraging advanced devices and technologies such as smart mobile terminals, IoT, and the Internet. These technologies provide seamless, omnipresent medical services. For example:

Tan et al. used IoT technology to obtain vital health signals from patients in remote areas where ambulances cannot reach, using biosensors, network cameras for real-time video, and WiMax/3.5G for wireless signal transmission to build an emergency medical service system [14]. Ajami et al. provided ubiquitous healthcare and medical advice for chronic obstructive pulmonary disease patients using an ontology knowledge base and rule reasoning [15]. Ali et al. developed an ECG signal processing algorithm for real-time low-energy heart activity monitoring using IoT and ubiquitous sensing technology, helping doctors monitor patients' physiological signals and daily activities [16]. Thaha et al. constructed a ubiquitous healthcare framework called "UbeHealth." They used deep learning, big data, and high-performance computing to predict network traffic, optimize data transmission rates, data caching, and routing decisions, identify different types of data with the same application protocol using edge computing, and collect and monitor biomedical signals and activities of patients using IoT [17].

Today, more and more hospitals and doctors are participating in the construction of ubiquitous medical services. By the end of October 2020, there were 900 Internet hospitals and over 5500 secondary-and higher-level hospitals providing online services in China. In the future, technologies such as cloud computing, big data, IoT, and AI will help create better and more comprehensive medical services.

1.4 Summary

This chapter introduces the fundamentals and current development of the discipline of medical informatics from the perspectives of the basics of information theory, the historical development of medical informatics, the growth of the medical information industry, and frontier research in medical information studies. With the development of medical information systems, medical data is experiencing explosive growth. The accumulation of vast amounts of data provides a crucial foundation for conducting medical information research and basic medical research. The rapid development of information technology offers essential technical support for processing medical data. However, due to the unique nature of medical data and the medical field, it is challenging to directly apply computer technology to medicine. Therefore, algorithms and technologies need to be adapted to maximize their benefits.

Despite the significant contributions of information technology in improving hospital environments and enhancing hospital management levels, many issues remain in the practical application of artificial intelligence technology in clinical settings. These issues include model generalization, model interpretability, and others. Additionally, the deepening of healthcare equity issues due to the widespread application of medical information technology is a topic of ongoing discussion among many medical experts.

References

1. Jingsong L. Biomedical informatics. People's Health Publishing House; 2018. p. 1–7.
2. Gallager RG, Claude E. Shannon: a retrospective on his life, work, and impact. IEEE Trans Inform Theory. 2001;47(7):2681–95.
3. Hersh WR. Medical informatics: improving health care through information. JAMA. 2002;288(16):1955–8.
4. Affairsc, Planning C. Medical informatics: an emerging medical discipline. J Med Syst. 1990;14(4):161–79.
5. Haux R. Medical informatics: past, present, future. Int J Med. 2010;79(9):599–610.
6. Rastegar-Mojarad M, Elayavilli RK, Li D, et al. A new method for prioritizing drug repositioning candidates extracted by literature-based discovery. Washington, DC: IEEE International Conference on Bioinformatics and Biomedicine (BIBM); 2015. p. 669–74.
7. Maryam LS, Nasser G, Rasoul MS, et al. A review of network-based approaches to drug repositioning. Brief Bioinform. 2018;19(5):878–92.
8. Elkin PL, Liebow M, Bauer BA, et al. The introduction of a diagnostic decision support system (DXplain) into the workflow of a teaching hospital service can decrease the cost of service for diagnostically challenging diagnostic related groups (DRGs). Int J Med Inform. 2010;79(11):772–7.
9. Feldman MJ, Hoffer EP, Barnett GO, et al. Impact of a computer-based diagnostic decision support tool on the differential diagnoses of medicine residents. J Grad Med Educ. 2012;4(2):227–31.
10. Jiang Y, Sereika SM, Dabbs ADV, et al. Using mobile health technology to deliver decision support for self-monitoring after lung transplantation. Int J Med Inform. 2016;94:164–71.
11. Rao GS, Sundararaman K, Parthasarathi J. Dhatri—a pervasive cloud initiative for primary healthcare services. In: 14th International Conference on Intelligence in Next Generation Networks; 2010. p. 1–6.
12. Tashzjian VC, Mosadeghi S, Howard AR, et al. Virtual reality for management of pain in hospitalized patients: results of a controlled trial. JMIR Ment Health. 2017;4(1):e9.
13. Nenonen M, Nylander O. A theoretical framework for health information systems. IJHCTM. 2002;4(6):467–77.
14. Tan TH, Munkhjarga G, Chen YF, et al. Ubiquitous emergency medical service system based on wireless biosensors, traffic information, and wireless communication technologies: development and evaluation. Sensors. 2017;17(1):202–16.
15. Ajam H, Mcheick H. Ontology-based model to support ubiquitous healthcare systems for COPD patients. Electronics. 2018;7(12):371–99.
16. Sodhro AH, Sangaiah AK, Sodhro GH, et al. An energy-efficient algorithm for wearable electrocardiogram signal processing, in ubiquitous healthcare applications. Sensors. 2018;18(3):923–43.
17. Muhammed T, Mehmood R, Albeshrl A, et al. UbeHealth: a personalized ubiquitous cloud and edge-enabled networked healthcare system for smart cities. IEEE Access. 2018;6:32258–85.

Electronic Medical Record Systems

2

Contents

2.1 Overview of Electronic Medical Record Systems ... 31
2.1.1 Electronic Medical Records and Electronic Medical Record Systems ... 31
2.1.2 Components of Electronic Medical Record Systems ... 31
2.1.2.1 Ward, Outpatient, and Emergency Physician Workstations ... 32
2.1.2.2 Ward Nurse Workstations ... 32
2.1.2.3 Test Systems ... 32
2.1.2.4 Inspection Systems ... 34
2.1.2.5 Treatment Systems ... 34
2.1.2.6 Surgical Anesthesia Systems ... 34
2.1.2.7 Pharmaceutical Assurance Systems ... 34
2.1.2.8 Case Management Systems ... 35
2.1.3 Current Research on Electronic Medical Record Systems ... 35
2.1.4 Case Studies of Electronic Medical Record Systems ... 36
2.1.4.1 The EPIC Electronic Medical Record System ... 36
2.1.4.2 The VA Medical System's Electronic Medical Record System ... 37
2.1.4.3 Donghua Digital Medical Information System ... 38
2.1.4.4 Haitai Electronic Medical Record System ... 40
2.2 Main Functions of the Electronic Medical Record System ... 41
2.2.1 Medical Order Processing ... 41
2.2.2 Medical Record Editing ... 42
2.2.3 Nursing Business Support ... 44
2.2.4 Medical Record Browsing ... 45
2.3 Frontier Research on Electronic Medical Record Entry and Quality Control ... 46
2.3.1 Intelligent Assisted Entry of Electronic Medical Records ... 46
2.3.1.1 Natural Language Processing in Intelligent EMR Entry ... 46
2.3.1.2 Knowledge Graph Technology in Intelligent EMR Entry ... 47
2.3.2 Voice-Enabled Electronic Medical Records ... 47
2.3.3 Intelligent Quality Control of Electronic Medical Records ... 49
2.3.3.1 Pre-Filling Default Values for Routine Items ... 49
2.3.3.2 Automatic Extraction and Entry of Established Item Information ... 49
2.3.3.3 Establishment of Various Knowledge Bases to Strengthen Professional Information Entry Guidance ... 49

J. Li et al., *Healthcare Information Systems*, Innovative Medical Devices,
https://doi.org/10.1007/978-981-97-9551-2_2

2.3.3.4 Empty Item Checks to Prevent Omissions of Key Items................ 50
2.3.3.5 Logical Checks to Improve the Accuracy of EMR Entry Information.. 50
2.4 Frontiers in Electronic Medical Record Data Integration and Application................ 51
2.4.1 Construction of Clinical Data Centers... 51
2.4.1.1 Data Extraction.. 52
2.4.1.2 Data Conversion.. 52
2.4.1.3 Data Loading... 52
2.4.1.4 Application Services.. 54
2.4.2 Clinical Data Center Services for Real-World Studies.............................. 54
2.4.3 Post-Market Research on Pharmaceutical Products Using Electronic Medical Records.. 56
2.4.4 EMR Services for Infectious Disease Early Warning................................ 58
2.5 Frontier Research on Information Sharing of Electronic Medical Records............... 59
2.5.1 Framework for Information Sharing in Electronic Medical Record Systems...... 59
2.5.1.1 System Interface Model... 59
2.5.1.2 Integrated System Model... 61
2.5.1.3 Integration Platform Model.. 62
2.5.2 Regional Medical Electronic Medical Record Transformation.................... 63
2.5.2.1 Middleware Design for Electronic Medical Record Sharing in Regional Medical.. 63
2.5.2.2 System Integration for Secure Electronic Medical Records in Regional Medical.. 64
2.5.3 Transformation of Electronic Medical Records for Internet-Based Healthcare... 65
2.6 Conclusion... 68
References.. 68

The medical record is a complete record of the medical process. When the information is recorded, stored and applied by electronic means, it is called electronic medical record. After going through the stages of electronic paper medical records, structured electronic medical records, and complete electronic medical records, the current electronic medical record system is not only able to provide assistance to medical staff by supporting information query, providing record templates, and intelligent auditing and reminding, in order to reduce and prevent the occurrence of errors and to enhance the safety of health care and service quality but also able to provide a high degree of sharing through the in-hospital, regional, and Internet multilevel data and information and carry out clinical medical services for single medical centers or multiple medical centers. It is also able to carry out clinical medical services for single medical centers or multiple medical centers through the high degree of sharing of data and information at multiple levels in hospitals, regions, and the Internet and to deeply explore and utilize the value of data [1].

2.1 Overview of Electronic Medical Record Systems

2.1.1 Electronic Medical Records and Electronic Medical Record Systems

Electronic medical record refers to the medical personnel in the process of medical activities, the use of medical institutions' information system generated by the text, symbols, charts, graphs, data, images, and other digital information, can realize the storage, management, transmission, and reproduction of the medical record, and is a form of medical record, including the outpatient (emergency) diagnosis of the electronic medical record and inpatient electronic medical record.

Electronic medical records, in chronological order, record the dynamics of disease development and clinical treatment during the patient's stay in the hospital, and this information exists in the form of data that can be retrieved and processed by computers, and the information is organically organized through the unified structural model of the medical record to form a highly structured and digitized database of medical record data. The collection and utilization of high-quality and reliable electronic medical record data cannot be separated from the use of electronic medical record systems.

According to the "Guidelines for Electronic Medical Record Management (Trial)," an electronic medical record system within a healthcare institution supports the collection, storage, and access of EMR information and online assistance. It aims to enhance medical quality, ensure medical safety, and improve medical efficiency through information processing and intelligent service functions. A complete EMR system typically includes clinical information systems used in wards, outpatient departments, and treatment rooms; laboratory systems that support clinical tests and pathology; diagnostic information systems supporting imaging and electrocardiography; pharmaceutical management systems ensuring adequate drug supplies; and blood management systems supporting blood supply.

The primary purpose of establishing an EMR system is to create a dynamic, continuous, comprehensive, and structured clinical data repository to standardize clinical diagnosis and treatment processes, provide clinical information services, and support clinical decision-making. By sharing EMR information, it promotes medical collaborative services across different institutions and departments, enhancing patient care. It also supports clinical research with continuous, reliable data and aids public health management by providing timely disease surveillance data, thus establishing an emergency response system for public health issues.

2.1.2 Components of Electronic Medical Record Systems

The EMR system is designed to manage and apply electronic medical records, primarily serving clinical department physicians. It consists of various information processing systems that integrate seamlessly through shared documents and messages [1]. Figure 2.1 illustrates the main medical information processing systems that comprise the EMR system.

2.1.2.1 Ward, Outpatient, and Emergency Physician Workstations

The workstation system of ward, outpatient and emergency doctor is used to support the daily medical work of clinicians. The system is based on the clinical application of the network, and realizes the mobile of electronic medical records, the execution of medical orders and the electronic management of medicine. Ward, outpatient, and emergency doctors' workstations mainly provide doctors with the functions of entering and issuing medical orders, applying for various examinations and tests, recording medical records, and checking historical medical records. The core function of doctors' workstations in wards, outpatient clinics, and emergency clinics is to issue all kinds of medical prescriptions. Ward, outpatient, emergency doctor workstation is the core of the whole electronic medical record system; the effective operation of the ward, outpatient, emergency doctor workstation system can improve the efficiency and quality of the work of the hospital, reduce the labor intensity of doctors, so that they have more time and energy to devote to the management of the patient and scientific research and exploration.

2.1.2.2 Ward Nurse Workstations

Ward nurse workstation is one of the important components of the electronic medical record system, which is used to assist ward nurses to complete daily nursing care for hospitalized patients. The main functions of this system are: ward management, including the management of patients' admission and transfer to and from wards, the management of bed utilization in wards, etc.; medical advice processing, including the entry, review, and execution of medical advice, etc.; nursing records, including the measurement of various vital signs and the records of various observation of patients' conditions, etc.; various operation and checking records, including the records of drug allocation, nursing operation execution and health education, etc.; cost management, including the query and printing of hospitalization cost lists, the application of refund for stopping and canceling medical advice, etc. The cost management includes inquiring and printing of hospitalization cost list, stopping and voiding medical advice and refund application. Ward nurse workstation is an important observation and execution record support system in ward medical treatment.

2.1.2.3 Test Systems

A test in a hospital is an examination that analyzes samples taken from a patient's body. Test system mainly includes laboratory information system (LIS) to support clinical testing and pathology information system (PIS) to support pathology department. The test system is mainly used to support data processing in all kinds of test work, the core function includes collecting, transmitting, analyzing, and distributing test data from test instruments, so that patients, laboratories, pathology rooms, medical units, and clinical examination centers and other modules are connected as a whole, thus providing patients with better quality services.

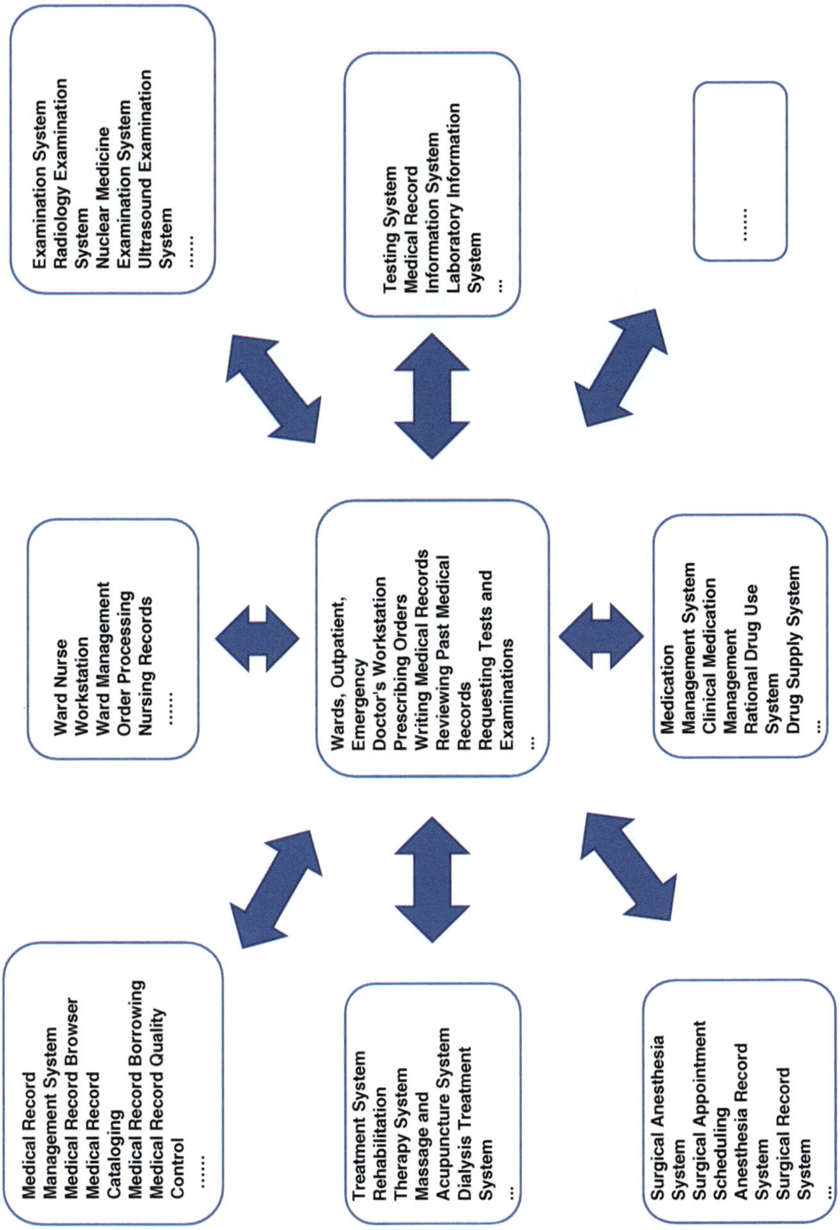

Fig. 2.1 Composition of the electronic medical record systems

2.1.2.4 Inspection Systems

The inspection system is mainly used to collect and process the information generated by the patients during the inspection process in the hospital. Common inspection systems include radiological information system (RIS), nuclear medicine inspection system, ultrasound inspection system, angiography inspection system, electrophysiology inspection system, and endoscopy inspection system. The core functions of these inspection systems include: inspection registration and booking, inspection data recording, inspection report processing, inspection image or graphic acquisition and management. Due to the large number of images generated by many inspections in the acquisition, exchange, storage, and reproduction processing have special requirements; therefore, hospitals often establish a specialized medical image processing system, the system is more powerful, data storage is more secure, and the speed of clinical access to the image is also faster.

2.1.2.5 Treatment Systems

In hospitals, aside from medication and surgery, there are many specialized treatment methods. The general model for an in-hospital treatment system includes modules for clinical application processing, treatment planning, treatment scheduling, treatment execution, treatment recording, and treatment record querying. Doctors in specialized treatment departments use this system to propose relevant applications based on the patient's condition. Treatment room technicians receive and verify these applications and payments, then develop treatment plans and prescriptions within the system and schedule appointments for the patients. Patients report to the treatment room according to the scheduled time for their treatments. During the treatment, the physician records the treatment data, issues medical orders, and prices the relevant items. Common specialized treatments in hospitals include radiation therapy, dialysis, rehabilitation therapy, hyperbaric oxygen therapy, acupuncture, and massage.

2.1.2.6 Surgical Anesthesia Systems

The basic idea of the surgical anesthesia system is to simplify the workflow of surgical anesthesia and realize the automated management of the whole process of surgical and anesthesia work. The functions of the system mainly include: surgical arrangement, preoperative visit, anesthesia record, surgical record, and other functions. Doctors will collect patients' vital signs data through anesthesia machines, respiratory machines, and various monitoring devices during patients' anesthesia and surgery. The surgical anesthesia system automatically acquires the patient's blood pressure, heart rate, respiration, and other data by connecting to these devices and manages and analyzes these data. The system can eventually realize automatic data acquisition, automatic report generation, and electronic medical records.

2.1.2.7 Pharmaceutical Assurance Systems

Drugs are special commodities for disease prevention and treatment, essential basic materials in medical activities, with both material and medical dual attributes, and an important part of hospital treatment and economic activities.

Pharmaceutical assurance systems is mainly used to support the use of outpatient and inpatient drugs, and its main functions include: receiving medical orders or prescriptions issued by clinicians, reviewing and analyzing the rational use of medication, preparing and dispensing drugs, distributing drugs, and recording adverse reactions. In the drug security system, it usually also includes drug inventory management and other material management functions.

2.1.2.8 Case Management Systems

Medical record management system is an important part of connecting medical work and medical management in electronic medical record system, which mainly provides medical record management personnel with a medical record management platform integrating medical record quality control, medical record sealing and unsealing, international classification of diseases code management, medical record borrowing management and medical statistics. Case management platform. The main functions of the case management system in the electronic medical record system are: real-time monitoring of the quality of patient records in the hospital, authorization management for the use of medical records, online sealing of medical records, data integration of various types of electronic medical records, general medical record browsing and reading support, and cataloguing of medical cases.

2.1.3 Current Research on Electronic Medical Record Systems

By 2022, electronic medical records have been developed for 50 years, and the development history of electronic medical record systems can be categorized into 4 stages from low to high according to the degree of functional perfection of electronic medical record systems.

The first stage is the electronicization of paper medical records. Paperless medical records are based on electronic files of scanned medical records or simply using the electronic medical record as a text editor, suitable for long-term storage of medical records.

The second stage is the standardized and structured electronic medical record stage. With the increase in medical data, healthcare professionals need to find effective information from the huge electronic medical record system, and structured data information is a prerequisite to ensure that the medical record information can be processed and retrieved by the computer. Healthcare professionals get the key information of the medical record by querying the structured data of the patient in the electronic medical record system and then find the specific medical record through the storage rules of the medical record.

The third stage is the electronic medical record stage that supports clinical decision-making. With the arrival of the medical big data era, the electronic medical record system gradually becomes a medical information resource base storing a large amount of medical data, which makes clinical decision support possible. In this stage, the electronic medical record system should not only be able to collect, integrate, and present all kinds of medical information about patients but also to process and analyze the data of the medical record data, extract and utilize the useful information to achieve the purpose of clinical decision support in the case of coexistence of structured and unstructured data.

The fourth stage is the highly shared stage of electronic medical records. With the continuous development of the electronic medical record system, a wide range of medical information such as hospital diagnosis and treatment information, community service information, pathology research, drug research, and so on are closely integrated. This requires that electronic medical records are no longer only shared between different departments in the hospital but should also be able to be shared between multiple institutions and departments such as regional health data centers, healthcare coordinating agencies, service guarantee agencies, regulatory service agencies, and residents' services, to break the original "information silos" of the hospitals and to realize the utilization of medical data [2] in a more efficient way.

With the rapid development of computer technology, countries like the USA, the UK, and Japan have increasingly recognized the importance of EMRs. In 2009, the incoming U.S. President Obama signed the American Recovery and Reinvestment Act (ARRA), aimed at promoting the widespread adoption of EMR systems across U.S. healthcare facilities. By 2018, EMRs were widely used in the USA. The UK's National Health Service (NHS) established a dedicated agency to develop and implement a national health information framework and EMRs, which are now extensively used in community primary care services. In the early 1990s, Japan's Ministry of Health began organizing research on data exchange standards, treatment standardization, and security among EMR organizations and institutions, culminating in a comprehensive report in 2005. Thanks to prolonged application and development, foreign countries have achieved significant results in EMR terminology standardization, interoperability, and privacy protection.

China's Ministry of Health (later integrated into the National Health and Family Planning Commission) officially initiated EMR pilot projects in 2009 and publicly issued the "Electronic Medical Record Pilot Work Scheme." Between 2017 and 2018, China's National Health Commission issued a series of documents such as the "Guidelines for Electronic Medical Record Management (Trial)," which significantly advanced EMR-related work from an administrative perspective. By the end of 2018, national level-three hospitals had largely completed EMR system construction, with the average implementation level rising from level 1 to nearly level 3, achieving internal data exchange within hospital departments and establishing cross-departmental shared information systems for certain medical business departments [3].

2.1.4 Case Studies of Electronic Medical Record Systems

2.1.4.1 The EPIC Electronic Medical Record System

The EPIC Electronic Medical Record (EMR) system is developed by Epic Systems Corporation, one of the largest EMR providers in the USA. The EPIC system covers a wide range of areas including emergency services, specialized care, inpatient

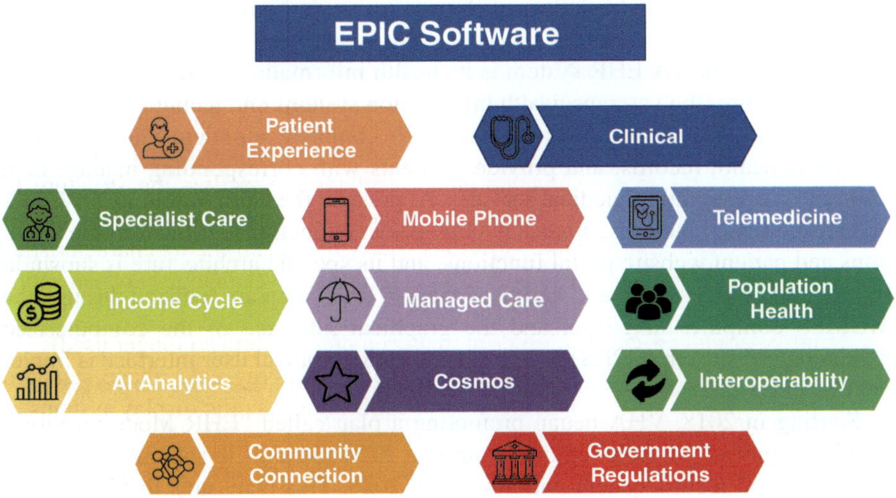

Fig. 2.2 Content and structure of the EPIC electronic medical record system

management, and patient management. The specialty system services include 24 specialties such as anesthesiology, cardiology, dermatology, obstetrics, otolaryngology, and radiology, among others. The system features highly specialized functions for each specialty, as detailed in the structure shown in Fig. 2.2.

The core of the EPIC system is the EpicCare software, focused on clinical care with numerous functional modules that can be flexibly configured. Doctors can easily access all patient records through this software, which integrates health analytics and decision support features to quickly and effectively identify potential risks to patients and provide appropriate intervention suggestions, enhancing the safety of patient visits. EpicCare also assists doctors in recruiting research participants for independent studies. Patients can use EpicCare for appointment scheduling, communication with doctors, and managing their health insurance. The software supports access via mobile phones and computers, facilitating patient appointments and allowing doctors to monitor patient conditions.

The EPIC EHR system also provides patients with a web-based EHR application called MyChart, which provides patients with real-time medical summary information about their case and helps them upload documents and images about their condition, thus changing the traditional medical reporting model, greatly increasing patient engagement in the medical process, and helping physicians to conduct patient follow-up visits.

2.1.4.2 The VA Medical System's Electronic Medical Record System

The Veterans Affairs (VA) electronic medical record system provided by the Veterans Health Administration (VHA), which focuses on U.S. veterans, is currently the largest public healthcare system in the nation and also received the 2016

National Electronic Medical Record System Survey's highest physician satisfaction rating.

The core of the VA EHR system is its health information systems and technology architecture (the veterans health information systems and technology architecture, VISTA). VISTA provides patients with complete inpatient and outpatient electronic health records, and provides patients with corresponding management tools and corresponding medical services. At present, the main functions of VISTA include clinical functions, financial management functions, infrastructure functions and patient website portal functions, and its specific architecture is shown in Fig. 2.3. The data storage and kernel of the VISTA system are realized through the MUMPS computer language, and the graphical interface of the computerized patient record system (CPRS) is also used. CPRS graphical user interface is implemented in Delphi.

Starting in 2018, VHA began promoting a plan called "EHR Modernization," which began trials in some regions in autumn 2020 and aims to roll out a new electronic medical record system nationwide by 2028. This plan aims to improve the care provided to veterans and enhance the experience of patients and healthcare providers across all institutions while changing the way VHA, the U.S. Department of Defense, the U.S. Coast Guard, and community care providers share health data. The new system is compatible with the existing electronic medical record system to ensure users can access complete patient records. It integrates the VA electronic medical record system with related data stored in a single electronic record system by the U.S. Department of Defense, eliminating the need for patients to carry paper records and enabling safer and faster patient data interaction. It also provides VA healthcare staff with long-term, complete patient treatment records.

2.1.4.3 Donghua Digital Medical Information System

The Donghua Digital Medical Information System, developed by Donghua Software Co., Ltd., is now used in over 40 tertiary hospitals nationwide. The system is divided into three major parts: hospital information services, public application services, and collaborative interaction support services, covering 80% of hospital operations.

Hospital information services are the most crucial part of the Donghua Digital Medical Information System solution and the core of full digital medical services, consisting of a basic business system and a comprehensive operation management system. The system application architecture is shown in Fig. 2.4.

The system management platform is the foundation of the digital hospital, a comprehensive representation of the technical framework and the command center of the entire system. The entire system is driven by the management tools provided by the system management platform, effectively operating all functional components, services, and permissions. The patient management system covers the main business processes of the hospital. The clinical management system includes all clinical business management systems, responsible for collecting and recording real-time clinical information data about patients. The hospital management system supports clinical systems and includes hospital-wide collaborative office systems,

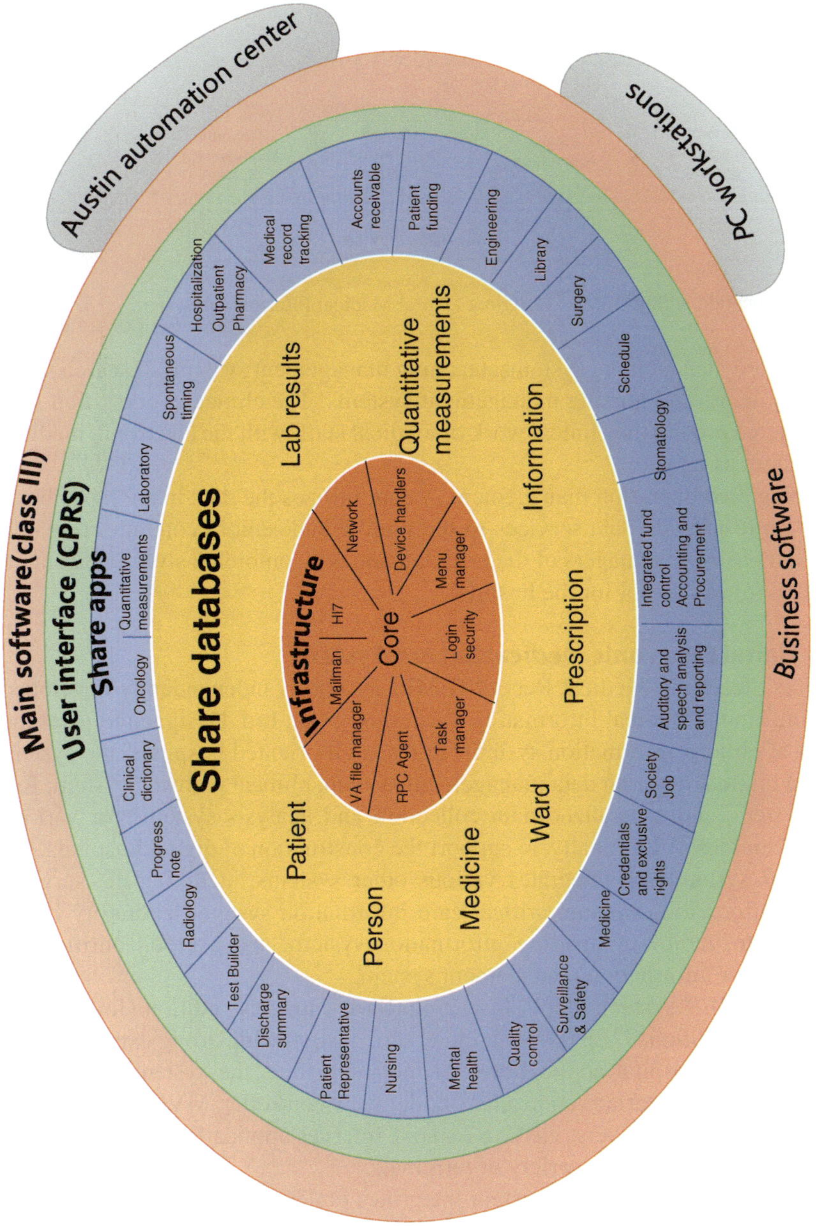

Fig. 2.3 VISTA system architecture

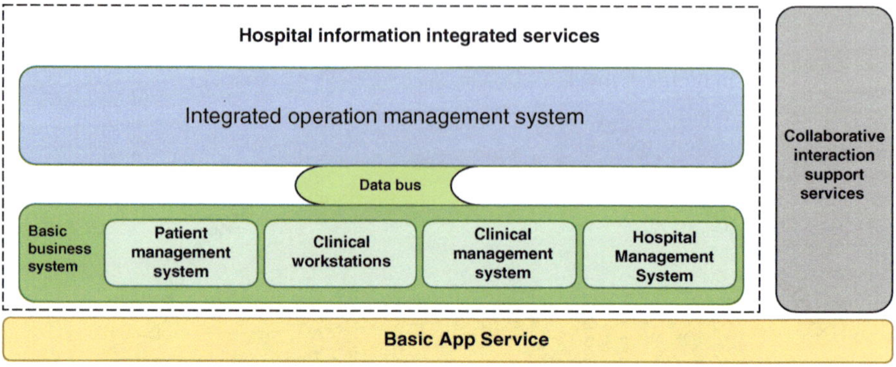

Fig. 2.4 Application architecture of Donghua Digital Medical Information System

medical record management systems, teaching management systems, research management systems, and nursing management systems. The clinical workstation system is centered around the clinical work of medical staff, with the electronic medical record system as its core.

The integrated operation management system utilizes the data in the basic business system to provide data services to the middle and senior economic, research and clinical business managers of the hospital, and is a comprehensive management and decision-making tool for the hospital.

2.1.4.4 Haitai Electronic Medical Record System

The Haitai Electronic Medical Record (EMR) system is independently developed by Nanjing Haitai Medical Information Technology Co., Ltd. Designed to meet the demands of clinical information systems in research-oriented hospitals, the system includes a clinical research data management system, clinical pathway system, follow-up system, and specialized data collection and analysis systems for various clinical specialties. Additionally, to support the construction of digital hospitals, the Haitai EMR system also integrates various other systems, including the surgical anesthesia information system, critical care information system, laboratory information system, radiology/imaging information system, and a blood purification treatment center information management system.

The Haitai HER system adopts Java 2 platform enterprise edition (Java 2 platform enterprise edition, J2EE) 3-tier architecture design, with strong expandability, support for large hospital applications. At the same time, the system follows the business model user interface controller (model view controller, MVC) architecture, compatible with Web servers, easy to expand Internet applications and telemedicine, and can be applied to a variety of terminals.

Relying on clinical data, the system integrates collection, storage, and analysis and can provide a complete solution for clinical personnel; it adopts knowledge base to collect clinical data of patients in real time; it adopts XML technology to store clinical data in a structured way; it provides researchers with a data analysis engine to support prospective and retrospective studies; at the same time, the system has a perfect quality management mechanism for medical records and a medical prescription management mechanism to ensure the safety of medication; the system can ensure the compliance of medical records with the state through an integrated platform. The system provides researchers with a data analysis engine to support prospective and retrospective studies; at the same time, the system has a perfect quality management mechanism for medical records and a medical prescription management mechanism to ensure that medical records comply with national regulations and ensure the safety of medication; the system, through the way of the integration platform, is capable of integrating the HIS, laboratory information system (LIS), pathology information system (pathology information system, LIS), and other information systems of the hospital into a single system, so as to ensure the safety of patients. The system can seamlessly integrate HIS, laboratory information system (LIS), pathology information system (PIS), radiology information system (RIS), and other systems within the hospital through an integrated platform to realize information sharing; the system supports the follow-up function to ensure that the clinical staff can observe the clinical data of the patients for a long period of time and modify the medical treatment plan according to the changes. The system supports the follow-up function, which ensures that the clinical staff can observe the patient's clinical data for a long time and modify the medical program according to the changes.

2.2 Main Functions of the Electronic Medical Record System

2.2.1 Medical Order Processing

Medical order processing is a core function within the electronic medical record (EMR) system, designed to support clinicians with the creation, modification, deletion, and discontinuation of medical orders. Based on the EMR, this process integrates clinical information with orders, outpatient services, diagnostics, lab tests, nursing records, infectious disease reports, antibiotic control approvals, a drug knowledge base, and more, to consolidate clinical information efficiently. This integration provides doctors with effective tools surpassing traditional paper records, enhancing diagnostics and treatments, improving healthcare professionals' efficiency, optimizing hospital workflows, reducing errors, and boosting medical quality.

Within the order processing system, predefined dictionaries facilitate the use of standardized medical terminology by doctors, ensuring consistency in subsequent diagnostic, therapeutic, and billing activities. The system is designed such that the items used in various medical orders correspond with those in systems for medications, diagnostics, treatments, surgeries, nursing, diets, etc., allowing for accurate information conversion. The foundational dictionaries typically include clinical drugs, dosing frequencies, administration methods, anesthesia techniques, skin test results, lab tests and templates, therapeutic medical orders, insurance mappings for drugs and diagnostic tests, local drug dictionaries, and herbal prescriptions.

Some electronic medical record systems also have the function of doctor's order set, which combines commonly used doctor's orders into a doctor's order set, and as long as the name of the set is entered, a series of doctor's orders can be automatically generated as defined, which greatly improves the efficiency of doctor's order processing. Some doctor's order processing systems also combine doctor's order sets with clinical path function, so that doctor's orders can be standardized, medical guidelines can be applied, and the efficiency of doctor's order processing can be improved. However, it is also believed that grouping of routine medical advice will easily lead to the dependence of some irresponsible doctors and cause similarity of medical advice among patients and unnecessary errors. In addition, many electronic medical prescription processing system also provides intelligent auxiliary functions, such as full sample prescription review, real-time audit warning, knowledge base prompts, and other functions, to fully support the "cross-departmental, cross-prescription, joint audit." The e-medical prescription system can audit the rationality of joint medication between the drugs prescribed by the doctor and other doctors when the doctor issues a prescription and make real-time warnings on unreasonable medication use in response to the patient's allergies, physiological status, diagnosis, test results, etc. The system can also provide suggestions for medication use in accordance with the diagnosis. The e-doctor's order system also supports the customization of rules for a variety of special groups (such as minors, pregnant patients, patients with liver, kidney and pancreatic injuries), and the pharmacy department can carry out risk management by combining real-time auditing and prescription review to try to prevent doctors from making mistakes when giving medical orders. The doctor's order will form a doctor's order record in the system. In the electronic doctor's order system, different doctor's orders are handled in different processes, which will produce different execution processes and correspond to the hospital subsystem. The realization of electronic doctor's order integrates various information systems in the hospitals at present, which makes the information transmission between the execution departments and executors involved in the processing of various kinds of doctor's orders more timely and tracks the status of the doctor's orders and controls the execution process of the orders, so that the medical quality management can be improved. It can track the status of medical advice and control the process of medical advice execution, so that the medical quality management can be changed from the management after the event to the real-time management before and during the event. The information transfer process of various medical instructions is shown in Fig. 2.5.

2.2.2 Medical Record Editing

A good performance and powerful medical record editor is a basic function in the electronic medical record system. For a long time, our country is accustomed to using pictures, text, tables, and other forms of medical records to record the medical

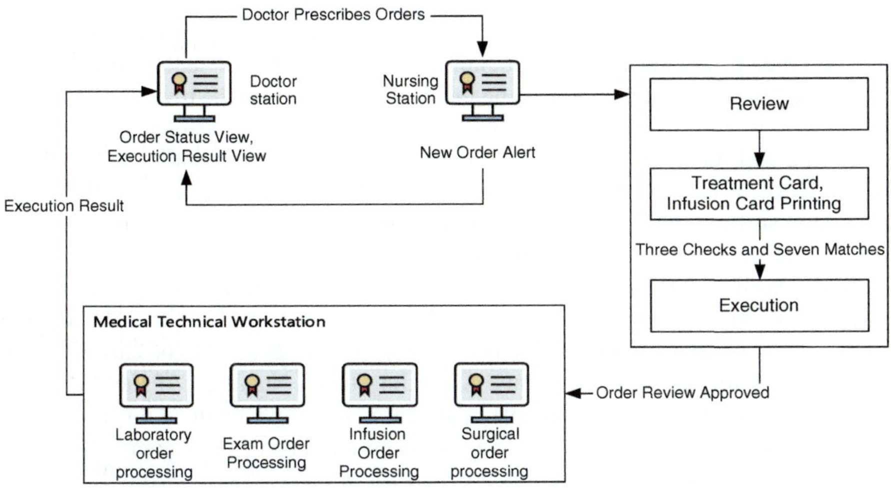

Fig. 2.5 Order information transmission process

process of history, symptoms, physical examination, examination, course of disease, surgery, anesthesia, discharge summary, and other free text information. Therefore, a feature-rich graphic editor is the basic function it must have and usually adopts the "What You See Is What You Get" editing process. Many medical record editors set up a user name and password login system, and at the same time, the whole hospital is divided into three levels of physicians: treating physicians, attending physicians and chief physicians. Each level of physician has different permissions, laying the foundation for the implementation of a three-tier medical record review system. The medical record editor can also introduce information such as medical orders, test results and inspection reports, and realize common editing functions, and insert buttons such as pictures, formulas, tables and special characters in the toolbar. The basic information of patients and other contents can be inserted in one block to avoid repeated input. For example, blood pressure, smoking status, time of onset and other information can be specially marked in the medical record, and these data can be directly extracted when consulting the medical record or conducting clinical research analysis; Support for calling the template to standardize doctors' medical records. Now there are also some medical record editors with intelligent auxiliary recording functions. For example, when the temperature recorded in the medical record is out of the normal value, the system is able to control it, and when the content of the medical record contradicts with the patient's gender and age, etc., prompts will be given in time; in order to realize intelligent prompts during the entry process, the medical record editing system needs to be designed with a special knowledge base for marking out the vocabulary, judgmental conditions, and processing logic that need to be handled during the entry process. Typically, the structured elements can be made to flexibly follow the healthcare information exchange standard HL7 (health level seven, HL7) or other standards. A three-tiered review system is in place, whereby the medical record submitted by the treating physician's records must be reviewed by the attending physician, as well as by the chief physician after the attending physician's review and approval. The attending physician cannot modify the medical record during the review, and no one is allowed to modify the medical record after the chief physician has finished reviewing and submitting the medical record. To ensure the originality and integrity of the medical record, trace retention is performed during the audit. All deleted content is still retained, but with appropriate marking. The trace retention function will ensure the implementation of the three-tier review system.

Since April 1, 2017, China's implementation of the "Electronic medical record Application Management Standards (Trial)" document stipulates that the writing and storage, use and storage of electronic medical records need to be carried out in accordance with relevant provisions. According to the standard: If the electronic medical record of outpatient (urgent) treatment is kept by a medical institution, the storage time shall not be less than 15 years from the date of the patient's last visit; Inpatient electronic medical records are kept for at least 30 years from the date of the patient's last discharge. Medical records generated by medical record editors are stored in many EHR systems in the form of files. For ease of exchange, the XML format for storing medical record files is the common format used today. In case of structured medical records, they are usually stored in relational databases. In the case of unstructured medical records with graphics or tables, these are usually also included in the file to be stored together; there are also some EHR systems with medical record editors that use non-relational databases to store descriptive medical records.

2.2.3 Nursing Business Support

China first applied computer technology to clinical nursing in the late 1980s, initially registering basic patient information and related costs. Over time, with the advancement of computers and the Internet, this evolved into more complex nursing workstation systems. The latest generation of mobile nursing systems combines fixed nursing stations with personal digital assistants (PDAs). These systems support identity verification, bedside real-time entry, data processing, order execution, vital signs monitoring, and health education, among other mobile nursing tasks. Based on networks and using PDAs as interfaces, these systems integrate HIS, LIS, and PACS, among others, into mobile terminals, extending hospital ward services and creating a paperless, filmless bedside execution system.

The mobile nursing system is based on mobile computing technology along with barcode or QR code recognition technology. It features the capability to identify and mark patient identities, medications, and biochemical specimens. Nurses can use PDAs at the bedside to scan and collect information, optimizing the nursing workflow. Upon admission, patients are issued specially designed wristbands. During treatment and nursing care, nurses scan these wristbands with a PDA to verify and confirm patient identities, enhancing the accuracy and efficiency of patient identification and ensuring the safety of all nursing and treatment procedures. For instance, before administering an infusion, a double barcode scan is mandatory to verify that the infusion recipient and the medication are correctly matched, preventing nursing errors and ensuring medical safety with precision and efficiency. The system also includes a new order reminder feature, which displays a reminder page in the relevant department as soon as a doctor issues a new order. This reminder repeats every five seconds until it is acknowledged, ensuring that medical staff can promptly process and implement the order without missing or delaying it. The system also provides an order verification function, requiring staff to verify new orders before execution: if verified as accurate, the order is approved for execution; if any errors are found, the order can be canceled or sent back to the doctor for reissuance. Additionally, after order verification, the operator must enter a verification password to complete the process, adding an extra layer of security to ensure the accuracy of the orders.

2.2.4 Medical Record Browsing

The medical record browsing reader is a function that must be provided in the electronic medical record system. Medical professionals need EHRs to be able to integrate multidimensional and multi-system data, provide multiple searching means such as patient search, time search, and keyword search in order to find the target medical records easily and quickly, and hope that they can provide more relevant medical records.

Integrating data from various systems within the EMR allows presenting all related data to healthcare professionals as needed. Typically, this data includes patient demographics, medical history, order records, diagnostic reports (including radiological reports), nursing records, vital signs, and surgical records, all displayed with relevant timelines. For data with periodic characteristics, appropriate visual representations can provide clearer insights, aiding in better treatment decisions.

According to the "Electronic medical record Application Management Standards (Trial)" document, the electronic medical record system should set the medical record access authority, and ensure that the medical staff to access the medical record needs to provide and complete the patient's electronic medical record data in a timely manner. The presented electronic medical record should show the patient's personal information, diagnosis and treatment records, record time and record personnel, and the name of the superior reviewer. The medical institution shall provide the applicant with copying services of electronic medical records. Medical institutions can provide electronic or printed version of the medical record. Copy of the electronic medical records should be available for independent reading of documents, printed electronic medical records of the paper version should be stamped with a medical institution medical records management seal. Conditional medical institutions can provide patients with medical imaging images, surgical video, interventional video, and other electronic data reproduction services.

2.3 Frontier Research on Electronic Medical Record Entry and Quality Control

2.3.1 Intelligent Assisted Entry of Electronic Medical Records

The electronic medical record system is an important tool for healthcare professionals to engage in diagnostic and therapeutic activities and records important information in the entire patient consultation process. Therefore, it is very important to ensure efficient and high-quality entry of electronic medical records. At present, there is still the phenomenon that most electronic medical record entry systems have a low degree of intelligence, and the majority of medical staff use the copy and paste input mode to pursue efficiency. This input mode leads to low quality electronic medical records. High-quality EHRs can promote the research of information extraction, while the results of information extraction research can promote the improvement of the degree of intelligence of EHR systems. Therefore, research on intelligent EHR input system is necessary.

Currently, some systems allow more than one type of data entry, with the most primitive method of guiding data entry through the use of static, predefined forms on paper or screen. This type of data entry is suitable for medical fields with predictable, patient-independent patterns of information needs, such as renal disease, orthopedic surgery, and other partially well-defined medical fields; however, in other medical fields, the pattern of data entry is difficult to predict in advance, such as general internal medicine. This requires dynamic types of data entry where the context of previously recorded information must specify the options for the next data entry. By providing adjustable input forms or menu options, the terminology combined with previous input is intelligently displayed. Another option combines free text data entry and natural language processing to arrive at the final medical expression and is by far the most flexible solution. This approach starts by temporarily storing medical records as free text, which is then transformed into a more unified medical expression by machine learning methods such as natural language processing. Choosing between these approaches is really a trade-off between ensuring the quality of the input and ensuring flexibility.

Intelligent assisted entry of electronic medical records is realized by using medical big data and machine learning methods, mainly applying natural language processing, knowledge graph, and other technologies as follows.

2.3.1.1 Natural Language Processing in Intelligent EMR Entry

Integrating medical knowledge into descriptive free text poses challenges for automated processing, making NLP and information extraction crucial for analyzing and mining EMRs. The semi-structured nature and linguistic features of medical texts bring new challenges and opportunities for NLP. The challenge lies in the distinct style of EMR texts compared to open-domain or other specialized texts, which might render standard tools like tokenization, part-of-speech tagging, and syntactic analysis ineffective. However, if the unique features of EMR texts are fully utilized, opportunities arise. For example, using extensive medical knowledge bases for information extraction is facilitated by the strong patterned expression common in medical language, making pattern mining relatively straightforward and reducing processing complexity due to the precise and unambiguous language. The structured organization of data also allows flexible implementation of information extraction methods and the use of structural relationships for inductive reasoning and inference. These features, if fully leveraged, can significantly enhance the accuracy and efficiency of EMR entry. NLP can humanize medicine, allowing doctors to spend more time communicating with patients. Some EMR systems have surpassed transcription bounds by searching existing records for structured information, such as annotating the administration date, supplier, batch number, and expiration of a previously administered flu vaccine.

2.3.1.2 Knowledge Graph Technology in Intelligent EMR Entry

The study of medical knowledge graphs, including their construction and application, has garnered increasing attention in the big data era. EMRs are replete with medical terminology, making medical dictionaries and knowledge bases crucial for building and utilizing EMRs. These resources can be used to mine entities and their relationships within EMRs, thus constructing extensive medical knowledge graphs. Employing medical knowledge graph technology can significantly enhance the professionalism and standardization of input information and intelligently link related professional terms, providing doctors with prompts to improve input quality and efficiency in subsequent searches.

Challenges in widespread adoption of intelligent entry systems remain significant. While intelligent EMR entry systems can enhance doctors' efficiency and the quality of medical records, they are not deemed essential by hospitals, resulting in low purchasing enthusiasm. Tech companies must collaborate with hospitals to access medical records and extract terminology, involving substantial communication and technical costs.

2.3.2 Voice-Enabled Electronic Medical Records

As artificial intelligence and big data continue to advance, the methods for inputting electronic medical records (EMRs) have become increasingly diverse and efficient. Current intelligent EMR systems have evolved to integrate speech recognition, natural language understanding, and speech synthesis technologies. These systems use an integrated hardware–software approach with voice input as the entry point, combining domain-specific noise-canceling microphones and intelligent mice for interactive voice-controlled input. They also provide various input methods, including flexible template editing and intelligent medical recommendation inputs, enabling doctors to complete medical record writing in real-time during consultations. This significantly enhances doctors' work efficiency and the EMR input experience. Moreover, it allows patients to promptly and quickly access their information through the voice EMR system while ensuring both efficiency and quality.

Under the severe situation of preventing and controlling the new coronavirus epidemic in 2020, the diagnosis and treatment workload of major epidemic prevention and sentinel hospitals has increased dramatically, and healthcare workers have a high workload and face a high risk of being infected. Yun Zhisheng's intelligent voice electronic medical record system has been applied to hundreds of new coronavirus sentinel hospitals in a timely manner. Cloud Knowledge is an intelligent voice electronic medical record system that has been applied since 2015. With the help of an intelligent medical language model built on the basis of deep learning, supercomputing, clinical knowledge map, and big data, the voice medical record entry recognition accuracy rate exceeds 98%, saving doctors nearly 2 h of work time in a single day's medical record entry and improving entry efficiency by 60%. The intelligent voice electronic medical record system can enter medical documents in real time for medical staff in multiple scenarios, such as outpatient medical record, inpatient medical record, and examination and test report record of medical technology department, through non-contact spoken language entry without touching office equipment. The hardware with anti-bacterial and anti-infective medical special noise-canceling microphone further reduces the risk of infection for healthcare staff.

iFLYTEK Healthcare's voice-enabled electronic medical record (EMR) system is another example. This system offers flexible multimodal assisted entry options to meet the varying documentation needs of doctors, significantly enhancing their work efficiency and the quality and experience of medical records while reducing the difficulty of hospital promotion. It specifically supports intelligent voice semantic entry, a rich template system for various specialties, and medical intelligent associative entry. The input modes include: (1) Intelligent voice semantic entry designed for different usage scenarios and doctors' habits, featuring three distinct voice input modes: tone, meaning, and word; (2) Template system entry, which can be flexibly used with different permissions; (3) Medical intelligent recommendation entry, where the system rapidly suggests rich content options in response to any keyword input. The system can also rapidly generate specialized medical vocabulary for common medical fields such as diagnoses, chemical formulas, and medical drugs through voice, having learned from a vast database of hospital records. On the hardware side, custom medical noise-canceling microphones are tailored to fit the environmental and operational characteristics of outpatient departments, addressing challenges like power endurance and wearability, offering antimicrobial treatment, and minimizing environmental interference to achieve higher accuracy in voice recognition.

The voice-enabled EMR system facilitates the entry of medical records for doctors, particularly in specialties requiring constant movement, such as dentistry, or where results are highly templated, like in sonography. This system allows doctors to devote more time and attention to patient care, though it also presents significant practical challenges. On the one hand, the difficulty of voice recognition necessitates the creation of comprehensive medical knowledge graphs, and the product's usage involves processes like signal collection, noise reduction, and model training, all supported by a robust technical team. On the other hand, the adoption of voice-enabled EMRs requires changing doctors' input habits and cultivating their ability to use multimodal assisted entry systems flexibly.

2.3.3 Intelligent Quality Control of Electronic Medical Records

Medical records are crucial medical documents reflecting a patient's condition, and the quality of electronic medical records (EMRs) is also an important indicator of the medical level of departments and hospitals. In the era of big medical data, it is more important to control the quality of data from multiple perspectives such as data generation, storage, and management to reduce the occurrence of "dirty"data.

From a system design perspective, EMRs can be specially designed for intelligent quality control in the following ways.

2.3.3.1 Pre-Filling Default Values for Routine Items

To prevent routine item vacancies and errors, some routine pending validation items are set to default values. For example, the quality grade of the medical record is defaulted to Grade A at the time of discharge submission, whereas the final medical record quality assessment grade information should be validated by the case management committee and then modified for entry.

2.3.3.2 Automatic Extraction and Entry of Established Item Information

The automatic entry function is key to improving the efficiency and accuracy of EMR entries. It can automatically extract and input partial basic information and medical conditions of patients through relevant modules of the hospital information system, thus reducing the arbitrariness of manual entries. For example, basic patient information can be automatically entered from identity documents read from the hospital admission module.

2.3.3.3 Establishment of Various Knowledge Bases to Strengthen Professional Information Entry Guidance

Professional data items in electronic medical records can be standardized by providing auxiliary input knowledge base to strengthen guidance and other means. Taking diagnostic items as an example, "diagnostic filling guidelines" provided by the system can be used to guide the input. When the doctor enters the diagnosis, the ICD 10 query and input window automatically pops up to assist the doctor to correctly enter the ICD 10 diagnosis information. On this basis, the ICD10 International Classification of Diseases, ICD9CM3 Classification of Surgical Operations, and Anesthesia for Surgery can also be maintained in the network auxiliary library according to the unified standards of the Ministry of Health, and doctors can only select standardized content when entering and cannot input characters at will.

2.3.3.4 Empty Item Checks to Prevent Omissions of Key Items

Adding an empty item check reminder function in EMRs can prevent the omission of key content. When doctors submit an EMR, the system automatically determines whether there are unfilled items such as patient information and main diagnoses. If there are unfilled items, the submission is not allowed, and the system prompts for the information that needs to be completed.

2.3.3.5 Logical Checks to Improve the Accuracy of EMR Entry Information

Customized quality control report function can be added to the electronic medical record system to improve data quality by customizing rules for quality monitoring and usage statistics in the process of diagnosis and treatment and realizing the logical verification function of the information to help the filler to quickly check in order to correct the entry errors. Custom quality control reports can be added to the EMR system. By setting custom rules, quality monitoring and usage statistics are performed during the diagnostic process to implement logical checking functions, which help the user quickly check and correct entry errors, thereby improving data quality.

From the point of view of standardization of entry by doctors, it is necessary to further strengthen the standardized training of doctors in entering information and to raise the importance of the entrants to the electronic medical record and their habits of mind and awareness of standardized entry. Regular training sessions and problem discussion meetings are held to improve and answer problems and questions in the use of electronic medical records. Improve users' proficiency in the electronic medical record system so as to achieve proficiency in the use of the system's detection mechanism in the process of using the system and reduce the occurrence of errors, so that doctors fully understand which parts need to be manually entered; whether there are any special requirements on the standardization criteria and scope of the manually entered parts; which parts can be intelligently retrieved directly from other modules; and which parts are more specialized and have to be guided by the assistance of the knowledge base to be Input. Through gradual familiarization and mastery, users can greatly improve the quality of data entry, thus reducing the occurrence of erroneous data from the source.

From the perspective of electronic medical record management, the electronic medical record system must be reviewed and modified by specialized personnel to ensure the security of medical record data, thereby guaranteeing the truthfulness, completeness, and validity of electronic medical records. Through the establishment of a security and confidentiality system for electronic medical records, a complete process of signing, tracking, filing, borrowing, copying, and altering systems, and a reasonable use mechanism, the corresponding access rights of medical personnel and relevant management personnel for accessing, copying, and printing of electronic medical records have been set up in order to manage and safeguard the security of electronic medical records. At the same time, data backup should be done well and stored off-site according to the regulations to prevent the loss and destruction of medical record information. The traditional medical management is mainly the final type of management, that is, a variety of medical indicators in the aftermath of the statistics, and then feedback medical process management, such management lags behind the medical process. In the electronic medical record system, all kinds of raw data can be collected in a timely manner during the medical process, forming management indicators and timely feedback to achieve the goal of link control. It adopts feasible technical ways to integrate various resources and effectively reminds and urges medical staff to complete medical record writing on time and in accordance with quality through statistics, analysis, early warning, and three-level quality assessment and other prior control means, so as to improve the quality of electronic medical records, enhance the pass rate of medical records, and thus enhance the comprehensive competitiveness of hospitals.

Currently, artificial intelligence technology is also being utilized for medical record quality control. To improve the efficiency of the quality inspection process of electronic medical records (EMRs) and to promptly reflect their quality, some EMR systems have made attempts, such as iFLYTEK Healthcare, which applies advanced natural language processing, machine learning techniques, and other AI algorithms. They have proposed an EMR quality inspection technology based on logical reasoning. This technology first conducts structured preprocessing of EMRs and then analyzes the structured medical record content, evaluating aspects such as content completeness, numerical standardization, and timeliness. This further assists in the formal quality inspection of medical records, helping doctors to complete the writing of EMRs, standardize and improve the quality of EMRs, and regulate doctors' diagnostic and treatment behaviors.

2.4 Frontiers in Electronic Medical Record Data Integration and Application

2.4.1 Construction of Clinical Data Centers

Electronic medical record (EMR) systems often involve extensive data sharing and exchange across different business processes to ensure that doctors can fully access patient information for accurate clinical decision-making. Additionally, hospitals need to track specific patient groups, monitor antibiotic usage, and manage emergency public health events, all requiring substantial data from various EMR functions.

To meet the needs of data sharing and exchange, hospitals must construct data centers. Known as clinical data repositories (CDRs), these are real-time databases. They standardize, integrate, and store diverse clinical data from patients, including laboratory test results, demographic information, pharmacy data, radiological reports, pathology reports, and details of admissions, discharges, and transfers. This aims to provide a comprehensive view of patient care within the hospital, facilitating data querying, analysis, and sharing, and easing the generation of medical reports and clinical research.

The process of establishing a CDR is shown in Fig. 2.6, involving data extraction, data transformation, data loading, and application services.

2.4.1.1 Data Extraction

The original data forms of the electronic medical record system are very redundant and complex, requiring the integration of a large amount of data, as well as the reconstruction of data tables. Therefore, according to the actual diagnosis and treatment process and application requirements, it is necessary to first determine the range of extracted data and construct different data forms and their fields. For example, the patient's personal information form, examination data form, visit record form, drug form, etc. The mapping relationship between different data tables and their corresponding clinical data sources should be determined, and then the corresponding data should be retrieved and extracted from the original data table of the EHR system.

2.4.1.2 Data Conversion

Data conversion is mainly to standardize data and store clinical data from different sources in a unified structure and standardized controlled terminology tables. First, standardized terminology forms and data exchange standards corresponding to different kinds of data are determined, for example, HL7 for message exchange between systems, HL7 clinical document architecture (CDA) for medical document exchange, digital imaging and communications in medicine (DICOM) for digital medical image transmission, Rx clinical drug standard nomenclature (RxDN) for drugs, communications in medicine (DICOM) for digital medical image transfer, RxNorm for drugs, ICD codes for disease classification, logical observation identifiers names and codes for laboratory tests (LOINC), and so on. Due to the different clinical record habits of different doctors, there are multiple descriptions of the same disease/drug, symptom, etc., and in the early days of the hospital, the degree of informatization was not high, and many records were written manually. Therefore, there are recording errors and inconsistencies in the clinical data, which require thorough cleaning of the raw data. For erroneous data, the constructor can fix it from other records of the patient, but considering that some of the data errors occurred many years ago and it is difficult to find the correct data, then it can be deleted to ensure the accuracy of the extracted data. For inconsistent data, the builder is required to convert it to consistent data, and if it cannot be repaired, then it can be deleted. The mapping tool is used to map the cleaned and completed data into the fields of different tables. Optimization measures such as adding indexes and counting can be applied to the mapped completed data to speed up the database retrieval efficiency.

2.4.1.3 Data Loading

CDR data loading involves determining the structure and integration mode of data loading. Currently, structures often used are star schema and snowflake schema. The star schema centralizes the core data tables surrounded by attribute tables like spokes of a star, linked by primary-foreign key relationships. This structure, simple

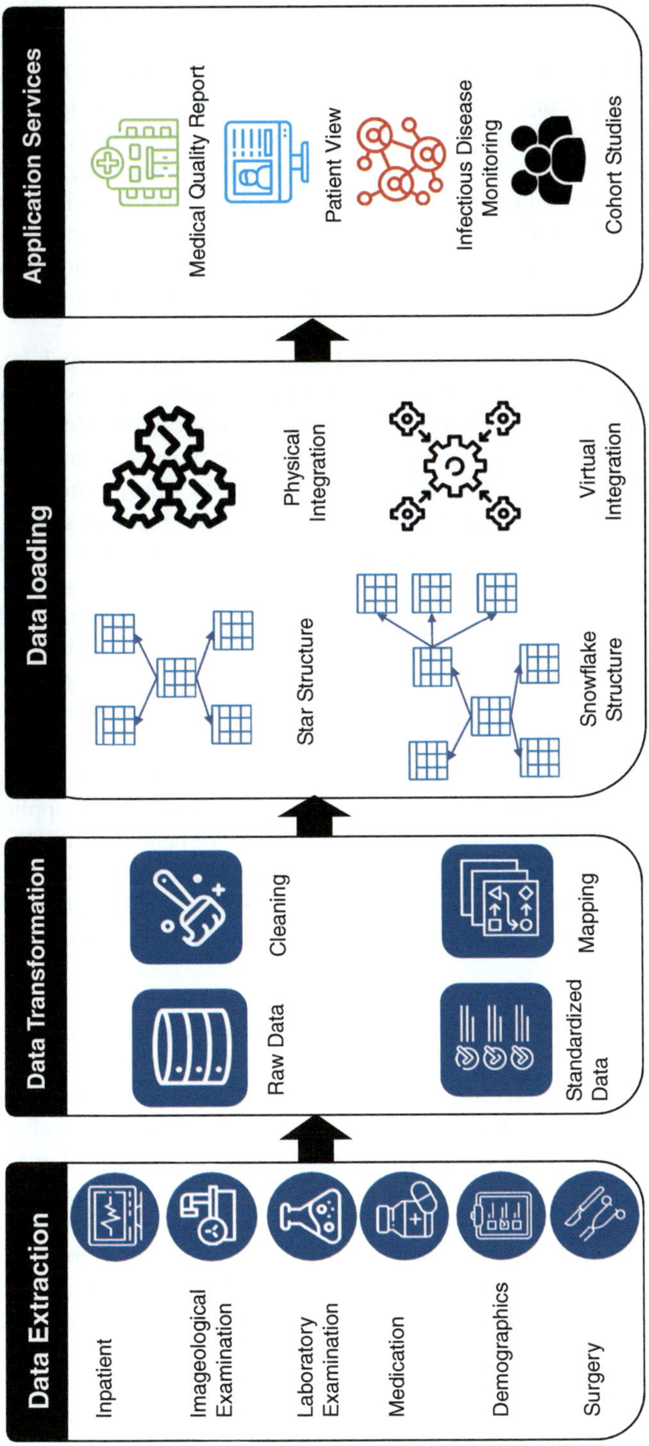

Fig. 2.6 CDR establishment process

in design, facilitates decision support for clinical standards but may involve data redundancy. Based on this structure, the National Institutes of Health (NIH) designed the I2B2 (Informatics for Integrating Biology and the Bedside) architecture, with a central fact table storing IDs for patient visits, clinical concepts, records, and primary physicians, while detailed information about patients, physicians, visits, and concepts is stored in attribute tables. The well-known open-source data warehouse tranSMART is built on this framework. The snowflake schema is similar to the star schema but includes multiple related tables for each attribute, creating a snowflake-like appearance. In reality, the star schema is a special case of the snowflake schema, which has low data redundancy and is suitable for storing high-dimensional data, but it is complex in design and inconvenient for querying.

Data integration methods are divided into physical and virtual integrations. Physical integration, where all data from various sources is consolidated in one place, is straightforward and feasible for single medical centers. However, for multicenter EMR systems, considering privacy and security issues, many medical centers might still need to control access to their EMR data. Thus, virtual integration is more appropriate for multicenter data. Virtual integration involves setting up a central site as an intermediary between users and data, with sub-sites at each medical center storing databases with sensitive information removed. Users access data from different medical centers through the central site. This method offers high security but requires the data models at all sites to align closely with the global data model, making it challenging to implement in reality.

2.4.1.4 Application Services

Medical application services are mainly based on the database to provide medical services for single or multiple medical centers. Common clinical application services include generating reports on the whole process of healthcare quality services, viewing a complete view of patient visits, detecting the use of antibiotics in hospitals, assisting in the detection of infectious diseases in hospitals, helping physicians to build patient cohorts to study the progress and management of diseases, and so on.

2.4.2 Clinical Data Center Services for Real-World Studies

Real-world study (RWS) refers to the collection of patient-related data in real-world environments (real-world data, RWD) and the analysis of this data to obtain clinical evidence of the usage value and potential benefits or risks of medical products (real-world evidence, RWE). The main types of research are observational studies, but clinical trials can also be conducted. RWS has currently become an important research method in the medical field. In 2016, U.S. President Obama signed the twenty-first Century Cures Act, which approved the Food and Drug Administration (FDA) to use RWE in appropriate circumstances to support regulatory decisions, allowing RWE to be used as evidence for the approval of new drug indications. In 2018, China's first RWS guideline, the Real World Study Guidelines, was published. In January 2020, China's State Drug Administration issued the Guiding

Principles of Real World Evidence in Support of Drug Research, Development, and Review (for trial implementation).

CDRs, centered around EMR systems, are undoubtedly an essential source of RWD, containing various interventions and outcomes related to patients, providing ample scientific evidence for evidence-based medicine. The process of serving real-world research through CDRs typically follows the steps shown in Fig. 2.7. Initially, a reasonable research hypothesis is formulated based on specific clinical questions; then, based on this hypothesis, a patient cohort construction plan and data collection scope are designed. Upon building the CDR, the collected patient data is analyzed. This data is not necessarily routine medical data from the past but can also include actively collected medical data, such as prospective cohort designs by doctors, stipulated patient follow-ups, and interventions, with these data registered in the EMR system. Current real-world studies using CDRs include disease risk prediction, drug repositioning, and detection of adverse drug events, as shown in Fig. 2.8.

Despite the many applications of RWS, it remains controversial, mainly due to the quality of RWD. Since RWD is collected in everyday environments rather than strictly designed laboratory settings, it contains many errors, making reliability assurance difficult. Moreover, compared to randomized controlled trials (RCTs), RWS places higher demands on user data analysis skills. If doctors lack sufficient statistical knowledge, it could lead to incorrect analysis results.

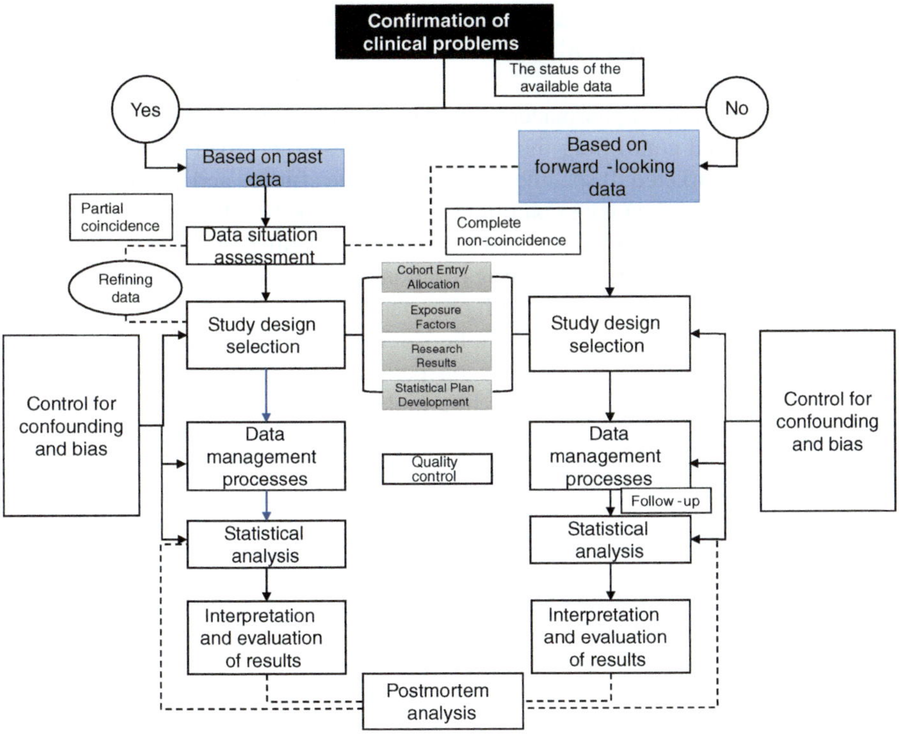

Fig. 2.7 Research ideas and processes in the real world

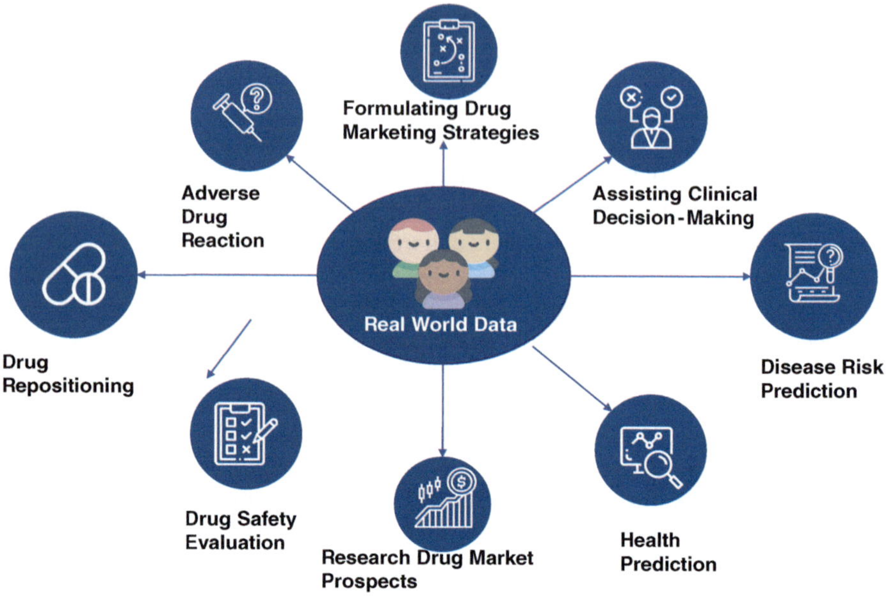

Fig. 2.8 Real-world research

2.4.3 Post-Market Research on Pharmaceutical Products Using Electronic Medical Records

Post-market research on pharmaceutical products is a critical method for identifying, assessing, and controlling the risks of drugs used in broad populations after they have been marketed. It specifically examines the efficacy and adverse reactions of drugs under widespread use conditions, evaluating the benefits and risks of drugs in general or special populations, and determining whether adjustments in dosing are necessary. Monitoring adverse drug reactions post-market plays a crucial role in identifying safety risks associated with pharmaceuticals and controlling these risks, serving as a vital means to ensure public safety in medication usage. EMR data, which contains complete information on patient medication and treatment processes, combined with other sources like mobile device health data and patient-reported outcomes, serves as real-world evidence to meet the aforementioned needs and is a primary data source for post-market safety studies [4].

Several common methods exist for identifying safety issues with drugs after they have been marketed:

1. Pre-market clinical and non-clinical trial studies.
2. Safety risk derivation based on pharmacological classifications, including understanding the mechanisms of drugs and risk derivation from drugs of the same type.
3. Monitoring the large-scale population medication usage post-marketing.

The first two methods may not capture real-time safety signals effectively, thus necessitating more reliable evidence from real-world data, which can be categorized into passive and active monitoring:

- Passive Monitoring: This involves healthcare professionals proactively reporting adverse reactions to regulatory authorities. This method has inherent limitations, such as low discovery rates and inaccurate evaluation results due to incomplete information.
- Active Monitoring: Initiated by a regulatory body, it requires, based on various methodologies, that healthcare institutions implement it.

The U.S. FDA has a long history of using real-world evidence to monitor and evaluate the safety of approved drugs, primarily through traditional risk assessment reports and adverse event reporting tools. In February 2015, the FDA accelerated the approval of palbociclib (brand name IBRANCE) in combination with letrozole for treating ER+/HER2-postmenopausal advanced breast cancer. A pharmacokinetics (PK) analysis conducted on 50 male and 133 female cancer patients during clinical trials indicated that gender differences had no significant impact on the drug's PK. In April 2019, Pfizer provided real-world evidence to the FDA based on the post-market electronic health records of male breast cancer patients, combined with Pfizer's global safety database and the IQVIA insurance database, demonstrating no safety difference in treating male and female patients with the same indications. The FDA approved the supplemental application for a new indication for palbociclib, in combination with aromatase inhibitors or the anti-tumoral drug fulvestrant for treating male patients with HR+/HER2-advanced or metastatic breast cancer.

As mentioned above, in order to guide and standardize the work related to the use of real-world evidence to support drug R&D and review and to safeguard the quality and efficiency of drug R&D work, China's State Drug Administration issued the Guiding Principles of Real-World Evidence to Support Drug R&D and Review (for trial implementation) in January 2020, which addresses the following for the support of real-world evidence for post-market drug regulation: "Real-world evidence is used to support drug regulatory decision-making, including providing evidence of effectiveness and safety for the registration and listing of new drugs, providing evidence for changes in the specification of marketed drugs, and providing evidence for post-marketing requirements or re-evaluation of drugs."

The National Adverse Drug Reaction Monitoring Sentinel Alliance is an alliance organization composed of monitoring sentinel sites identified by the State Drug Administration Drug Evaluation Center (SDA DEC), which is committed to exploring the active monitoring mode of adverse drug reactions, conducting key monitoring and post-marketing evaluation and other research, promoting rational use of medicines, and safeguarding the public's safety of medicines. The National Center for Adverse Drug Reaction Monitoring officially launched the identification of national ADR monitoring sentinel sites (medical institutions) and the deployment and implementation of the Chinese hospital pharmacovigilance system (CHPS) in April 2017, which is based on the electronic medical record system of medical institutions to establish a corresponding database. With the help of adverse drug reaction (ADR) rules knowledge base and search engine technology, CHPS realizes intelligent search and active monitoring of ADR prescription events in hospitals and directly completes the system management functions of generating, auditing, reporting, feeding back, and analyzing ADR information in medical institutions, thus changing the original mode of reporting ADR reports. This can change the limitations of the original ADR reporting model, such as high omission rate, strong reporting arbitrariness, and incomplete reporting information.

2.4.4 EMR Services for Infectious Disease Early Warning

It is estimated that at least 25% of the 60 million annual deaths worldwide are related to infectious diseases, with neglected infectious diseases claiming over 500,000 lives each year and causing chronic infections in at least one billion people. To mitigate the immense trauma caused by various infectious diseases, rapid identification and diagnosis of disease outbreaks and pathogens are necessary to effectively allocate and utilize resources for effective and timely responses.

Since the outbreak of SARS in 2003, infectious disease risk assessment and prediction have become focal points in disease control efforts. China's national infectious disease automatic early warning system has been operational since 2008. By early 2018, it could issue alerts for 33 types of infectious diseases and had become the largest infectious disease monitoring network globally, covering 70,000 healthcare institutions with nearly 150,000 authorized users. The system employs fixed threshold and moving percentile methods to statistically analyze reported cases and automatically generate and promptly send alert signals while also swiftly gathering information related to the alert processes. Additionally, the system has transformed the traditional method of monthly, graded reporting by county, by establishing the National Infectious Disease Reporting Information Management System and its core subsystem, the National Infectious Disease Direct Reporting System. This integration with hospital information systems (HIS) has simplified the process for clinicians to fill out infectious disease report cards.

As the workload of medical institutions increases and the demand for medical services grows, this infectious disease monitoring and early warning system struggles to operate efficiently, presenting several issues: (1) The current extensive reporting of infectious diseases by clinicians using paper materials, with preventive healthcare physicians entering the data into the system on their behalf, leads to low reporting rates, timeliness, and accuracy, with high error and underreporting rates, and imposes significant work pressure on healthcare workers; (2) With the advancement of hospital informatization, hospital information systems centered around electronic medical records have developed significantly, but these capabilities are yet to be fully utilized in infectious disease reporting; (3) Current disease early warning models mainly target specific infectious diseases and are insufficient for monitoring emerging, rare, or undiagnosed diseases.

In September 2014, Shanghai piloted the Infectious Disease Epidemic Reporting and Management Information System project, supported by the Chinese Center for Disease Control and Prevention (CCDC), with Songjiang District serving as the pilot area. Based on residents' health records and hospital electronic medical records, a data exchange platform was built. This platform intelligently collects infectious disease-related information from medical institution EMRs, generates infectious disease report cards, supplements information, and sequentially uploads it to district and city databases, ultimately pushing it to the National Infectious Disease Network Direct Reporting System, establishing a matching data management approach. Practical verification has shown that the platform can accurately and timely extend infectious disease reporting information to doctor workstations through the regional platform, truly achieving real-time reporting and significantly enhancing the quality and efficiency of hospital infectious disease reporting.

2.5 Frontier Research on Information Sharing of Electronic Medical Records

2.5.1 Framework for Information Sharing in Electronic Medical Record Systems

To provide patients with the most comprehensive and accurate diagnostic and treatment services, physicians often need to integrate information from multiple systems within electronic medical records. To ensure that every aspect of the medical process or various departments can fully and timely understand the patient's condition, grasp the upstream and downstream diagnostic and treatment information, and leverage the powerful capabilities of hospital informatization, information sharing between different electronic medical record systems is necessary.

There are several approaches and technological architectures for achieving information sharing and system interoperability among electronic medical record systems. Currently, there are three main models: system interface model, integrated system model, and integration platform model.

2.5.1.1 System Interface Model

During the development of electronic medical record systems, hospitals often incorporate products from different vendors, and domestic vendors develop professional electronic medical record systems with different standards, development methods, and data formats. Different systems need to share information through data exchange interfaces. In the actual diagnostic and treatment process, there is a need for extensive information exchange and interoperability among related systems, including sharing various result documents and exchanging various messages. If there are N professional systems that constitute the electronic medical record and each system has interfaces with each other, theoretically, up to $N \times (N-1)$ interfaces may be needed. If a hospital adds a new professional system, N additional interfaces are required. In the actual application of electronic medical record systems, the demand for shared information is mainly concentrated between clinical physician workstations and various medical and support departments such as inspection, testing, treatment, and pharmaceutical services. The interface requirements between different inspection systems and treatment systems are less frequent, as illustrated in Fig. 2.9.

Adding data exchange interfaces between various systems requires substantial investment and also involves the cooperation of developers of each system to modify the systems. Common interface methods include: using the interface service program provided by the counterpart for synchronous data exchange; systems on both sides of the connection use agreed data exchange standards; asynchronous data exchange interfaces using a shared middle database. To solve the information sharing between different systems, it is often necessary to specifically agree on the interface methods and data exchange standards. Currently, many organizations have developed various levels of standards for hospital information systems to exchange data, such as HL7 V2, HL7 V3 for inter-system message exchange, HL7 CDA for exchanging medical documents, DICOM for digital medical image transmission, LOINC for standardizing laboratory observations, ICD10 for unified diagnostic classification, and SNOMED CT for structuring various medical terminologies. Due to the abundance of standards, selecting which standard to use for data exchange between different professional systems of electronic medical records can sometimes be challenging. Consequently, the medical information system integration (Integrating the Healthcare Enterprise, IHE) standard emerged, which consolidates the basic information framework of medical processes and some major inspection and treatment processes and specifies which information standards to choose in these processes.

Since each system may be designed by different system developers with different system architectures and software environments, the types of interfaces between systems can be very complex, and once the structure of a particular system changes, the interfaces to the systems connected to it need to be adjusted. This model will

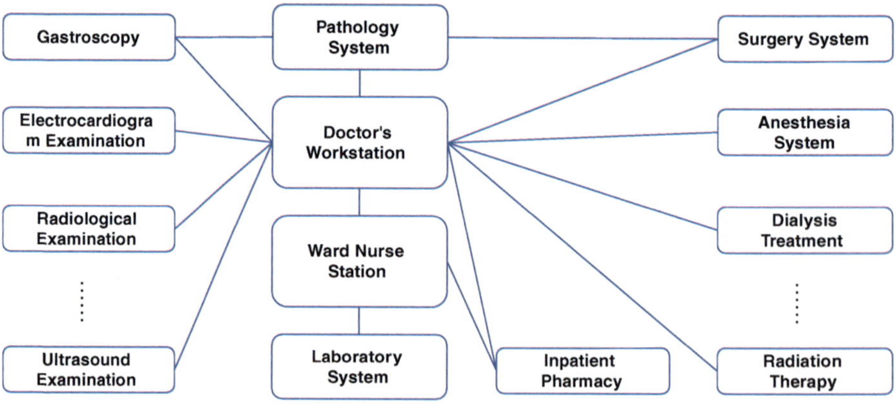

Fig. 2.9 System interface mode for information sharing among various electronic medical record systems

result in a high degree of inter-system coupling requirements and poor maintainability when the system becomes complex, and the operating costs of the system will become very high and the software maintenance will be more difficult at a later stage.

2.5.1.2 Integrated System Model

The integrated system model is a form of data sharing based on standards. Medical business processing systems such as physician workstations and inspection systems are established under the same technical framework. Except for a few systems integrated from other frameworks, information sharing between systems in the same technical system is usually done through an internal database, as shown in Fig. 2.10. This system adopts an integrated approach, unifying system design planning and technical standard requirements, thus achieving interface-free transmission of information between system modules and high-level information sharing. The advantages of this system include low cost, high efficiency, good system integration, and a consistent user interface. The corresponding medical processes of various systems are designed according to a more standardized procedure, usually aligning well with regulations. However, this model of electronic medical record systems also has disadvantages, such as the functionalities of various professional systems not being detailed enough and not fitting tightly with special processing procedures. In real-world settings, integrated electronic medical record systems are usually developed by the same system developer, making the construction process relatively simple and coordination work minimal for hospitals, but at the same time, it also affects the range of products hospitals can choose.

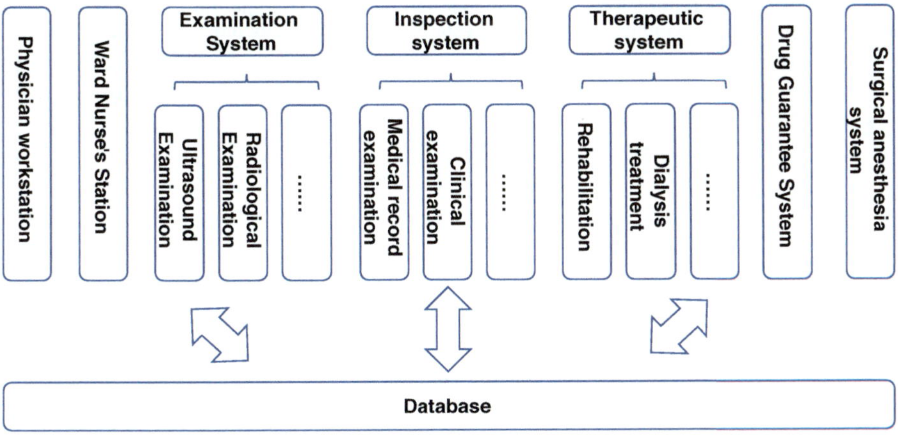

Fig. 2.10 Integrated system model electronic medical record system sharing mechanism through database

2.5.1.3 Integration Platform Model

The integrated platform model refers to the effective integration of the various specialized systems of the electronic medical record in accordance with standardized medical information standards and technologies, so as to realize information sharing and data interoperability among the systems. Figure 2.11 gives a schematic diagram of how each specialized system is connected under the integrated platform model. The integration platform for information systems usually includes functions such as instant message exchange, document exchange, and data integration. The integration platform also establishes interfaces between specialized information systems according to common standards, among which the relevant standards and key technologies are the HL7 standard, the CDA standard, the middleware technology based on the HL7 standard, and the electronic medical record storage and conversion technology based on XML. The HL7 standard mainly defines the standard format and communication protocols for the exchange of clinical and managerial data in the healthcare industry. The standard supports file and data sharing among multi-application systems, which enables the HIS and clinical information system in the hospital's electronic medical record system to achieve seamless and complete exchange of medical data and information, and the hospital information management system between different platforms can also communicate smoothly. CDA standard is an XML-based clinical document structure standard for the medical industry. It standardizes the file format of electronic medical records, which makes the medical record documents easy to be parsed and converted by computers, and easy to be retrieved and used. The combined use of CDA standard and HL7 standard provides an effective way for information sharing among different platforms in the

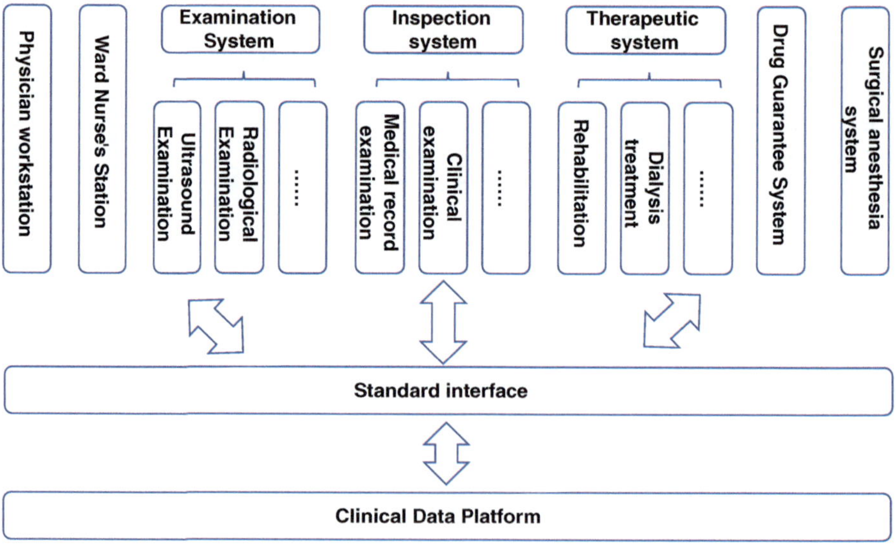

Fig. 2.11 Integration platform model connecting various professional systems through standard interfaces for sharing

electronic medical record system. However, the current data exchange standards mainly define the high-level data exchange methods and usually lack the underlying data exchange specifications. Therefore, the actual construction also requires relevant interface modifications for specific integration platforms. In addition, each specialized system in the electronic medical record system should have corresponding data exchange interfaces with the integration platform, which is a prerequisite for the integration platform mode to integrate the whole electronic medical record system. However, in the actual application process, adding standard data exchange interfaces for each specialized system will increase the cost of building the EHR system.

2.5.2 Regional Medical Electronic Medical Record Transformation

The concepts of medical community and medical consortium have to be mentioned when it comes to the transformation of regional healthcare-oriented electronic medical records. Among them, medical community is short for medical community, which is a subset of medical consortium, while medical consortium is short for medical joint, and both concepts come from the Guiding Opinions of the General Office of the State Council on Promoting the Construction and Development of Medical Consortiums, which was released by the State Council in 2017. The document proposes four organizational modes of medical consortia, which are the formation of medical groups mainly in cities, the formation of medical communities (county medical communities) mainly in counties, the formation of specialty alliances across regions, and the development of telemedicine collaboration networks in remote and impoverished areas.

In part 4 of the document, "Promoting the Up and Down Connectivity of Quality Medical Resources within the Medical Consortium," it clearly stated the need to achieve continuous recording and information sharing of electronic health records and electronic medical records and to achieve interconnectivity of diagnostic and treatment information within the medical consortium. The medical consortium shares the health information data of residents within the region, facilitating services such as appointment diagnostics, bidirectional referrals, health management, and telemedicine, making it convenient for patients to seek medical care and enhancing the level of medical scientific research and technology.

In response to national requirements and standards, many related practitioners have actively engaged in the transformation of electronic medical records for regional medical purposes, considering multiple aspects and angles of how to transform electronic medical records. Below are two typical cases.

2.5.2.1 Middleware Design for Electronic Medical Record Sharing in Regional Medical

There are various methods to achieve electronic medical record sharing, but most require the transformation of the hospital's original information system combined with joint debugging, involving many intermediate links and limitations such as response time and invocation methods in the data interaction process. Independent third-party middleware with few functions and simpler implementation can improve operational immediacy. Hu Hongyu and others adopted this approach, designing an electronic medical record sharing file middleware named EMRSMW, and introduced a NoSQL cluster storage mechanism to ensure system reliability and significantly enhance performance.

The middleware uses an independent application programming interface (API) to provide connection interfaces to the hospital's original information systems such as HIS and EMR. Considering that the data in the hospital's original information systems is held by multiple parties and presented in different data types and characteristics, it is challenging to use a unified framework for direct connection. Therefore, the middleware is designed to adapt to different types of information and information sources, providing specialized interface types and data processing methods for the original information systems of various hospitals. Also, considering the continuous advancement of hospital informatization, the hospital's original information systems might change in capacity, type, and functionality. Thus, the middleware also emphasizes scalability and flexibility. The final design of the middleware effectively implemented data collection, data conversion, and document query functions, promoting information sharing of electronic medical records within the region.

2.5.2.2 System Integration for Secure Electronic Medical Records in Regional Medical

There are various approaches to realize the sharing of electronic medical records, among which the well-known one is the cross-enterprise document sharing (XDS) technology proposed by the Integrating the Healthcare Enterprise (IHE) specification. The framework of cross-enterprise document sharing (XDS) technology is well-known. However, the current system adopting this approach can only export ordinary media for patients to carry and keep by themselves, and this system generally adopts fixed encryption and decryption algorithms when obtaining EHRs from different organizations, which makes the media easy to be cracked and has the risk of information leakage. Zhang Guanjing et al. designed a regional medical electronic medical record security integration system, which realized the dynamic adjustment of electronic medical records and dynamic encryption and decryption algorithms.

The realization of the system is divided into the following steps: first, create an electronic medical record template, sort and number the column names in the electronic medical record template, create storage columns corresponding to the sorting number in the database, and then randomly select an encryption algorithm and send it to a hospital information system. The encrypted electronic medical record is obtained from the hospital information system, the encryption algorithm is invoked to decrypt the encrypted electronic medical record, the column names in the decrypted electronic medical record are parsed, and the column names corresponding to the encrypted electronic medical record are matched with the column names in the electronic medical record template. Second, a new electronic medical record template is generated based on the matching results, the column names in the new electronic medical record template are reordered and numbered, a storage column corresponding to the reordered and numbered columns is created in the database, the data in the acquired electronic medical record is stored in the storage columns corresponding to the reordered and numbered columns in the database, and a new electronic medical record is generated. Finally, an index number is established for all the new electronic medical records and an encryption algorithm is invoked to encrypt the new electronic medical records with the established index numbers. Dynamic adjustment of the electronic medical records is realized by this way of matching the names of the electronic medical record columns, and the security is also improved by applying the randomized encryption and decryption algorithms to the transmitted electronic medical records.

In addition to the above two schemes, many other methods can also achieve continuous recording and information sharing of electronic medical records, which will aid the further development of smart healthcare and telemedicine in China. With the assistance of smart healthcare, the system can intelligently output relevant patient information, allowing medical staff to comprehensively understand the patient's condition. Medical staff can also directly obtain accurate information from the system, saving diagnostic and treatment time. With the assistance of telemedicine, patients in regions with relatively backward medical resources can undergo examinations locally, and then experienced doctors can diagnose through the electronic medical record sharing method, ensuring the health of residents in remote areas. As researchers continue to transform electronic medical records for regional medical purposes, the transformed electronic medical records will play an increasingly important role in the health of the entire population.

2.5.3 Transformation of Electronic Medical Records for Internet-Based Healthcare

The domestic medical informatization industry has gone through three developmental stages:

1. HIS Stage: The aim was to enhance hospital management efficiency, with the focus on HIS construction. HIS primarily managed the comprehensive administration of hospital human resources, logistics, and financial flows, including modules like outpatient registration, outpatient billing, admission and discharge management, and pharmacy management.
2. Clinical Information System (CIS) Stage: The main focus was on various clinical applications, centering around patient-oriented management of diagnostic and treatment processes. Key modules included EMR, PACS, LIS, and anesthesia surgery systems.
3. Interoperability and Integration Stage: As the informatization of various hospital departments matured, on the one hand, internal data interoperability improved hospital management and clinical decision-making through data sharing and

value mining. On the other hand, data interoperability between different medical institutions facilitated collaborative work and enhanced overall efficiency.

The future of medical informatization will enter an intelligent phase, transitioning from informatization to intelligence, utilizing technologies like big data and artificial intelligence to achieve assisted diagnostics and health management, addressing the core issue of medical resource scarcity.

In the interoperability and integration stage, how to securely and effectively share electronic medical record information is a current research focus and a crucial step toward advancing future intelligent medical development. Thus, it is necessary to transform electronic medical records in line with current Internet medical trends to use the Internet to promote information interoperability across different regions and medical institutions.

Given the imbalance in domestic medical resource distribution and the aging trend versus the increasing medical and health demands of the public, the construction of Internet medical services is of significant importance:

1. Internet medical services allow consumers to enjoy services such as online appointment scheduling, consultation, payment, lab result viewing, and home medication delivery, providing convenience.
2. The Internet as a medium can provide more dimensional information about residents' health status, living environments, and social interactions, aiding in more accurate diagnoses.
3. Gathering more information facilitates more timely and accurate public health and epidemic prevention activities.
4. The Internet enables easier access to medical health information and promotes communication between patients and doctors.
5. Internet medical services also allow health regulatory authorities to access more, more accurate, and more timely information, improving transparency and regulatory standards. Moreover, Internet medical services are crucial for implementing tiered medical diagnosis and treatment and enhancing the efficiency of the medical system, which refers to assigning patient care based on the severity and treatment difficulty of conditions, with different levels of medical institutions handling different diseases, gradually moving from general to specialized medical processes.

While Internet healthcare brings benefits, it also faces data security issues. The privacy and security of health care data are not only related to the life and health of patients but also to the safety and security of national health insurance systems. Both Europe and the USA have strict healthcare privacy rules that focus on secure encryption of data, especially during the transfer of data between computers. According to statistics, more than 100 million people in the USA have been affected by breaches of EHR security, and the stolen medical data has been used to fraudulently invoice insurance companies for counterfeit care. Sales of electronic medical record information on the "dark web" have surpassed credit card data. One of the most significant challenges facing the healthcare industry today is how to share critical medical data with stakeholders while maintaining data integrity and protecting patient privacy. While healthcare data standards are more complete, EMR data can still be compromised by issues such as inconsistent workflows and lack of ownership, which can severely impact decision-making and data accuracy while in turn impacting patient treatment and care. There is now a growing emphasis on coordinated care and encouraging greater patient involvement, with participants accessing, viewing, editing, and sharing EMR data at every stage of treatment while ensuring accurate documentation of medication use and diagnosis.

To address these issues, one of the most advanced and effective methods currently is integrating electronic medical records with blockchain technology. Given the sensitivity of personal health data and numerous issues in its sharing process, using blockchain is highly pertinent. EMR information and information shared on blockchain's distributed ledger are updated and protected for use by any authorized individual. Blockchain-based EMR solutions will also reduce the time needed to access patient information, improve data quality, and enhance interoperability. Additionally, using blockchain for electronic health records can reduce overhead costs, especially in software development and health record system maintenance. The advantages of managing EMR with blockchain include standardized digital health data management, which has been a long-standing goal. Hospitals and care providers will no longer need specific software or databases to access patient data. For instance, a decentralized blockchain can facilitate information sharing without relying on private networks between local hospitals, avoiding conversions to the data organization structures of other institutions, and securely sharing electronic medical record metadata to gather statistical information, understand patient health trends, and improve patient care quality. Seamless, accurate, real-time information sharing in the healthcare industry is an inevitable direction for the development of future intelligent medical systems, but security concerns and regulatory compliance must be considered. Moreover, Internet medical data sharing will significantly improve collaboration between medical institutions, also enhancing diagnostic accuracy and enriching patient treatment options, thus heralding an era of cost-effective proactive care. This is where blockchain plays a key role, addressing issues related to data ownership and providing secure, responsible peer-to-peer sharing without troubling the patients.

Blockchain can real-time collect, store, protect, and share health data, facilitating access for healthcare professionals and researchers to a vast number of anonymized patient records for research, thereby increasing sample sizes and enabling researchers to better understand diseases and treatment options. Blockchain-based electronic medical records can also provide personalized health advice to patients through apps or emails and generate supplementary data via wearable devices and mobile apps, meaning doctors can monitor patients' post-surgery or illness conditions in real-time, promptly identifying issues related to diet, exercise, and vital signs like heart rate without the need for face-to-face consultation diagnostics.

Many forward-thinking healthcare organizations have recognized that blockchain technology can save time and money and fundamentally change their operational methods. More importantly, standardizing the management and access to electronic medical records through blockchain will elevate patient care to new heights of intelligent medical care. Patients will receive more accurate diagnoses, significantly reducing the likelihood of medical errors, and will be able to actively manage their entire digital health records. The secure organization and coordination of electronic health metadata can be used to grasp health trends, improve treatment methods, and eradicate diseases.

On top of blockchain technology to ensure data security, the vigorous development of cloud computing technology brings huge opportunities for data sharing in Internet healthcare. Cloud computing can greatly increase mobility and efficiency. New electronic medical record systems provide interfaces that can access patient data, and healthcare professionals can use any device to directly access patients' electronic health information (EHI). This is a major shift in the way patient information is handled, breaking the tradition of keeping patient information only on the hospital LAN. Cloud-based data sharing models allow healthcare data to be tracked anywhere, anytime, no matter where we are, making data entry into and retrieval from EMRs more efficient.

2.6 Conclusion

The existing medical processes often involve multiple specialized systems which, while effectively improving the efficiency of medical staff, also restrict the efficient flow of data between systems [5]. Electronic medical record (EMR) systems are designed to record all types of information throughout the medical process, incorporating these specialized systems to fully leverage patient treatment data and knowledge bases to enhance medical safety and quality.

With strong national support and promotion, the informatization construction of medical institutions has made significant advances. However, current EMRs still face issues related to data standardization and volume, data storage, data security, and system stability. To address these issues, continued collaborative efforts from the government, medical institutions, and system developers will be necessary in the future.

References

1. Shortliffe EH, Cimino JJ. Biomedical informatics. Science publishing Company; 2011. p. 213226.
2. Ralph JJI. A comprehensive review of an electronic health record system soon to assume market ascendancy: EPIC. J Healthc Commun. 2016;1(4):3644.
3. Xianqun F. Internet + medical health. People's Health Publishing House; 2020. p. 5663.
4. Declerck G, Hussain S, Daniel C, et al. Bridging data models and terminologies to support adverse drug event reporting using EHR data. Methods Inf Med. 2015;54(1):2431.
5. Hecht J. The future of electronic health records. Nature. 2019;573(7775):114116, S114.

Laboratory Information Systems 3

Contents

3.1 Overview of Laboratory Information Systems 70
3.1.1 Introduction to Laboratory Testing and Laboratory Testing Systems 70
3.1.2 Development History of Laboratory Information Systems 72
3.1.3 Current Research Status of Laboratory Information Systems Both Domestically and Internationally 74
3.1.3.1 System Integration 74
3.1.3.2 Immediate Test 75
3.1.3.3 Decision Support 75
3.1.3.4 Analysis Report 75
3.1.3.5 Molecular and Genetic Testing 75
3.1.3.6 System Improvement and Evaluation 76
3.2 Main Framework and Workflow of Laboratory Information Systems 76
3.2.1 Main Framework of Laboratory Information Systems 76
3.2.1.1 Pre-analytical Stage 76
3.2.1.2 Analytical Stage 79
3.2.1.3 Post-analytical Stage 80
3.2.2 Workflow of Clinical Laboratory System 81
3.2.2.1 Test Request and Registration 81
3.2.2.2 Sample Management 81
3.2.2.3 Sample Testing 82
3.2.2.4 Result Review and Verification 82
3.2.2.5 Project Review and Approval 82
3.2.2.6 Report Issuance 82
3.3 Case Analysis 83
3.3.1 Neusoft Smart Laboratory Information System 83
3.3.2 Shanghai Ruimei Examination Information System 85
3.4 Frontier Research on Clinical Laboratory Systems 86
3.4.1 Clinical Biological Sample Library 86
3.4.2 Miniaturized and Portable Point-of-Care Testing Equipment and Systems 90
3.4.2.1 Mobile Imaging Platform for Digital Influenza Virus Counting 91
3.4.2.2 Lung Cancer Diagnostic Kit 92
3.4.2.3 Portable Pencil Like Immunosensor Platform 92
3.4.3 Regional Test Center 93

J. Li et al., *Healthcare Information Systems*, Innovative Medical Devices,
https://doi.org/10.1007/978-981-97-9551-2_3

3.5 Summary........ 94
References........ 94

Laboratory Information Systems (LIS) is a laboratory information management system designed specifically for hospital laboratory departments, which utilizes computers to comprehensively manage various laboratory information. LIS can receive, process, and store information generated during the testing process, enabling the automation of tasks related to laboratory work. LIS can also promote communication between laboratory departments and clinical doctors, accelerate the delivery of patient test reports, and play a key role in improving testing quality, reducing information transmission errors, shortening the generation cycle of test results, and improving patient diagnosis and treatment outcomes. Starting from the framework and workflow of LIS, this chapter explores its development history, research status, and cutting-edge research.

3.1 Overview of Laboratory Information Systems

3.1.1 Introduction to Laboratory Testing and Laboratory Testing Systems

Laboratory testing is the testing of samples of a patient's blood, body fluids, secretions, excretions, and debris through visual observation, physical, chemical, instrumental, or molecular biology methods. It emphasizes the adoption of strict quality management measures throughout the entire testing process (before, during, and after analysis) to ensure the quality of the test and provide valuable experimental data for clinical use.

LIS is the practical application of information technology in the field of medical testing, used to achieve and strengthen the transmission of information during the testing process. It connects laboratory analytical instruments through computer networks and establishes a distributed management system centered around the laboratory. LIS establishes a comprehensive quality assurance system based on scientific laboratory management theory and database technology, achieving networked sharing of testing data, paperless recording, resource and cost management, and quantitative assessment of personnel, providing advanced technical support for the overall improvement of laboratory management level and comprehensive management of the laboratory. It is a crucial part of clinical testing today, helping to obtain high-quality data and reliable results.

The document provided by the Public Health Informatics Institute (PHII) lists 19 core functions of LIS: Laboratory Test Processing; Test Scheduling; Proactive Specimen/Sample Collection (Prescheduled Tests); Specimen and Sample Tracking/Chain of Custody; Media, Reagent, Stains, Controls, etc.; Manufacturing; Inventory Control Including Kits & Forms Management; General Laboratory Reporting;

Statistical Analysis and Surveillance; Billing for Laboratory Services; Contract and Grant Management; Training, Education and Resource Management; Lab Certifications/Licensing; Customer Concerns/Suggestions; Quality Control (QC) and Quality Assurance (QA) Management; Laboratory Safety and Accident Investigation; Laboratory Mutual Assistance/Disaster Recovery; Core IT Services: Hardware and Software; Budgeting and Funding; Policies and Procedures

The lifecycle of LIS is divided into three main stages: preanalytical, analytical, and post-analytical. In the pre-analytical stage, LIS can greatly improve the security of sample data, ensure data validation, and prevent data damage or loss. It does not simply automate manual processes, but focuses on redesign of the process. In the pre-analytical stage, the main tasks of LIS are as follows: login management; Ensure correct identification of samples; Create a patient database; Create and maintain a unique sample ID; Help identify samples with incorrect markings; Generate sample barcodes. In the analytic phase, the main tasks of LIS include: using pre-analytical data to ensure the correct identification of samples; Assists in work management by automatically capturing instrument results; Reduce transcription errors from instrument data; Verify the laboratory results; Assist in quality control management. LIS can play a role in process monitoring, workflow, instrument interfaces, and quality assurance. In process monitoring, LIS can continuously mark the position and status of each sample throughout the entire laboratory process. It also has the ability to monitor workflow metrics, such as monitoring the turnover time of samples. In the workflow, LIS establishes rules to ensure that users follow the correct process and notifies users through alerts when needed. In terms of instrument interface, LIS imports data directly from the instrument through a targeted interface, which can reduce data transcription errors and accelerate the analysis process. In more advanced LIS, bidirectional interfaces can be used to send data to the instrument, and the instrument's laboratory results and QC data can also be automatically returned to LIS. In terms of automated quality assurance, LIS can automatically track and generate QA reports, including sample rejection, sample transfer, error operation log table, communication log, event management log, analyzer usage and maintenance requirements, and instrument operation status. In the post-analysis stage, the focus is on submitting the laboratory data to different recipients based on the testing purpose. The test results can be presented as independent results with relevant equipment or geographical location annotations. Meanwhile, additional information can be submitted as needed, including cut-offs or surveillance limits, to support decision-making.

The data exchange standard for clinical systems is HL7 (Health Level 7) health information exchange standard. In the past, LIS was mainly an independent system, with laboratory generated data managed by the laboratory department. LIS is highly coupled and participates in all stages of the diagnostic testing process, from generating test orders to issuing reports. Later, the situation changed and LIS had to interact with numerous healthcare systems to operate effectively. LIS must exchange data with practice management systems, hospital information systems, electronic health record systems, and billing systems. The connection between the laboratory and other hospital systems relies on standardized message formats and communication protocols. The data exchange between various information systems is carried out through application programming interfaces, which include software, protocols, and connections that support electronic data exchange from one system to another. Common message formats and communication protocols are used to standardize data exchange between applications. HL7 is a standard message format used for data exchange between information systems. HL7 is commonly used to send orders from the order input system to LIS, and to send LIS results to clinical information systems. It is also used to register the system for transmitting relevant demographic data and patient status information. HL7 defines the types of messages that can be sent and the data that can be exchanged within the message. The data is encoded into Extensible Markup Language (XML) for storage, display, and transmission. XML has become a standard in many industries. HL7 message types include inspection orders, inspection results, and registration notification messages. In addition, HL7 defines how to exchange messages and provides error communication guidelines. Each HL7 message is divided into segments, which are further divided into one or more fields.

LIS can bring many benefits. LIS can improve laboratory data management, enhance laboratory efficiency, and enhance quality, providing a basis for laboratory data aggregation, analysis, and management. The laboratory can collect information from LIS and provide timely reports for monitoring, managing, and formulating health policies. At the same time, the entire inspection process and data management have been improved, providing better QC/QA. By adopting international laboratory standards, accurate and complete information can be provided to laboratory staff and management in a timely and efficient manner, supporting information tracking, collection, storage, and analysis in workflow and testing processes, issuing reports to patients and other institutions, and improving data security.

3.1.2 Development History of Laboratory Information Systems

In the early 1960s, advances in computing technology prompted people to experiment with data management related functions in healthcare environments. Bolt Beranek Newman collaborated with Massachusetts General Hospital to create a system. The system includes time-sharing and multi-user technologies, which later had a significant impact on the implementation of modern LIS. Around the same time, GE announced a plan to build HIS, although the plan ultimately failed. The first era of LIS was created by large technology companies with little or no knowledge of hospital operations. There were many reasons for the lack of successful LIS cases in this era, but the most important ones were the lack of suitable programming languages and computing technologies.

Pappalardo and Marble developed a MUMPS high-level programming language in the mid-1960s. This language not only introduces very advanced programming concepts. For example, interfaces for multiple concurrent users and tools for porting database drivers from one instruction set architecture to another also integrate a hierarchical database file system for persistent storage. In other words, MUMPS was one of the first hierarchical database management systems in computing history. However, the development team behind MUMPS is small, only using relatively inexpensive hardware and requiring close collaboration with clinical staff to a large extent. The development of MUMPS has a promoting effect on the development of LIS, as it has a multi-user interface and a layered system for persistent data storage. However, its advanced and decentralized use across multiple entities, as well as extracting and analyzing data from databases, were still challenging for the information technology of the time. Therefore, there are very few healthcare and clinical testing systems developed based on MUMPS.

The second generation LIS in the late 1960s and early 1970s was marked by a rapid improvement in technological level. Although almost all of these systems are implemented on the basis of MUMPS, their implementation details differ greatly. The World Health Organization developed its own LIS in 1970 to improve the efficiency of data management and reporting. These LIS require a significant amount of time and resources to implement. With the advancement of technology, some laboratories purchased customized systems in the 1970s.

By the 1980s, the emergence of Structured Query Language (SQL), relational database management systems, and HL7 protocol facilitated software developers to expand the functionality and interoperability of LIS, enabling business analysis and intelligent technology to be applied to clinical data. Technology companies such as Intel and IBM began relentlessly improving their semiconductor manufacturing technology, allowing available computing power to double every year or two, a phenomenon now known as Moore's Law. Standardized and highly portable programming languages designed for ease of use and powerful functionality, such as Pascal and C/C++, emerged and were recognized by the industry, leading to the third-generation LIS. The exponential growth of computing power means that MUMPS can be replaced by a high computational cost but user-friendly relational database management system. In the next decade, laboratory instrument manufacturers began developing commercial LIS solutions aimed at improving system efficiency. However, these software instrument solutions still have limitations and require special customization for specific scenarios, which can result in significant implementation costs and time.

With information technology and processors becoming more advanced and cost-effective in the 1990s and early twenty-first century, informatics developers created universal and flexible LIS, reducing the need for customization compared to previous generations. In addition, developers have built an open-source system that provides multiple systems for laboratories to choose from to track, analyze, and store laboratory data.

After 2010, network based and database centric LIS changed the way people interact with data. Network driven data formatting technologies such as Extensible Markup Language made the interoperability between LIS and EMR a reality. Subsequently, cloud computing technology further changed the implementation of LIS, while also raising new issues related to security and stability.

Modern LIS has entered an unprecedented new era, supporting configurable clinical decision support rules, system integration, testing extension tools, and point-of-care testing (POCT) functions. The LIS module has also begun to appear in electronic medical records, providing hospitals with enterprise level solutions covering multiple departments.

3.1.3 Current Research Status of Laboratory Information Systems Both Domestically and Internationally

Under the influence of the current information age and economic globalization, LIS has shown a trend of globalization, characterized by simplicity and ease of use, the ability to widely connect and control instruments, sample collection and processing, providing rich chemical structures, and the application of multimedia recording. It has been applied in clinical testing. Currently, many workflows in the laboratory are very complex. Therefore, LIS has also become complex and comprehensive, including advanced features to improve clinical care and patient safety (such as patient queue matching, duplicate monitoring alerts, extended support, advanced decision support, rich analyzer interfaces, sample tracking, quality control, and quality assurance). A more comprehensive LIS will eliminate the need for middleware, as this feature is already included in LIS.

In addition, many existing functions in LIS will continue to improve with use, such as the improvement of human–computer interaction to make the use of LIS more intuitive. The updated graphic properties have a clearer and richer appearance, and the larger button design makes it easier for users to see highlighted content when making choices. With the rapid development of decision support, laboratory efficiency and productivity have been improved, specifically manifested as: automatic verification of results and order input; Reflection testing cascading provides the most suitable testing for the laboratory and can improve utilization; Sample tracking can track each sample throughout the entire laboratory process from sample collection to processing. By scanning the sample barcode, the sample can be linked to patient information within the system; Data analysis and dashboards are used to monitor important indicators that have an impact on the laboratory. For example, antibiotic management and bacteria associated with hospital-acquired infections. Currently, LIS has added more modules and middleware from the era of intelligence. For example, speech recognition, intelligent scheduling, intelligent billing, etc., to meet the special needs of certain laboratories.

In addition, LIS continues to expand into new fields, such as adding molecular testing and POCT. The era of intelligence requires LIS to quickly integrate new features to keep up with market changes. At present, LIS has the following research hotspots.

3.1.3.1 System Integration

The interface between LIS and other systems is becoming increasingly important, such as analyzers, public health laboratories, tumor registration offices, billing systems, and EHR. With the increasing attention paid to interoperability systems, constantly updating experimental methods, and constantly changing analyzers, this integrated demand will continue to exist. Petrides et al. summarized ten challenges during the implementation of EHR-LIS interface in a medical center with 777 beds [1]: selection and harmonization of test codes, detailed training for providers on test ordering, communication with EHR provider champions during the build process, fluid orders and collections, supporting specialized workflows, sufficient reports and metrics, increased volume of inpatient venipunctures, adequate resources during stabilization, unanticipated changes to laboratory workflow and ordering specimens for anatomic pathology.

3.1.3.2 Immediate Test

The demand for POCT in healthcare systems is constantly increasing, as POCT can accelerate diagnosis, shorten treatment cycles, save time and costs in many cases, thereby improving patient satisfaction and continuity of diagnosis and treatment.

3.1.3.3 Decision Support

Matthias et al. designed and developed LIS in the Coronavirus disease (COVID-19) epidemic scenario to solve the key bottleneck in the pre-analytical and post-analytical stages [2]. Provide decision support in the pre-analytical stage to enable the laboratory to automatically notify and proactively guide sample preparation and transportation procedures. The system calculates the minimum number of blood vessels required to perform all analyses through algorithms (considering not only the total volume of blood, but also the sample processing and packaging methods in the laboratory), and then notifies the blood sampler of the optimal sampling strategy. The tool also prompts the blood collector to provide packaging instructions and explain the triple packaging requirements. In the decision support of the post-analysis stage, patients are classified as non-suspected COVID-19 cases, suspected but not confirmed COVID-19 cases (test results to be determined), and confirmed COVID-19 positive cases based on the test results. According to this classification, patients of different categories are hospitalized in different units to minimize the spread of diseases within the hospital. LIS quickly and effectively transmits the test results to EHR, and the "COVID-19 Status" button is displayed on the EHR homepage of each patient. This button displays real-time laboratory test results and allows doctors to quickly classify patients based on polymerase chain reaction (PCR) and computed tomography results.

3.1.3.4 Analysis Report

LIS needs to track multiple internal analysis indicators for the laboratory, such as test utilization, personnel level, and quality control, and provide detailed reports. LIS can also track certain disease states of patients, such as diabetes and anticoagulation monitoring.

3.1.3.5 Molecular and Genetic Testing

The increasing attention and technological progress toward personalized healthcare have driven the demand for molecular and genetic testing. This requires LIS to support complex molecular detection workflows, algorithms, as well as the storage and processing of massive data. Charles pointed out through investigation that LIS and many molecular instrument software lack some necessary functions, which can have an impact on the test workflow, efficiency, and safety. Therefore, there is still a lot of work to be improved in the field of LIS.

3.1.3.6 System Improvement and Evaluation

Yusof et al. proposed a new LIS evaluation framework to identify error events, contributing factors, and providing preventive measures for errors and delays in testing. This reduces errors and improves inspection efficiency, while effectively simplifying the inspection process [3].

3.2 Main Framework and Workflow of Laboratory Information Systems

3.2.1 Main Framework of Laboratory Information Systems

The core of clinical laboratory information management is LIS. This section elaborates on the main framework of LIS from three stages: pre-analytical, analytical, and post-analytical. In the pre-analytical stage, LIS participates in sample registration, sample collection, and sample processing. During the analytical phase, LIS needs to transfer the samples to the corresponding analyzer, process the data received from the analyzer, and generate test results. In the post-analytical stage, LIS is responsible for result transmission, report generation, key value identification, and document storage. The main framework of LIS is shown in Fig. 3.1.

3.2.1.1 Pre-analytical Stage

The pre-analytical stage refers to the stage that occurs before analyzing the sample. The pre-analytical stage includes patient identification, sample collection and transportation, sample registration, sample reception, and sample identification. The errors generated in the pre-analytical stage are estimated to account for 40–70% of laboratory errors. The occurrence of these errors is mainly due to manual operations, including errors in paper applications, manual registration, and manual data input. By deploying LIS correctly, errors generated during the pre-analytical phase can be prevented. LIS can ensure quality and safety by providing an electronic interface for registration, inventory collection, barcode sample identification, and standardization.

Patient Identification

Medical records rely on unique and permanent patient identifiers. Patient identification information (such as a combination of name, date of birth, and medical insurance number) must be entered into the system before requesting verification. In most healthcare systems, the registration process involves obtaining patient demographic information. Patient demographic data includes patient name, date of birth, address, phone number, ethnicity, and gender. Using the above patient information,

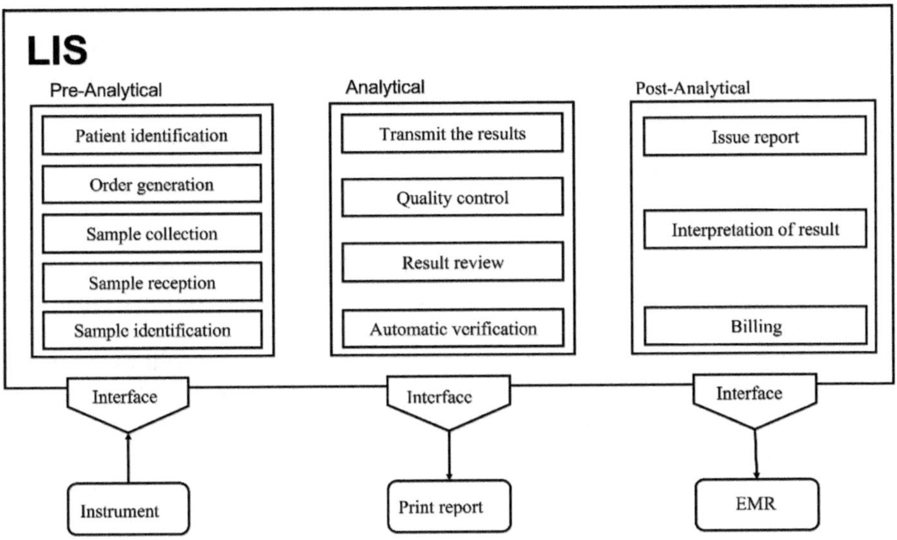

Fig. 3.1 LIS framework

the registration system assigns a unique medical record number to the patient (or retrieves it from the database), and transmits the patient information to downstream systems according to HL7 standards. For example, pharmacy information systems, clinical information systems, and LIS; Patient information can also be manually entered into LIS. Regardless of the scale and input method used, LIS relies on patient identifiers and demographic information to generate report results.

Order Generation

The staff manually input paper medical orders into LIS or generate test orders through the computerized physician order entry system (CPOE, also known as electronic prescription system). The CPOE system provides a clinical order set and nursing methods for doctors to choose based on the patient's clinical status. Due to the fact that doctors can only choose from the available options. Therefore, electronic order input can filter out expired inspection options and provide clinical decision support. From the perspective of workflow and error reduction, CPOE can reduce misunderstandings and errors.

Sample Collection

Sample collection can be driven by batch collection of LIS (such as morning centralized collection) or temporary collection based on individual orders (such as outpatient collection or patient bedside collection). Before collection, LIS will print sample labels containing at least two patient identifiers and sample types (such as test tube types). For temporary collection orders, sample labels are made on demand at the patient's bedside using professional software and portable devices that can scan the patient's wrist strap barcode and print sample labels in real-time. These, also known as "instant" barcodes, are portable devices that load electronic orders, print appropriate labels, and provide relevant instructions on the type and quantity of containers required for the order. For outpatient sample collection, print labels and collect detailed information according to order requirements. Under normal circumstances, samples are labeled with order, test, and patient information and sent to the laboratory for analysis.

Sample Reception

Whether it is through electronic transmission in the order input system or manual input by inspection personnel, the sample will be marked with a unique code (referred to as the sample number) when received. This code is used to track samples throughout the entire testing process. The sample number will associate the inspection order and patient information with the sample. In order to keep the sample number short, some LIS will cycle through the sample number, and some LIS will attach dates to the sample number or use other methods to maintain the uniqueness and permanence of the sample number. In LIS, the sub samples of the sample (such as three different tubes extracted for a patient) are identified by container identification (CID). CID is a unique number that can clearly identify sub samples within a given sample. CID is a key identifier that links the order and result data in the analyzer and LIS. The use of a unique CID is crucial for achieving automation and sample retrieval.

Sample Recognition

Samples are crucial for accurately reporting results. Manual transcription may be the most important source of laboratory errors, with errors occurring approximately once every 300 manual inputs. Sometimes, errors such as digit or decimal misalignment that are particularly difficult to detect may ultimately lead to false positives in the results. During the pre-analytical phase, CPOE transferring orders to LIS is an important means of reducing manual transcription and related errors. In addition, barcodes are extensively used in the laboratory to prevent transcription errors, as well as to identify and track samples throughout the entire testing process. In most systems, each test tube of the sample is uniquely labeled with a barcode. Using an automatic barcode scanner or manually scanning barcode labels by laboratory staff can simplify sample tracking throughout the entire laboratory. Most highly automated instruments integrate barcode scanners into the instrument, supporting automatic recognition and tracking of barcode samples. Radio frequency identification (RFID) is a relatively new automatic identification technology that uses radio waves to identify objects. The RFID system uses small electronic tags that are read by RFID scanners, similar to the way barcode scanners read and print barcodes. RFID tags are composed of small integrated circuits. The data of the marked object is stored in the memory of the integrated circuit. The radio frequency signal generated by the RFID scanner is wirelessly transmitted to or from the RFID tag. RFID tags can store a large amount of information, are very stable, and there is no need for angle matching between the reader and the tag. RFID tags are very suitable for many scenarios in the test process, including sample tracking and patient wristband recognition. Several automation suppliers are currently using RFID technology as the foundation for their automated sample tracking systems.

3.2.1.2 Analytical Stage

During the Analytical phase, LIS transmits results through instrument interfaces, while also conducting quality control and assurance, result review, and automatic verification.

Input Result Information from Instrument Interface

Connecting automated instruments to LIS can greatly improve productivity and reduce errors. To connect the instrument, it is necessary to use device drivers or medical device interface software to enable communication between LIS and the instrument. Instrument manufacturers usually provide interface specifications to LIS suppliers before the introduction of instruments. The instrument interface can be unidirectional or bidirectional. The one-way interface only sends results from the analyzer to LIS, and this type of data transmission can also be referred to as data "upload." In a unidirectional interface, no data is transmitted from LIS to the instrument. Therefore, it is necessary to input order and sample identification information into the analyzer using other methods. At this point, CID can serve as an identification link in these scenarios, as the CID in LIS is associated with patient demographic data. In addition, due to the barcode on the sample tube, having the analyzer scan the barcode on the sample tube can provide a simple way to provide sample identification information to the analyzer. The bidirectional interface allows LIS and analyzer to send data to each other. Through a bidirectional interface, LIS sends patient/sample identifiers and commands to the analyzer, which then sends the results to LIS. Transferring sample identifiers and detection instructions from LIS to the instrument is called "download" (the instrument downloads information from LIS).

Quality Control and Quality Assurance

Quality control is crucial fortest. LIS provides the data required to detect turnaround time (TAT) as it adds timestamps to key events: order time, collection time, receipt time, and result time. In addition to TAT reports, LIS also provides various other management reports, including test volume, workload statistics, and billing. LIS provides views and reporting tools so that staff can easily create reports to query important management and clinical issues.

Result Review

Result validation is an important feature of LIS. After the preliminary results of the detection are marked as "executed," LIS will provide an interface where technicians can review the results. To ensure that only valid results are published, LIS will apply rules to compare with laboratory indicators, including analyte reference ranges or critical value limitations. In addition, the current results can be compared with the patient's previous results (incremental examination) to alert technicians to potential errors. The rules and calculations required for result reporting are usually also located in LIS, such as the calculation of international standardized ratios, anion gaps, and glomerular filtration rate.

Automatic Verification

Traditional technicians rely on individual results or local result groups for result validation, and personal judgment may lead to errors. Automatic validation refers to the process of verifying laboratory results using computer-based algorithms without the scrutiny of technical experts. The most common automatic verification algorithm is to identify and verify the range of results. Carefully designed automatic verification algorithms can improve TAT and enhance operational efficiency. Because humans cannot view thousands of results in a short amount of time while identifying potential errors and other details.

3.2.1.3 Post-analytical Stage

In the post-analysis stage, LIS will report and interpret the test results as well as conduct billing and sample tracking.

Issue a Report

The best report not only relies on data availability, but also on intuitive, efficient, and clear presentation of results. A carefully designed electronic reporting application can improve retrieval efficiency and clarity by highlighting recent results, grouping relevant tests, customizable user-friendly charts, and convenient and fast filtering methods. Special attention should be paid to the labeling of abnormal results, reference intervals, and remarks in laboratory reviews.

Interpretation of Results

As the options and complexity of testing increase, many clinical doctors lack sufficient knowledge to explain all the complex test results in clinical situations. LIS can provide explanatory support for complex test results and create personalized interpretation reports by attaching annotations. This report can be transmitted to medical records and displayed together with the test results. An explanatory laboratory report includes a description of the diagnosis, relevant details that may affect the test, and additional testing recommendations. In several studies, such interpretation reports have had a positive impact on doctors, patients, and hospitals.

Billing Function

LIS needs to report accurate cost statistics for all laboratory tests to the financial system. For each order, LIS typically reports to the billing system on the tests performed, patient demographics, medical orders, visit information, and patient diagnosis. If LIS cannot accurately collect and report this information, it may violate regulatory regulations.

3.2.2 Workflow of Clinical Laboratory System

The LIS workflow can be summarized as follows: outpatient doctors and inpatient workstations submit testing requests and register them, generate corresponding patient barcode labels for laboratory tests, and match the patient's basic information with the testing instruments while generating the laboratory test form; manage the collected test samples, record and maintain the chain of supervision for laboratory samples and reagents; manage and apply corresponding testing equipment to conduct experimental testing on samples; review and verify the results generated by the testing instruments, and the system will automatically match the testing data with patient information through data interfaces and result approval based on corresponding relationships; Review and approve the samples, experiments, and studies after testing; Provide a final report for use by doctors and patients. The LIS workflow is shown in Fig. 3.2.

The functional details implemented by LIS in each process of the workflow shown in Fig. 3.2 are as follows:

3.2.2.1 Test Request and Registration

LIS provides a method for assigning unique identifiers to entities. For example, LIS stores the supplier identifier of the sample as a unique identifier in a barcode or RFID. Unique identifiers should be able to appear in necessary records, files, and reports referencing these entities. Record the collection details of the corresponding registered samples, including container size and type, container quantity, collection date and time, collector name, batch number, storage location, storage method, collection method used (standard and non-standard), safety issues and retention period, and allow the addition, modification, and deletion of new and customizable inspection items. In case of errors, the adverse or unexpected characteristics of the submitted samples can also be recorded.

3.2.2.2 Sample Management

LIS accurately identifies physical samples in the system through barcode or RFID technology. Record and maintain the chain of custody for laboratory standards and reagents, including recording the first opening date, storage location, quantity,

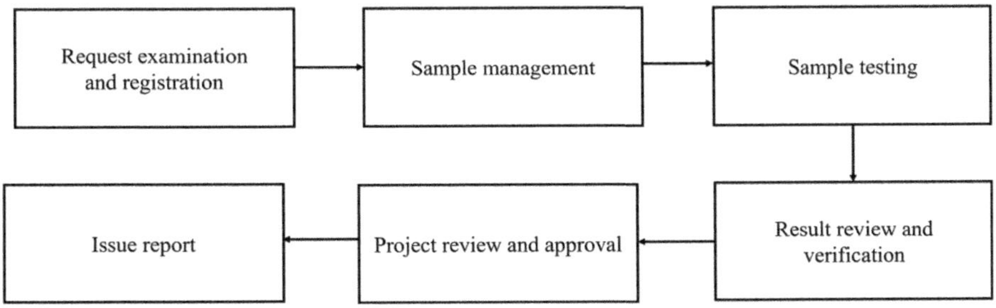

Fig. 3.2 LIS workflow

status of samples and reagents, and grouping logically associated samples together based on relevant metadata (such as sample type, testing method, designated user, and status). Testing methods can also be linked to specifications, standards, and reagents to create personalized sampling and testing, such as representative sampling, calibration testing, quality control testing, preventive maintenance testing, stability testing, sterility testing, compatibility testing, identity testing, availability testing, and service event related testing.

3.2.2.3 Sample Testing

Users can choose approved and unexpired samples and reagents for testing and experimentation. At the same time, the system can detect whether there are expired items and retest with new samples to prevent expired samples, reagents, or other media from participating in the inspection process. It can also check the physical, control, and specification limitations of instrument samples. Users can input all tests related to a single sample, and can also customize the input method. For example, when uploading from a spreadsheet, LIS can intelligently remind users to create and reassign inspection work when inputting unqualified inspections. LIS fully records all data created during testing or experimentation, including instruments used, calculations performed, as well as relevant graphics, charts, and spectra. Records can also capture the signatures of personnel conducting tests or experiments, as well as those reviewing records for compliance purposes.

3.2.2.4 Result Review and Verification

Compare the results of the inspection with predefined data ranges. When the results exceed these data ranges, LIS will clearly remind users, while maintaining a complete audit trail of the operation to modify the test results.

3.2.2.5 Project Review and Approval

LIS accurately records detailed information on the final disposal of samples, providing corresponding functions for specific sample states such as "approved" and "rejected," including processing retesting, resampling, recalculating, responding to non-conforming items, and handling. At the same time, authorized personnel are allowed to view the relevant metadata of the test results during the review and approval process, including the instruments and reagents used, the original data of the instruments, and related reports.

3.2.2.6 Report Issuance

After the authorized personnel verify and approve the results and related metadata, the system accurately generates various sample inspection reports, including detection and analysis certificates, pending samples, samples and reagents that exceed standards, instrument calibration information, expired reagent processing, and trend charts of laboratory performance. LIS uses analytical certificates to verify the status of results, including unique identifiers, analytical procedures used, reference intervals, environmental conditions, testing personnel, other precautions, inspection opinions and explanations, as well as detailed information such as supplier information, applicable time and date, and exports report files in computer-readable formats (such as unformatted spreadsheets, CSV files or XML files, PDF formats) and links them to standards, reagents, and test samples. It also marks possible test results that may not meet specifications or expectations. Reports that have been changed, modified, or reissued should be clearly labeled, and the content and reasons for the information changes should be clearly identified in the report. In addition to standard reports, the system can also provide methods for custom reporting, including but not limited to sample registration reports, work and backlog lists, laboratory performance reports, instrument reports, statistical analysis reports, regulatory reports, accident reports, regulatory chain reports, quality assurance reports, service reports, inventory analysis reports, and investigator reports.

3.3 Case Analysis

3.3.1 Neusoft Smart Laboratory Information System

The Neusoft Smart Laboratory Information System (see Fig. 3.3) aims for comprehensive quality control and rich IoT, serving as a standardized, intelligent, and integrated work platform for medical laboratories. It serves laboratory physicians, technicians, nurses, clinical doctors, patients, and department managers, providing a series of business support such as sample process management, report release, and department management. The system has complete functions and strong equipment connection capabilities, making it the best work platform for modern hospital laboratory business operation and department management. The system fully supports the ISO 15189 specification and meets the evaluation and rating requirements for interconnectivity and electronic medical records.

The bottom layer of the product consists of various data analysis equipment, such as blood analysis equipment, body fluid analysis equipment, mass spectrometer, blood culture equipment, and other assembly line equipment. In the LIS business process, samples are used as units to fully support the collection, measurement, and analysis of turnaround time (TAT). Various tests can be performed on all samples include clinical testing, microbiological testing, biochemical testing, bone marrow examination, body fluids testing, molecular testing, immunology tests, and assisted reproductive technology, to meet the requirements of large hospitals. The system can also be integrated with the MYLA system for microbiological testing and supports POCT bedside testing scenarios, meeting the needs of patients or samples who are not convenient to move for real-time testing. At the same time, the sample flow is also complementary to the overall management module of the system, especially in quality control management, knowledge base, environmental management, reagent management, and equipment management.

Overall, it complies with the ISO 15189 quality standard, fully meets quality control requirements, and meets certification requirements such as the China National Accreditation Service for Conformity Assessment (CNAS) and Level 7 electronic medical records. At the same time, LIS's business has also been extended

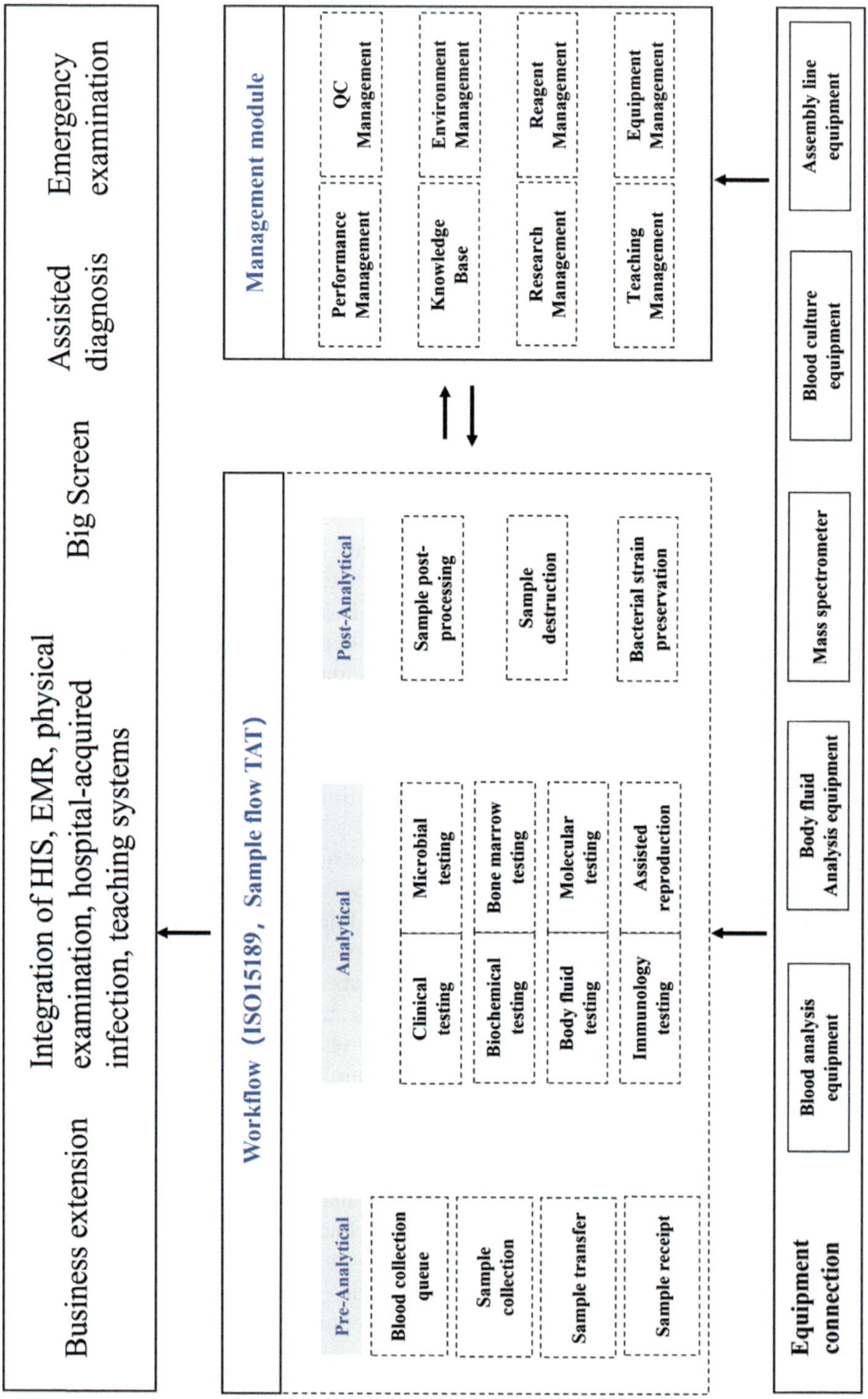

Fig. 3.3 Neusoft smart laboratory information system architecture

to other hospital information systems, such as integration with HIS, EMR, physical examination, blood transfusion, and hospital-acquired infection systems, to assist doctors in auxiliary diagnosis and rapid testing of emergency patients. At the same time, testing information can also be presented on the hospital's command and control screen, allowing everyone to conduct intuitive analysis.

The information system of Neusoft Smart Laboratory has been applied in many large hospitals, including Shengjing Hospital of China Medical University, Zhongnan Hospital of Wuhan University, Jiangsu Province Hospital, Zhongda Hospital Southeast University, and the First Affiliated Hospital of Guangzhou Medical University. It can be seen that hospital informatization is receiving increasing attention, not only in the testing itself, but also in a series of links such as scientific research and teaching.

3.3.2 Shanghai Ruimei Examination Information System

Shanghai Ruimei Computer Technology Co., Ltd. specializes in laboratory information management and has completed cooperation with laboratory departments of dozens of hospitals in Shanghai, Zhejiang, and other regions. Overall, it can be divided into testing network workstations and blood collection sub systems ward application module, director office module, blood bank management system, consumables and reagents management module, outpatient report printing center, and queuing and calling module. The entire clinical testing workflow is shown in Fig. 3.4.

The clinical laboratory network workstation in Fig. 3.4 mainly covers the basic information, examination items, and examination results of patients, and is manually reviewed by specialized physicians to track the patient's samples in real time and avoid simple errors. The inspection items can also be automatically reviewed

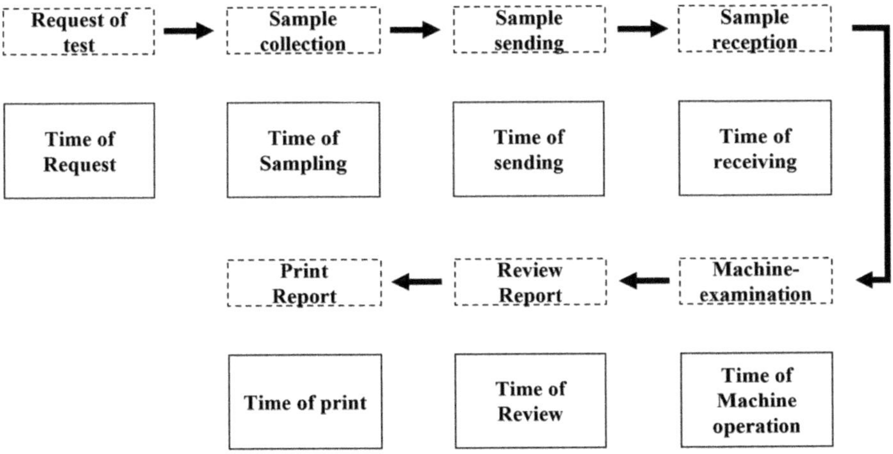

Fig. 3.4 The whole workflow of clinical testing workflow

and diagnosed in medicine through an intelligent knowledge base, timely reminding users and improving the accuracy and timeliness of the inspection. The operation is relatively simple, and through integrated input, it is convenient for users to get started and use. The blood collection system, as a subsystem of the inspection information system, mainly realizes functions such as patient fee verification, automatic bill splitting, barcode printing and comparison, blood collection standards, and patient receipts.

The ward application module is mainly aimed at hospitalized patients, and doctors can directly complete the request, ordering, and cancelation of the items that need to be tested by the patients at the hospital. At the same time, the system is also connected to HIS, and doctors can directly view the status and result monitoring of tests in this module, and form trend statistics for the same item of tests in patients, providing doctors with more accurate clinical diagnostic basis.

The director's office module mainly realizes attendance management for various departments of the laboratory, and also provides a complete understanding and control of the usage and work progress of various instruments.

The blood bank management system queries and statistically analyzes data such as blood in and out management, blood preparation, blood type testing and review, blood cross testing, and patient blood use, and indirectly exchanges data with HIS. The consumables and reagents management module is responsible for maintaining consumables data, including inventory, inquiry, statistics, automatic deduction of reagents, and automatic prompts for minimum inventory levels.

The outpatient report printing center is designed to enable report queries at any location throughout the hospital. Patients can independently obtain reports through card swiping, barcode recognition, network, and other methods. The queuing and calling module sorts and calls the patients who need to be tested, standardizes the testing process, reduces the risk of cross infection among patients, and shortens the time for patients to seek medical treatment.

3.4 Frontier Research on Clinical Laboratory Systems

3.4.1 Clinical Biological Sample Library

At present, various types and forms of clinical biological sample libraries have been gradually established worldwide and have become an important component and research platform for life science and related disease research in the medical system. Clinical biological samples are scarce and cannot be updated, and their research results and conclusions are in line with the actual situation of human pathology, effectively reflecting the characteristics of the disease and providing reference for clinical diagnosis and treatment. In addition, clinical biological samples have become a valuable resource for exploring the pathogenesis of diseases, mastering the laws of disease development, developing medical methods, and developing pharmaceuticals.

The establishment, operation, and management of clinical biological sample banks should be scientific, systematic, and comprehensive. The collected clinical samples of patients include body fluids, blood, pathological tissues, nucleic acids, and proteins. To establish a reasonable clinical biological sample library, the following requirements need to be met: (1) In order to ensure the updating and supplementation of samples, there needs to be a stable source of samples; (2) In order to ensure the timeliness and reliability of the samples, it is necessary to have a standardized biological sample collection process and complete clinical diagnosis and treatment conditions; (3) Laboratory staff must possess clinical medical knowledge; (4) Need for improved medical facilities and sample information management software systems; (5) Necessary post-processing techniques for samples to ensure their suitability for research in cell biology and molecular biology [4].

With the gradual increase in sample size and sample information, and the dynamic changes in both, it is increasingly important to establish a safe, reliable, stable, efficient, and fully functional biological sample information collection and induction biological sample library management system. The registration of biological sample information includes the following three aspects: first, basic information of biological samples, such as quantity, type, quantity, date, location, storage location, usage time, situation, personnel, and research; The second is the citizen information, medical history, family genetic information, diagnosis and treatment indicators and measures, as well as follow-up information of the sample patients; The third is to provide feedback on experimental results and data, such as analysis, collection, tracking, sample allocation and cooperation, correlation research, research topics, etc., to reduce repetitive work.

In the use of samples, the clinical biological sample library should have standardized and comprehensive management measures to prevent unexpected situations such as sample loss and contamination caused by improper management or operation. In order to meet the needs of reuse, samples are packaged to ensure their storage, a scientific and reasonable biological sample storage system is established, as well as subsequent processing and validation technologies such as cell separation, cell identification, cell detection, and nucleic acid extraction technology, which can ensure the quality of the extracted products provided to laboratory personnel. Regular sampling inspections should be conducted on stored biological samples to ensure their activity, reduce losses, improve work efficiency, and ultimately achieve the goals of biological research.

Clinical biological sample resources should be carefully protected and utilized in conjunction with the patient's condition, diagnosis and treatment results, routine testing, and treatment methods. Specifically, it is necessary to observe and study the occurrence and development of diseases, and comprehensively evaluate the different levels of organs, tissues, cells, and molecules; Adopting new medical technologies in difficult cases can help improve medical quality and accumulate medical experience. In addition, it provides a large number of confirmed samples of single and multiple diseases for medical research and teaching, which can reduce research time and facilitate targeted research work.

Due to the rapid development of high-throughput biotechnology, omics technology, and big data analysis, the process of personalized healthcare has accelerated in recent years. Translational medicine, precision medicine, and chronic disease specialties have become important components of China's medical science and technology strategy. The development of medical research urgently requires a large number of high-quality clinical biological specimens. Therefore, the speed of establishing different levels of human biological resource banks worldwide is getting faster and faster. Human biobanks can be divided into population oriented biobanks and disease oriented biobanks, the latter of which is also known as clinical biobanks. As early as 1994, China established the Immortal Cell Banks of Chinese ethnic groups. In 2003, the China National GeneBank started construction. After 2005, China has sparked a wave of construction of biological sample banks. Beijing, Shanghai, and Shenzhen have all established regional biological sample banks with the support of national and local government scientific projects, becoming the leading forces in this field. Clinical biological sample banks, due to their complexity, usually originate from medical institutions and are often built within hospitals, with independent operating spaces and various management systems.

In May 2016, a closed anonymous questionnaire survey was conducted on 42 active clinical biological sample libraries from provinces and cities such as Beijing, Shanghai, Jiangsu, and Guangdong. The results showed that in terms of the age of clinical biological sample inventories, clinical biological sample libraries with 2–5 years, 6–9 years, and more than 10 years accounted for 35.7%, 40.5%, and 11.9%, respectively. In terms of the scale of clinical biological sample banks, 57.1% of clinical biological sample banks have a sample size of over 6000 that meet the research conditions; 40.5% of clinical biological sample banks have a sample size of over 10,000 cases; Clinical biological sample banks with over 30,000 and over 100,000 specimens account for 64.3% and 40.5%, respectively. In terms of storage facilities, clinical biological samples are mainly stored independently in hospitals, accounting for 85.7%.

At present, there has been rapid growth in the top-level design and management organization of clinical biological sample libraries. Due to the fact that the clinical biological sample library of hospitals heavily relies on the information department, clinical department, laboratory department, and infrastructure department, the attention and coordination ability of superiors, as well as the cooperation relationships between departments, affect the development of the entire clinical biological sample library. In addition, the shortage of personnel has also limited the effective operation of some clinical biological sample banks.

The development of clinical biological sample banks is aimed at meeting the growing demand for high-quality medical research. According to a study by Rand Corporation, collecting clinical biological samples has been present in the USA for over 100 years. Therefore, the goal of clinical biological sample banks should be oriented toward the needs of medical research. The research results indicate that the utilization rate of clinical biological sample banks in China is relatively low. This is sometimes similar to the usage rates in other countries. For example, a blood bank in France reported a usage rate of only 0.025%. The speed at which medical researchers utilize these resources lags far behind the speed at which biological samples are collected. According to research findings, the reasons for the low utilization rate of clinical biological sample libraries in China are as follows: lack of top-level design in inclusion and collection standards, resulting in difficulty in ensuring resource quality, limited sharing and application; Research foundation and research ability may also affect the speed of resource utilization; Different standards and insufficient sharing mechanisms pose challenges to the ability to achieve resource sharing. This makes it impossible to integrate more resources and restricts the development of research projects. Finally, as funding mainly comes from hospitals, clinical biological sample banks are more likely to be used by researchers from the same hospital.

In recent years, although China has made certain progress in improving standards, personnel training, and quality control system construction, there is still a relative lack of clinical data quality control in the domestic clinical biological sample library. In addition, due to personnel and financial constraints, the quality control system is often not fully implemented. Therefore, based on a clear perspective and design, the focus of China's clinical biological sample library construction should be on improving execution, detail, and validation.

The most prominent feature of information platforms is the ability to obtain rich clinical data and systematically integrate new research data. Therefore, an information management system for clinical biological sample libraries is essential. At present, most clinical medical data is unstructured, and hospitals use a wide variety of information systems with different functions. These factors pose many challenges to the data integration, data standards, data tracking, data management and other functions of information systems. According to the survey, the information management system currently used in clinical biological sample banks in China can basically meet the needs of most biological sample bank construction. However, the contribution of this information management system in the construction of clinical biological sample libraries and clinical research is relatively weak. The uncertainty of data integrity standards restricts the integration of medical big data. Compared with more mature systems for sample management, clinical data collection systems still have shortcomings in automatic population data collection, data tracing, and data management.

Meanwhile, clinical biological sample banks face inevitable medical ethical issues. In the past, researchers often needed to select and test clinical samples based on the research subjects. However, the collected samples are only for research purposes, and the collection and preservation of biological samples end with the completion of the experiment. Researchers and sample providers often dispose of the remaining samples as medical waste after clinical diagnosis and treatment. In the process of collecting clinical cases and operating clinical biological sample banks, relevant staff need to pay attention to the review and constraint of medical ethics issues, mainly including the following three points.

1. The benefits and risks of clinical biological sample banks, as well as the determination of ownership of biological samples

There is a significant difference between in vitro studies of biological samples and clinical studies directly involving the human body, and there is almost no harm to the sample provider. When samples and their information are included in the clinical biological sample library, the individual attributes of these samples are to some extent transformed into the population biological attributes of disease types or sample types. Therefore, individual samples become public scientific research resources, thereby achieving the sharing of individual and social interests of sample providers.

2. Protecting the privacy of biological sample providers and the security of samples

In the practical operation of clinical biological sample banks, in order to prevent privacy leakage of sample providers and ensure the objectivity and accuracy of research, encrypted samples are usually used to identify unique codes, and anonymous methods are applied to protect the privacy of sample providers, thereby ensuring that sample providers are not affected by the study. At the same time, different levels of access permissions should be established to clarify the relevant information of visitors. When external or foreign organizations are involved, corresponding protection measures need to be formulated to prevent the leakage of clinical biological samples and sample providers, in order to prevent the loss of disease information and ethnic heritage information.

3. Content of informed consent for setting up clinical biological sample banks

The basic principles of informed consent are full knowledge, full understanding, independent choice, personal decision-making, etc. Its content includes signed consent and verbal consent. When designing and determining the content of informed consent, it is necessary to fully inform the functions of the biological sample library and the obligations of researchers, clarify risks and potential accidents, and emphasize that sample providers have the right to terminate informed consent at any time. In addition, regulations need to be set to restrict researchers, including their qualification levels. Biobanks and regulatory authorities effectively regulate biological samples to ensure that they are only used for medical research and to ensure that the personal information and privacy of sample providers are not disclosed. This not only benefits the protection of the rights of sample providers, but also enhances their participation. On the basis of fully understanding and accepting the content of the informed consent form, the sample researchers independently choose to sign the consent form and are authorized to use biological samples and related information under the review of the ethics committee.

3.4.2 Miniaturized and Portable Point-of-Care Testing Equipment and Systems

In recent years, due to the intensification of China's aging population, the coverage of medical insurance has been continuously expanding, residents' income and per capita medical and health expenses have increased, and the demand for medical services has sharply increased. The prospects of the in vitro diagnosis industry are broad, and the point-of-care testing (POCT) industry has also grown rapidly. In vitro diagnosis (IVD) refers to products and services that obtain clinical diagnostic information by testing human samples (blood, body fluids, tissues, etc.) outside the human body, in order to determine diseases or body functions. According to the classification of detection methods, in vitro diagnosis usually includes biochemical diagnosis, immune diagnosis, and molecular diagnosis. POCT is a hot topic in in recent years for in vitro diagnosis. It improves traditional in vitro diagnostic equipment into portable automated instruments, omitting many manual steps of traditional laboratory testing. This means that in the future, in vitro diagnosis will develop toward automation, miniaturization, and real-time direction. The difference between POCT and traditional laboratory testing is that POCT uses portable instruments for analysis, eliminating the necessary steps for laboratory testing such as sample transportation and processing. At the same time, the equipment also has lower requirements for operators, reagents, and samples. Although due to technical reasons, the accuracy of POCT testing is difficult to match that of large-scale testing equipment, it greatly simplifies the requirements for time and location in laboratory testing, and reduces medical costs. With the introduction of immune response and molecular biotechnology, the convenience and application range of POCT have been improved. At present, the most widely used fields include blood sugar, pregnancy and ovulation, cardiac markers, blood gas and electrolytes, infectious diseases, tumor markers, drugs and alcohol, etc. Meanwhile, the main methods for evaluating the presence of biomarkers for viruses and other diseases, while effective, are expensive, especially considering specific economic and regional factors. This method is very difficult to apply in many cases.

3.4.2.1 Mobile Imaging Platform for Digital Influenza Virus Counting

In 2019, Minagawa et al. from the University of Tokyo in Japan created and tested another miniaturized system that utilizes low-cost components and a smartphone for digital biological analysis detection [5].

The mobile imaging platform uses a simple optical device to achieve low noise fluorescence imaging, allowing detection of the fluorescence of individual bovine alkaline phosphatase (bALP) molecules or individual influenza virus particles encapsulated in the air-lift reactor. Although the images obtained using mobile imaging platforms are distorted due to spherical aberration, and the spatial resolution of mobile imaging platforms is lower than that of traditional microscopes, mobile imaging platforms enable quantitative digital biometric determination of bovine alkaline phosphatase molecules and digital influenza virus counting (DIViC). Compared with traditional fluorescence microscopy, the detection efficiency of mobile imaging platforms for digital influenza virus counting is 60%. Nevertheless, the sensitivity of digital influenza virus counting combined with mobile imaging platforms is still 100 times higher than commercial rapid influenza diagnostic tests.

These results indicate that digital influenza virus counting with mobile imaging platforms is suitable for the next generation of real-time detection, enabling extremely sensitive detection of influenza viruses and diagnostic testing in the early stages of infection. The experimental evidence of clinical samples supports this result.

However, further development of diagnostic testing still faces several technical challenges. Firstly, it is necessary to optimize the optical system to improve spatial aberration and resolution. This will make image analysis require more dense array reactors and smaller volumes to obtain a wider dynamic range and faster analysis. Even if significant background signals are found in the analysis of clinical samples, reliable diagnostic testing is still necessary for clinical samples.

3.4.2.2 Lung Cancer Diagnostic Kit

Lateral flow assay (LFA) is one of the most popular point-of-care detection tools, widely used as a portable biological detection strip due to its low cost, fast detection speed, and selectivity toward target biomarkers. Shandong Normal University developed a low-cost, easy-to-use, and highly sensitive lung cancer diagnostic kit (LCDK) in 2020, which can quickly identify non-invasive lung cancer using clinical salivary gland and urine samples [6].

The design of this detection platform consists of three parts: (1) Adaptor modification for screening and concentrating exosomes Fe_3O_4@SiO_2 nanoparticles (Fe_3SO_4@SiO_2-aptamer nanoparticles, FSA); (2) Double specific nuclease (DSN) used to achieve reporter gene hydrolysis triggered by exosomal miRNA; (3) A horizontal flow test strip used to read data. This POCT system based on test strips has successfully utilized clinical salivary gland and urine samples to achieve true non-invasive diagnosis of lung cancer, with high sensitivity and selectivity. The results are comparable to the standard real-time polymerase chain reaction (qRT PCR) method. Meanwhile, LCDK has been shown to have high sensitivity to miRNA205 at concentrations as low as 7.76×10^{-12} mol/L. In addition, the specificity of LCDK detection depends on the sequence of the adapter and reporter DNA, which can be transformed into any sequence. Therefore, it seems that LCDK can be used to diagnose other diseases, and it is expected that this kit will be widely used in clinical diagnosis.

3.4.2.3 Portable Pencil Like Immunosensor Platform

Portable immunoassay devices have a high demand for POCT of biomarkers. In 2020, Northeast Normal University released a powerful portable pencil like immunosensor (PPS) platform for detecting three inflammatory markers, including interleukin-6 (IL6), procalcitonin (PCT), and C-reactive protein (CRP) in human serum samples. The PPS platform consists of a unique pencil shaped fiber optic immunosensor, a series of pencil cap shaped reagent bottles, and a battery powered photon counting detector for recording chemiluminescence. The PPS pencil shaped fiber optic immunosensor moves from one reagent bottle to another by insertion/extraction and completes the immunoassay steps. Each pencil shaped fiber optic immunosensor in the PPS platform can perform up to ten consecutive detections by simply pushing the complete probe into the reagent bottle. The PPS platform is integrated into a portable handheld device (32 × 23 × 11 cm), with a mass of only 3 kg. Experiments in various environments have shown that the sensor has good repeatability, good linear relationship, and effective dynamic range. The experimental results were compared with clinical methods, and the results showed that the method has high accuracy and precision. The PPS platform is versatile, operable, and requires minimal instruments and technology, simplifying the immunoassay process. Therefore, it has broad prospects in POCT of biomarkers [7].

3.4.3 Regional Test Center

Regional Medical Testing Center, also known as Regional Testing Center, refers to a large medical laboratory established within a certain region to provide high-quality testing services to medical institutions at all levels in the region, achieve sharing of testing resources, homogenization of testing quality, standardization of testing services, mutual recognition of testing results, and undertake certain tasks such as talent cultivation, teaching, and scientific research.

The construction of regional medical testing centers was carried out earlier in foreign countries. For example, Quest Diagnostics in the USA has the top two independent medical laboratories and is the most well-known provider of in-depth medical device testing, with business coverage in over 130 countries and regions worldwide. Quest Diagnostics not only provides a large number of clinical testing services, clinical trial services for treatment consultation, diagnosis, monitoring, and treatment of diseases and health conditions, but also involves other fields, including manufacturing and selling diagnostic kits, POCT products, providing pre-clinical research and testing services, and providing risk assessment services for insurance companies. Quest Diagnostics was listed on the New York Stock Exchange in 1996 and currently has 31 regional large diagnostic centers, 155 rapid response laboratories, and over 2100 patient service centers in the USA. It has over 3500 testing items and diagnoses over 100 million samples annually.

Since the General Office of the State Council issued the "Notice on the Comprehensive Reform Pilot of County level Public Hospitals" in 2012, which first proposed "exploring the establishment of inspection and testing centers," China has successively issued more than ten policies to promote the development of regional medical inspection centers in order to achieve graded diagnosis and treatment and promote regional resource sharing. The construction of regional medical inspection centers has become an important direction of medical policies. As a third-party industry apart from hospitals, the overall penetration rate of regional medical testing centers in China is still relatively low. Compared with developed countries such as Japan, due to the limited number of large hospitals in Japan, the penetration rate of regional medical testing centers has reached 67%; There are many large general hospitals in the USA, but the penetration rate also reaches about 35%. However, in China, it is only about 5%, which provides a broad market space for the construction of regional medical testing centers. According to statistics, with the support of national policies, the number of third-party testing centers has reached 1275 in the first half of 2018, but it is still in the early stages of development, especially in terms of size and number of testing items, there is still a significant gap. The number of testing items in China is generally around 2600, while the number of Quest Diagnosticscan reach 3500.

The development of regional medical testing centers in China has shown a diversified trend. In terms of nature, there are private third-party medical laboratories (such as Jinyu Medicine, Dian Diagnostics, etc.), as well as regional medical testing centers established based on public hospitals (such as the Luohu District Medical Testing Center in Shenzhen); From a disciplinary perspective, there are comprehensive regional medical testing centers, specialized regional medical testing centers, as well as chain regional medical testing centers and independent laboratories in various regions.

Regional medical testing centers play an important role in improving the national hierarchical diagnosis and treatment system and enhancing regional medical capabilities. In response to the problems of rudimentary testing equipment, limited testing items, lack of technical personnel, and insufficient clinical diagnostic ability in grassroots medical institutions, regional medical testing centers have professional talents, specialized testing equipment, and testing items to provide effective medical testing services for grassroots medical institutions, which can to some extent solve the problem of difficult medical treatment for patients. At the same time, regional medical testing centers have a large scale in the procurement of reagents, consumables, and equipment, thus having price advantages. All nonemergency work in hospitals can be carried out by regional medical testing centers, thereby reducing the clinical testing pressure on hospitals, reducing unnecessary supply and labor costs, ensuring uninterrupted doctor services, improving turnover time, and enhancing regional medical capabilities.

3.5 Summary

As an indispensable part of hospital information systems, LIS is constantly expanding its functions with the continuous improvement of hospital informatization level. In addition to completing basic laboratory related tasks, LIS is playing an increasingly important role in hospital information management, diagnostic capabilities, talent cultivation, and scientific research.

With the development of mobile healthcare and telemedicine, LIS is no longer limited to hospitals. The emergence of regional testing centers and POCT has expanded the service area of LIS, better improved the diagnosis and treatment results of patients, optimized the national hierarchical diagnosis and treatment system, and enhanced the level of medical services within the region.

References

1. Petrides AK, Tanasijevic MJ, Goonan EM, et al. Top ten challenges when intervening a laboratory information system to an electronic health record: experience at a large academic medical center. Int J Med Inform. 2017;106:916.
2. Weemaes M, Martens S, Coypers L, et al. Laboratory information system requirements to manage the COVID-19 panel: a report from the Belgian national reference testing center. J Am Med Inform Assoc. 2020;27(8):1293–9.

3. Yusof MM, Arifin A. Towards an evaluation framework for Laboratory Information Systems. J Infect Public Health. 2016;9(6):766773.
4. Li H, Ni M, Peng W, et al. A survey of the current situation of clinical banks in China. Bioreserve Biobank. 2017;15(3):248–52.
5. Minigawa Y, Ueno H, Tabata KV, et al. Mobile imaging platform for digital influenza virus counting. Lab Chip. 2019;19(6):2678–87.
6. Zhou P, Lu F, Wang J, et al. A portable point of care testing system to diagnose lung cancer through the detection of exosomal miRNA in urine and saliva. Chem Commun. 2020;56(63):8968–71.
7. Nie R, Huang J, Xu X, et al. A portable pencil like immunosensor for point of care testing of flammatory biomarkers. Anal Bional Chem. 2020;412(13):3231–9.

Picture Archiving and Communication Systems

4

Contents

4.1 Overview of Picture Archiving and Communication Systems 98
4.1.1 Introduction to Picture Archiving and Communication Systems 98
4.1.2 Development History of Picture Archiving and Communication Systems 100
4.1.3 Current Research Status of Picture Archiving and Communication Systems at Home and Abroad 102
4.1.4 Technological Development of Picture Archiving and Communication Systems 103
4.1.4.1 Standardization of Internal Storage Format to DICOM 3.0 103
4.1.4.2 Adoption of Standard Compression Algorithms to Compress Image Files 104
4.1.4.3 Transition from Three-Tier Storage Model (Online, Nearline, and Offline) to Two-Tier (Online and Backup) 104
4.1.4.4 Intelligent Medical Imaging Platform 104
4.2 DICOM Standard 104
4.2.1 Overview of the DICOM Standard 104
4.2.1.1 Basic Concepts of the DICOM Standard 104
4.2.1.2 Scope of the DICOM Standard 105
4.2.1.3 Domains of Application of DICOM 105
4.2.2 Development History of the DICOM Standard 105
4.2.3 Introduction to DICOM 3.0 Standard 107
4.2.3.1 Principles of DICOM 3.0 Standard 107
4.2.3.2 Basic Content of DICOM 3.0 Standard 108
4.2.3.3 DICOM 3.0 Standard Data Structure 110
4.3 Main Functions and Key Technologies of Picture Archiving and Communication Systems 111
4.3.1 Main Functions of Picture Archiving and Communication Systems 111
4.3.1.1 Examination Information Registration 111
4.3.1.2 Image Acquisition Function 112
4.3.1.3 Image Transmission and Storage Function 114
4.3.1.4 Image Display and Processing Function 114
4.3.1.5 Report Management Function 114
4.3.1.6 System Management Function 115
4.3.2 Key Technologies of Picture Archiving and Communication Systems 115
4.3.2.1 Workstation Displays 116

J. Li et al., *Healthcare Information Systems*, Innovative Medical Devices,
https://doi.org/10.1007/978-981-97-9551-2_4

4.3.2.2 Network ... 117
4.3.2.3 Storage ... 118
4.4 Cutting-Edge Research in Picture Archiving and Communication Systems ... 120
4.4.1 Miniaturized and Mobile Imaging Devices and Systems ... 120
4.4.1.1 Mobile CT Scanner ... 120
4.4.1.2 Mobile MRI Scanner ... 121
4.4.1.3 PET ... 121
4.4.2 Image Reconstruction and 3D Printing ... 122
4.4.3 Regional Imaging Center ... 123
4.4.3.1 Significance of Constructing Regional Imaging Centers ... 124
4.4.3.2 Principles for Constructing Regional Imaging Centers ... 124
4.4.3.3 Data Storage Methods in Regional Imaging Centers ... 125
4.4.3.4 Case Studies of Regional Imaging Center Construction ... 125
4.5 Summary ... 126
Reference ... 127

The use of digital medical imaging systems in healthcare institutions has been widely promoted, becoming one of the most valuable tools for supporting clinical decisions and diagnostic treatments. Compared to traditional film-based analog systems, storing and retrieving images in a Picture Archiving and Communication System (PACS) show significant advantages. The "Opinions of the General Office of the State Council on Promoting the Development of 'Internet + Healthcare'" issued by the General Office of the State Council in 2018 pointed out that "It is encouraged for higher-level medical institutions within medical consortia to utilize technologies such as artificial intelligence to provide services like telemedicine consultation, remote ECG diagnosis, and remote imaging diagnosis to grassroots levels. This will promote real-time access, mutual recognition, and sharing of examination and test results among medical institutions within the medical consortia." The construction of PACS can comprehensively improve work efficiency, reduce operating costs, and create excellent opportunities for telemedicine, remote work, and collaborative work environments.

4.1 Overview of Picture Archiving and Communication Systems

4.1.1 Introduction to Picture Archiving and Communication Systems

PACS, also known as Medical Imaging Information System or Picture Archiving and Communication Systems, is an integral part of the hospital information system and is generally used in the radiology departments of hospitals.

The routine tasks of this system involve digitizing various types of medical images produced daily by different instruments (including MRI, infrared devices, CT scanners, ultrasound machines, X-ray machines, microscopes, etc.) through different interfaces (network, DICOM, analog, etc.). This method of storage is both fast and has a large capacity, allowing for quick retrieval when needed. Additionally, some PACS systems include auxiliary diagnostic management functions.

In today's medical industry, PACS refers to a comprehensive application system that integrates high-performance servers, networks, and storage devices as the hardware support platform, and uses large relational databases as the storage management tools for medical imaging data. It combines applications such as image acquisition, image transmission, image storage, image management, image diagnostic management, and report querying into one integrated system.

PACS has several advantages over previous physical storage methods, specifically:

1. Cost savings on materials

   Compared to physical storage methods like paper and film, PACS's digital storage method saves a significant amount of material costs.
2. Reduction in hospital management costs

   Digitally stored images do not degrade over time and occupy very little physical space, saving substantial costs related to film storage and management.
3. Increased efficiency for doctors

   The digital storage method introduced by PACS allows doctors to easily access and view imaging data from various locations without long waits or significant manpower, greatly improving their work efficiency.
4. Improvement in medical standards for doctors

   With digital storage, doctors can use various image processing technologies to detect small lesion areas more easily and can also conveniently access previous medical records to reference past experiences, leading to more accurate diagnoses.
5. Enhancement of hospital resource accumulation

   The images and reports of medical records within a hospital are valuable resources. With the introduction of PACS, distortion-free digital storage and standardized reports provided by hospital doctors become valuable technical assets for the hospital.
6. Optimal resource utilization

   The introduction of PACS not only advances the development of telemedicine and expands the service range of imaging equipment but also promotes technical exchanges between hospitals, facilitating joint progress and development.

4.1.2 Development History of Picture Archiving and Communication Systems

With the continuous advancement of medicine and the constant introduction of various medical imaging diagnostic technologies, hospitals and other medical institutions are increasingly relying on imaging data (such as ultrasound, CT, X-rays, etc.) for diagnosis. Traditional medical imaging management still uses physical storage methods, organizing and piling up films, pictures, and other materials. As the number of imaging examinations for patients continues to increase, the amount of imaging data that needs to be stored also increases, creating numerous difficulties in organizing, storing, and retrieving the data, and sometimes leading to loss of information. This physical storage method has become increasingly outdated compared to advanced medical imaging diagnostic technologies, leading to the emergence and rapid development of digital medical imaging management methods, named PACS.

The above introduction outlines the origins of PACS development. Next, the development process of PACS will be detailed according to the history of technological innovation. Scholars generally divide the development process of PACS into three stages: emergence, development, and perfection.

The first stage is the initial emergence stage, generally considered to be from the mid-1980s to the mid-1990s. During this stage, computer performance was relatively low and prices were relatively high. Most related research focused on using limited computer resources to handle large volumes of digital images, achieving certain results in hardware acceleration and algorithm optimization. There was no unified digital image transmission standard at this time, and images from different devices could not be exchanged. Therefore, PACS systems of this period were mainly based on a single computer, without involving multiple computers, and were relatively slow, with limited functionality and low image display quality, failing to meet the needs of the time and leading to low recognition of PACS. PACS was mainly used in radiology departments, connecting to some equipment, with the primary goal of digitizing films. The typical feature of PACS in this period was "users find the data." After data entered PACS, users needed to provide search conditions to query and find the corresponding images and related data, requiring significant manual participation to fully utilize PACS functions, resulting in limited usefulness.

The second stage is the development stage of PACS, generally considered to be from the mid-1990s to the late 1990s. Over time, computer and network technologies greatly improved, particularly the performance of machines, significantly enhancing the processing speed and performance of PACS user terminals. Image display technology also saw significant breakthroughs during this period, with the emergence of display quality control software meeting the needs of film reading, leading to increased recognition and some clinical application of PACS. Subsequently, the need to reasonably store diagnostic reports and other information led to the creation of RIS (Radiology Information System). The goal of this system was to optimize the workflow management in radiology departments, covering the entire process from appointment, consultation, image generation, film output, report writing, review, to film distribution. By this point, it had become a consensus in hospitals to use electronic devices to optimize workflows and save manpower. Consequently, various medical imaging devices began to be used clinically. The interaction of different devices introduced workflow issues, such as ensuring communication between PACS and RIS during diagnosis, registration, storage, and image acquisition. Over a period of time, the DICOM (Digital Imaging and Communications in Medicine) standard gradually formed and became complete, defining a medical image format that met clinical needs and facilitated data exchange. With all conditions met, various PACS emerged, with Full PACS being particularly important. Full PACS aimed to connect all imaging networks within a hospital, gradually including non-radiology images such as electrocardiograms, ultrasounds, and pathology into the PACS scope, and began sharing some information with other hospital systems. This method further increased the speed of film reading and facilitated the use of clinical departments. The typical feature of PACS in this period was "data find the devices," as PACS introduced the concepts of data pre-fetching and auto-routing. When data entered PACS, it was automatically sent to predetermined devices based on rules set by the user and information from other systems.

The third stage is the perfection stage of PACS, generally considered to start from the late 1990s and continue to the present. During this stage, display quality control software further developed, new models of display devices emerged, and technical factors such as temperature and lifespan had negligible effects on display quality. Many clinical software tools were also introduced into PACS to assist in diagnosis and treatment. As hospitals progressed toward being film-less, system integration and fusion became the development direction. With the widespread recognition of the DICOM 3.0 standard, RIS and PACS began to fully integrate with systems like HIS (Hospital Information System), gradually blurring the boundaries between systems and integrating workflows, increasingly emphasizing holistic medical solutions, resource sharing, and unified process operations. In addition to the integration and connection of PACS with other systems, PACS from different regions also began to integrate and connect with each other. This enabled the sharing of medical information on a larger scale, truly realizing the function of telemedicine consultation. The typical feature of PACS during this period is "information and images find the user," similar to the second stage's "data find the devices." This is based on pre-set rules and information from external systems to automatically transmit the corresponding images and related data to designated devices, and then distribute them to specific users. The close integration and connection between PACS and other external systems successfully achieved the automated workflow of information and images finding the user, thereby successfully realizing the automation of PACS operations.

In conclusion, since the 1980s, PACS has emerged but was not widely recognized due to the lack of high-speed computer networks, high-performance display devices, and large capacity storage devices. With the development of computer graphics and network communication technologies in the 1990s, PACS matured, gradually became popular, integrated with other systems, and perfected, meeting clinical diagnostic needs with the added advantage of remote diagnosis.

4.1.3 Current Research Status of Picture Archiving and Communication Systems at Home and Abroad

The development of PACS abroad began relatively early and is comparatively mature. In contrast, research and application of PACS in China started late and developed relatively slowly. However, after decades of development, PACS has become relatively perfected both domestically and internationally. Currently, PACS is almost fully implemented in hospitals, enabling comprehensive sharing of imaging data within departments such as radiology, ultrasound, endoscopy, and pathology.

As the application of PACS deepens both domestically and abroad, some issues have gradually emerged. For instance, to improve the accuracy of patient diagnosis, the clarity of imaging data within PACS needs to be enhanced, leading to larger storage space requirements. Hospitals need to store patient imaging data for extended periods, which makes traditional medical imaging storage structures and methods inadequate for further PACS development, necessitating the development of newer, more rational storage structures and methods. Globally, the standards for developing medical and other systems are not uniform. Different development companies produce products with different structures, databases, and operating systems, resulting in varying degrees of standardization for PACS implemented in hospitals worldwide. There is a need for a globally unified system development standard. Additionally, PACS lacks sufficient antivirus software. If the stored imaging data contains viruses, it could infect terminals and potentially cause the entire PACS to collapse, risking the loss of substantial imaging data. Therefore, enhancing the security capabilities of PACS, such as data backup and storage redundancy, is necessary.

The above introduction highlighted some issues encountered during PACS operation. Addressing these issues to fully leverage PACS's functionalities is the current focus of PACS research. Besides, with the continuous emergence of new technologies, another major research direction is how to enhance PACS's performance and better integrate it with modern times, for example, by leveraging the currently popular cloud storage technology.

Cloud storage is a new storage method that uses distributed file systems, cluster applications, network technologies, and other functions to combine various types of storage devices on a network to work together, forming a platform that provides data storage and business access externally. Integrating cloud storage technology with PACS eliminates concerns about storage expansion due to unlimited storage capacity. Lifecycle policies can be set on the cloud storage platform to balance efficiency and cost. The hierarchical system on the cloud storage platform can provide different permissions to different hospital staff, offering certain security protection technologies for hospital imaging data.

"Mobile + Internet" is another current hotspot. With the continuous development of mobile internet technology and the improvement of various information transmission technologies, the transmission speed of images has become faster, achieving full coverage of imaging data within departments and even hospitals in PACS. Coupled with the proliferation of smart mobile terminals such as smartphones and medical carts, PACS can operate more efficiently and flexibly, allowing patients to conveniently access and transmit some imaging data online and enabling some experts to diagnose diseases online.

Currently, PACS has some issues but also unique advantages in certain aspects. With the passage of time and continuous technological development, future PACS may achieve breakthroughs in the following areas:

1. Modularization of functional systems:
   As PACS becomes more sophisticated, its functionalities increasingly exhibit modular characteristics. Generally, it can be divided into six parts: examination information registration module, image acquisition module, image storage and transmission module, image display and processing module, report management module, and comprehensive information management module. Through module division, different modules can be quickly located, thereby meeting users' various needs.
2. Medical imaging teaching:
   In the past, medical imaging teaching was conducted using film and slides, which was relatively rudimentary. The number of medical imaging films was limited, and slide clarity was low, leading to less-than-ideal teaching outcomes. Establishing a teaching platform through PACS can improve students' independent learning abilities and enhance the richness and practicality of the entire teaching process while making it easier to access imaging data.
3. Regional platform sharing:
   Although PACS has achieved comprehensive coverage within hospitals and inter-departmental linkage, inter-hospital linkage has not yet formed. A regional PACS sharing platform can be established to achieve resource sharing between hospitals, enhancing doctors' work capabilities and efficiency.

4.1.4 Technological Development of Picture Archiving and Communication Systems

The technological development of PACS is mainly reflected in the following aspects:

4.1.4.1 Standardization of Internal Storage Format to DICOM 3.0

Currently, almost all advanced PACS manufacturers in Europe and the United States use the formal DICOM 3.0 file format to store images. Some older PACS designs still use ACRNEMA 2.0 or SPI, and only very old PACS systems use manufacturer-defined formats. Using the DICOM 3.0 format has many advantages. For instance, when replacing PACS in the future, there is no need to rely on the old PACS manufacturer to convert data. More importantly, using the DICOM 3.0 file format allows for the addition, subtraction, and modification of image file content at any time, whereas traditional fixed-field-length image formats require a complete overhaul for any partial modification.

4.1.4.2 Adoption of Standard Compression Algorithms to Compress Image Files

The new generation of PACS mostly adopts standard compression algorithms supported by DICOM, such as JPEG, JPEG Lossless, JPEG 2000, JPEG LS, and Deflate. The use of manufacturer-defined algorithms to compress images is becoming increasingly rare.

4.1.4.3 Transition from Three-Tier Storage Model (Online, Nearline, and Offline) to Two-Tier (Online and Backup)

Currently, advanced PACS manufacturers in Europe and the United States are promoting a two-tier storage system: online and backup. The backup is only for emergencies, such as fires or earthquakes. Online storage uses hard disks with redundant array of inexpensive disks (RAID) plus network-attached storage (NAS) or storage area network (SAN). A few years ago, the most common PACS storage model was a three-tier image storage mode: online, nearline, and offline. New images were stored online on hard disks, slightly older images were stored nearline on network servers, and even older images were stored offline on magneto-optical disks (MOD) or tapes.

4.1.4.4 Intelligent Medical Imaging Platform

The intelligent imaging IT platform is the main development direction of hospital information systems. The ability to quickly obtain all diagnostic information is the only standard for evaluating the quality of an imaging workstation. Syngo.via is the world's first "thinking" imaging workstation platform, which changes the traditional concept of image post-processing. It abandons the software-oriented traditional CT workstation work mode and initiates a new work perspective oriented toward anatomical or disease diagnosis. It breakthroughly becomes an imaging workstation platform that directly serves disease diagnosis, freeing doctors from the tedious post-processing of images and allowing them to focus on medical diagnosis.

4.2 DICOM Standard

4.2.1 Overview of the DICOM Standard

4.2.1.1 Basic Concepts of the DICOM Standard

DICOM (Digital Imaging and Communications in Medicine) is a standard specifically developed for the storage and transmission of medical images by the National Electrical Manufacturers Association (NEMA) and the American College of Radiology (ACR). This standard has been widely accepted by medical equipment manufacturers and the medical community. As long as the DICOM standard is followed, different types of digital imaging equipment produced by different manufacturers can communicate through PACS. The emergence of MRI, CT, and ultrasound devices with DICOM standard interfaces is of crucial importance to the digital networking of medical information systems.

4.2.1.2 Scope of the DICOM Standard

According to the DICOM standard manual, the DICOM standard facilitates interoperability between medical imaging equipment by specifying the following:

1. For network communication, the DICOM standard defines a set of protocols that all devices complying with the DICOM standard should follow.
2. These protocols allow the exchange of command syntax, semantics, and related information.
3. For media communication, the DICOM standard defines a set of media storage services and specifies a file format and medical directory structure for accessing images and related information on exchange media. Devices claiming DICOM standard compliance must adhere to these specifications.
4. The DICOM standard must provide information about the implementation of compliant solutions.

The DICOM standard does not specify the following:

1. Implementation details of any features on devices claiming DICOM standard compliance.
2. Overall characteristics and functions of a system integrated from a set of DICOM standard-compliant devices.
3. Evaluation-related testing and verification processes.

4.2.1.3 Domains of Application of DICOM

According to the DICOM standard manual, the DICOM standard pertains to the field of medical informatics, addressing the issue of information exchange between medical imaging equipment and other systems. Since medical imaging equipment needs to interact with other medical devices and information systems, the DICOM standard overlaps with other areas within medical informatics. However, the DICOM standard does not explicitly define the extent of this overlap.

The DICOM standard primarily focuses on diagnostic medical imaging practices in radiology, cardiology, pathology, dentistry, ophthalmology, and related disciplines and imaging therapies (e.g., interventional radiology, radiotherapy, and surgery). However, it also broadly applies to various image and non-image-related information exchanges in other medical contexts, such as clinical research.

The DICOM standard enhances the interoperability of systems in a multi-vendor environment that demands consistency, but the DICOM standard itself does not guarantee interoperability.

4.2.2 Development History of the DICOM Standard

In the 1970s, with the emergence of CT equipment and other digital diagnostic imaging devices, along with the increasing use of computers in clinical applications, the American College of Radiology (ACR) and the National Electrical

Manufacturers Association (NEMA) began to recognize the need for a unified standard for the various image formats produced by different manufacturers. This led to the necessity of establishing a standard for transmitting images and related information between devices from different manufacturers.

In 1983, ACR and NEMA formed a joint committee to establish such a standard with the following objectives:

1. To facilitate the communication of digital image information between different equipment manufacturers.
2. To promote the development and expansion of PACS, enabling PACS to interact with other hospital information systems.
3. To allow the creation of diagnostic information databases accessible across different regions.

In 1985, ACR and NEMA released the ACRNEMA 1.0 standard, designated as 3001985. This standard was subsequently revised twice: Revision 1 in October 1986 and Revision 2 in January 1988. The standard established a hardware interface, a minimal set of software commands, and a set of consistent data formats.

In 1988, ACR and NEMA released the ACRNEMA 2.0 standard, designated as 3001988. This version included the original ACRNEMA 1.0 standard, the published revisions, and additional revisions. The 2.0 standard also introduced new content for command support for display devices, a new hierarchical scheme for image identification, and additional data elements to improve image description differentiation.

In 1993, ACR and NEMA significantly revised the original 300 standards, which were replaced by the DICOM 3.0 standard. Compared to the previous ACRNEMA standards, DICOM 3.0 included several major enhancements:

1. Network Environment Compatibility: DICOM 3.0 was designed to work in network environments, whereas ACRNEMA was only for point-to-point communication. To operate in a network environment, DICOM 3.0 required the addition of a Network Interface Unit (NIU) and supported operations using industry-standard network protocols like TCP/IP.
2. Offline Media Exchange: DICOM 3.0 supported offline media exchanges, whereas ACRNEMA did not specify file formats or physical/logical storage options. DICOM 3.0 allowed the use of industry-standard media such as CD-R, DVD-R, USB, and common file storage systems.
3. Service-Oriented Protocol: DICOM 3.0 established a service-oriented protocol that defined the semantics of commands and related data, and how DICOM-compliant devices should respond to them. This included services for managing the workflow in imaging departments, unlike ACRNEMA, which only specified data transmission services.
4. Consistency Levels: DICOM 3.0 defined different levels of consistency requirements, whereas ACRNEMA only specified minimal compliance. DICOM 3.0 provided clear descriptions for implementers on how to construct optional consistency declarations.

In 1995, with the support of the American Heart Association, DICOM 3.0 added image support for cardiology and formally reorganized the ACRNEMA Joint Committee into a broader collaborative organization known as the DICOM Standards Committee, encompassing a wider range of professionals in the medical imaging field.

4.2.3 Introduction to DICOM 3.0 Standard

4.2.3.1 Principles of DICOM 3.0 Standard

International Applicability and Localization Principle

DICOM 3.0 is a global standard applicable to any region. It provides mechanisms for handling data to accommodate different cultural needs, such as various writing systems, character sets, languages, and structures for addresses and names. It supports different workflows, processes, and policies in biomedical imaging fields across different regions and medical practices.

Localization means meeting national or regional health and workflow policy requirements without deviating from the standard. This might involve specific code sets (such as workflow codes) or configuring the use of data elements (including specifying allowed local values and making optional elements in the standard mandatory for local use). Localization and configuration can be specified through mechanisms outside the DICOM standard, such as integration profiles for healthcare enterprises. However, configurations must not contradict each other; they can add requirements but must not conflict with the DICOM standard, as this would make it impossible for devices to comply with both the DICOM standard and the profiles.

Continuous Maintenance Principle

DICOM 3.0 is maintained according to the procedures of the DICOM Standards Committee, meaning it is constantly evolving. In addition, the DICOM Standards Committee encourages users of the DICOM 3.0 standard to actively submit various enhancement proposals. These proposals can be submitted to the secretariat. Several times a year, there are votes and approvals for supplements and revisions to the DICOM 3.0 standard. Once the final supplement and revision texts are approved, each change is officially published individually and takes immediate effect. Periodically, all approved supplement and revision texts are consolidated and published in updated versions of the standard. Once changes are integrated into the latest version of the standard, individual change documents are no longer maintained, and the committee directs readers to use the merged version of the standard.

The basic requirement for updating the standard is to maintain compatibility with previous versions. The maintenance process may involve deprecating certain versions. Deprecation does not mean that these functionalities cannot be used, but the DICOM Standards Committee will no longer maintain the documentation for these deprecated functions. Readers can refer to previous versions of the DICOM 3.0 standard for information on deprecated functionalities. The committee discourages using deprecated functions for new implementations and recommends using alternative methods retained in the standard.

Information Objects and Unique Object Identification Principle

Many DICOM 3.0 standard services involve exchanging persistent information objects (e.g., images). Instances of such information objects may be exchanged among many systems and organizational environments over time. While some organizations may make minor modifications to instance attributes to facilitate processing (e.g., enforcing local patient ID values), the semantic content of the instance remains unchanged.

Each instance is tagged with a globally unique identifier that is preserved during all exchanges. Any modification to the semantic content of an instance is considered the creation of a new instance, which is then assigned a new globally unique identifier.

Consistency Principle

Consistency in the DICOM 3.0 standard is declared within the Service Object Pair (SOP) class. This class provides services for operating on types of information objects (e.g., CT or MRI images) and specifies how generated instructions apply to information objects. SOP classes are modified in a forward and backward-compatible manner. Consistency declarations and requirements refer to the SOP class identifier, not the DICOM 3.0 standard version. Each implementation should provide a conformance statement in a structured format to improve interoperability between different products.

Information Model Consistency Principle

DICOM 3.0 defines numerous information objects following a common composite information model, with entities representing patients, studies, series, equipment, reference frames, and specific instance data types. These models are abstractions of concepts and behaviors in the real medical imaging environment. For acquisition, "study" resembles an ordered process, while "series" is akin to a protocol type for displaying data. In other fields, like radiotherapy, "study" and "series" may not have a clear relationship with real-world entities or behaviors but still require consistency. This simplified model is sufficient for practical needs in managing images and related data in daily practice.

4.2.3.2 Basic Content of DICOM 3.0 Standard

According to the latest DICOM 3.0 standard manual, the DICOM 3.0 standard includes the following content:

1. Introduction and overview: A brief introduction to the concepts, composition, basic content, and evaluation of the DICOM standard.
2. Conformance: Defines the principles to be followed for implementing the DICOM standard, including conformance requirements and declarations.

However, it does not set any test or verification procedures to evaluate conformance implementation.

3. Information object definitions: Defines a series of information object classes, providing abstract definitions of real-world entities for digital medical imaging and related information (such as waveforms, structured reports, radiotherapy doses, etc.). Each information object class definition includes attribute definitions and purpose descriptions but not the values of the attributes. It defines the real event model and corresponding information model, with future versions potentially expanding the content to support new functionalities.
4. Service class definitions: Defines a series of service classes that associate one or more information objects with one or more commands to be executed on these objects. Specifies the requirements for specified elements and how to apply generated instructions to information objects. Specifies the requirements for communication service providers and users. Defines the common characteristics of all service classes and how conformance statements construct each service class.
5. Data structures and encoding: Explains how to construct and encode the information objects in Part 3 and the service classes in Part 4. Addresses the encoding rules needed to construct the data stream for conveying information in Part 7. Defines the syntax for many common methods of information objects. Specifies the encoding rules for international character sets used in the DICOM standard.
6. Data dictionary: A centralized registry defining the geometry of all DICOM standard data elements used to represent source information. Defines elements for exchange media encoding and lists unique identifiers assigned by the DICOM standard. Specifies unique tags, names, value types, value counts, and whether an element is deprecated for each element. Specifies characteristic values, names, and types for each identifier.
7. Message exchange: Specifies the services and protocols for exchanging messages between applications in a medical imaging environment, defined in Part 8. Specifies the operations and notifications that service classes defined in Part 4 may use. Specifies the rules for establishing and terminating communications defined in Part 8 and the impact on incomplete transactions. Defines rules for controlling command requests and responses. Constructs the encoding rules needed for command streams and messages.
8. Network support for message exchange: Specifies the required communication services and upper-layer protocols.
9. Point-to-point communication message exchange services support (no longer used)
10. Media storage and file format for media exchange: Specifies a new media image information storage model for removable storage. Specifies a hierarchical model for storing medical images and related information on storage media. Specifies a DICOM standard file format that supports encapsulation of any information object. Specifies a secure DICOM standard file format. Specifies DICOM standard file services. Specifies various concepts of media storage.

11. Application configurations for media storage: Specifies a subset of application-specific implementations with DICOM standard conformance declarations.
12. Formats and physical media for media exchange: Specifies the structure to describe the relationship between the media storage model and specific physical media and media formats. Specifies specific physical media characteristics and associated media formats, facilitating information exchange between applications in medical environments.
13. Point-to-point communication print management support (no longer used)
14. Grayscale standard display function: Specifies the grayscale image standard display function, providing a method for calibrating specific display systems to present images consistently across different display media.
15. Security and system management profiles: Specifies security and system management profiles for implementations declaring conformance. Security and system management profiles are defined by referencing externally developed standard protocols (such as DHCP, LDAP, etc.). This section does not address security policy issues.
16. Content mapping resources: Specifies templates for structuring documents into DICOM standard information objects. Specifies the terminology sets used in information objects. Defines and maintains the terminology vocabulary by the DICOM standard. Provides translations of coded terms for specific countries.
17. Explanatory information: Specifies informative and normative appendices containing explanatory information.
18. Web services: Specifies methods for retrieving or storing DICOM standard objects using web services.
19. Application hosting: Specifies an API for DICOM standard-based medical information systems, allowing programs written to this standard interface to become plugins for medical information systems.
20. Imaging report using HL7 clinical document architecture: Specifies templates for encoding imaging reports using the second edition of the HL7 Clinical Document Architecture standard (CDA R2), forming an implementation guide for CDA.
21. Transformation between DICOM standard protocols and other representations: Specifies transformations between DICOM standard representations and other representations for the same information.
22. Real-time communication: Specifies a service for real-time transmission of DICOM standard source data.

4.2.3.3 DICOM 3.0 Standard Data Structure

A DICOM medical file consists of a DICOM file header and a DICOM dataset. The overall structure of a DICOM file is shown in Fig. 4.1, including the file preamble, prefix, file meta-elements, and data elements. Here is a brief introduction to the DICOM standard data structure.

Fig. 4.1 DICOM file structure

DICOM File Header	Preamble (128B)
	Prefix (4B)
	File Meta - Element
DICOM Dataset	Data Element
	......
	Data Element

DICOM File Header

Each DICOM file must contain a DICOM file header, comprising three parts: preamble, prefix, and file meta-elements. The preamble occupies 128 bytes, and the file prefix occupies 4 bytes. The file preamble in the DICOM file header can store certain explanatory information, with specific values determined by the device manufacturer, or set to 00H if not applicable. The 4-byte file prefix contains the string "DICM," which can be used to determine if a file is a DICOM file. The file meta-elements consist of several data elements with group numbers 0002, defining a series of global information for DICOM.

DICOM Dataset

Following the DICOM file header is the DICOM dataset, composed of multiple data elements. Each data element can appear only once in a DICOM dataset, but can be repeated in nested data formats. The DICOM dataset includes the main information of the DICOM file. Parsing a DICOM dataset requires using the data dictionary defined in the DICOM standard, as previously introduced.

4.3 Main Functions and Key Technologies of Picture Archiving and Communication Systems

4.3.1 Main Functions of Picture Archiving and Communication Systems

PACS has become one of the most important digital imaging tools in the global field of radiology. As mentioned in Sect. 4.1, adopting PACS not only leads radiology into a film-less era but also reduces material costs, physical storage space, and manual labor associated with traditional radiology films. Additionally, it helps improve communication between radiologists and other clinicians. The workflow of PACS is shown in Fig. 4.2.

The main functions include examination information registration, image acquisition, image transmission and storage, image display and processing, report management, and system management.

4.3.1.1 Examination Information Registration

Medical staff at the hospital radiology front desk register the patient's basic personal information and examination application information. If the hospital has a HIS and it is connected with PACS or RIS, patient information can also be retrieved

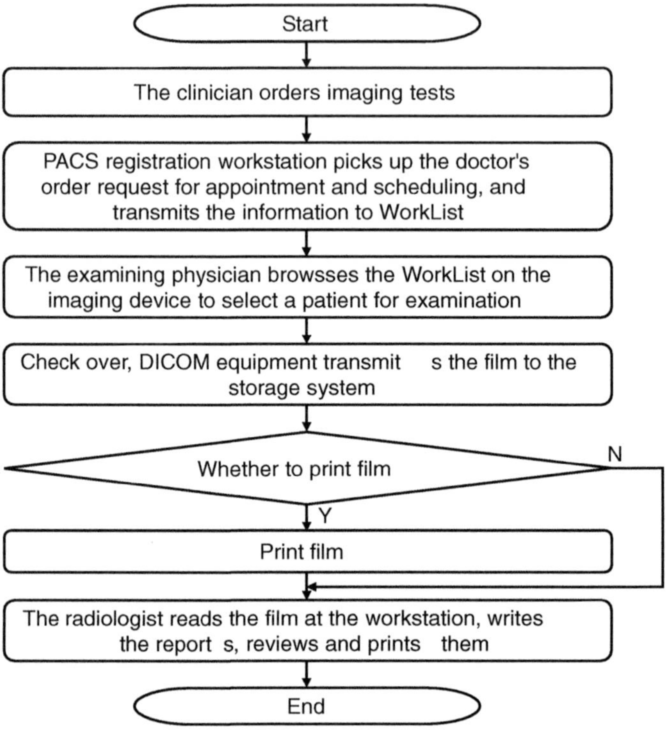

Fig. 4.2 PACS workflow

from HIS for automatic entry. Once the patient information is entered, other workstations can call the corresponding patient information from the PACS main database, eliminating the need for manual re-entry. For medical imaging equipment with WorkList service, doctors can directly extract the patient's basic information from the server; if not, doctors need to manually enter the patient's basic information through the workstation or retrieve it from the triage desk.

After registering the patient's basic information, medical staff can further perform tasks such as triage registration, follow-up registration, scanning application forms, printing application forms, and arranging triage.

4.3.1.2 Image Acquisition Function

Image acquisition is the foundation of PACS, referring to obtaining images with clinical diagnostic and reference value through medical imaging equipment (e.g., CT scanners, ECG machines). Data acquisition mainly involves radiology imaging equipment and can connect to other departments' equipment like pathology, ultrasound, nuclear medicine, or endoscopy if needed. Image acquisition equipment in radiology department generally includes instruments for CR, DR, DDR, DSA, CT, and MR. Most of the acquisition equipment is equipped with digital interface, while analog images transmitted by non-digital interfaces need conversion to digital images through specific analog-to-digital conversion equipment like video cameras or scanners.

A acquisition computer (gateway) is needed between the image acquisition equipment and the PACS network. The gateway's primary functions are: (1) Acquiring image data from imaging devices. (2) Converting the data into a standardized DICOM format. (3) Transmitting the standardized data to the PACS controller. Figure 4.3 shows the data flow from medical equipment to the clinical PACS workstation.

Standardized access to PACS ensures the standardization and validity of image files, facilitating medical image researchers in parsing and extracting information. Medical images can be divided into static and dynamic images based on their nature. Dynamic medical images, captured in frames and converted into image data, include angiography and echocardiography. Static images generally fall into three categories:

1. Digitized data compliant with DICOM 3.0 can directly connect to PACS computers.
2. Non-DICOM 3.0 compliant digital data requires PACS administrators to obtain data structures and interface protocols from imaging equipment manufacturers to convert to DICOM 3.0 compliant data.
3. Non-digital data, such as films and video images, can be converted to standard digital data using specialized scanners or captured frame-by-frame using cameras from medical equipment monitors.

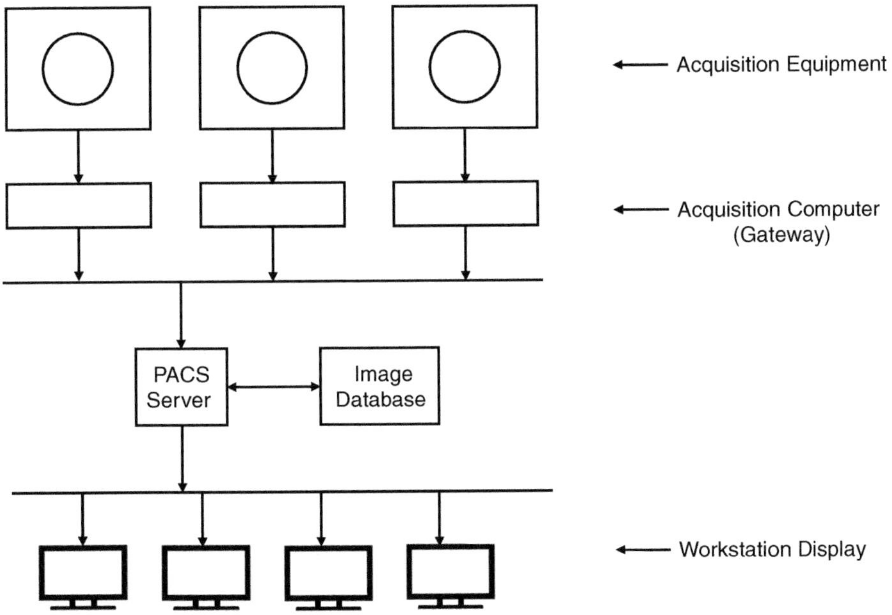

Fig. 4.3 The data flow from medical equipment to the clinical pacs workstation

4.3.1.3 Image Transmission and Storage Function

Image transmission is a key part of PACS, enabling image information sharing within departments, between different hospital departments, and even between different hospitals. Images are transmitted via digital communication devices, considering factors like communication standards, speed, security, fault tolerance, and maintenance costs. Based on communication speed, digital communication networks can be divided into low-speed Ethernet, medium-speed fiber distributed data interface, and high-speed asynchronous transfer mode.

After being transmitted via digital communication devices, images directly enter the storage management system. Medical image storage in PACS is generally divided into offline and online methods: offline storage is used for image data that will not be needed in the near future and can be stored on relatively inexpensive storage devices; online storage is for data that will be used soon and is usually stored on local disks, which can be accessed without a network connection and are managed directly by the database. Designing the storage management system involves addressing two core issues: data integrity and system efficiency. Data integrity means that PACS must not lose images acquired from the acquisition devices, while system efficiency refers to minimizing the data access time for image workstations.

The storage management system, the core of PACS, comprises a communication network, database system, archive server, and optical disk library. Acquisition computers (gateways) and display workstations connect to the storage management system via the network. Images from acquisition devices are first sent to the archive server, then to the optical disk library, and finally to designated workstations through the network.

4.3.1.4 Image Display and Processing Function

PACS can parse image and related patient information from acquired image files and display them to doctors via monitors. After completing imaging examinations, doctors can immediately review the images and make clinical diagnoses. PACS retrieves image data from the primary server's disk array or connected front-end servers based on preset paths, making image review more efficient and convenient compared to traditional film review. PACS also provides various image processing functions.

Doctors can perform multiple processing operations on images via monitors. Medical image processing involves using image processing techniques to acquire, enhance, and segment medical images to obtain required human and biological information. These techniques allow doctors to adjust image brightness and contrast, window width/level, measure density values, lesion sizes and volumes, flip images, resize, crop, annotate, and perform 3D reconstructions.

4.3.1.5 Report Management Function

Hospitals assign professionals to evaluate and analyze medical image quality. For images that pass quality assessment, doctors can write and edit reports online. The report writing interface includes a comprehensive module library to assist in generating accurate diagnostic reports. Doctors can use common diagnostic templates to reduce the burden of medical record writing. During report writing, doctors can compare multiple cases for the same or different patients to arrive at accurate diagnoses and generate reports.

Reports follow a hierarchical review system, requiring lower-level doctors' reports to be reviewed and approved by higher-level doctors before publication. Typically, levels range from intern, examination technician, report doctor, review doctor, to chief doctor. If high-level doctors find inaccuracies in image diagnoses during the review, they can void the report, re-diagnose the images, and rewrite the report. During the review, changes can be tracked and compared, and reports can be saved as typical cases for reference by other doctors and departmental learning.

4.3.1.6 System Management Function

The system management function includes managing patient and medical staff accounts, setting permissions, departmental management, and configuring PACS parameters. This module allows administrators to manage and maintain the system from any location within the hospital, integrating management and configuration information for normal hospital operations and storing it in the database. This standardizes system operation processes and reduces errors in daily work.

This module simplifies various PACS tasks, such as user management, basic parameter configuration, and report form definition. Designing PACS functionality modules as convenient visual operation windows improves the speed of retrieving, analyzing, and diagnosing patient image data across departments, and facilitates efficient PACS management.

PACS improves workflow, efficiency, and productivity, saving time and enhancing medical service efficiency. Integration with other hospital systems also improves communication efficiency between radiologists and clinicians. However, PACS implementation still faces challenges, such as difficulty integrating multiple PACS units within and between hospitals, limited storage capacity, incomplete backup and recovery solutions, and data migration issues. Solutions like multi-site PACS integration, open-source PACS, and multimedia use can address some of these issues. Research suggests that web-based PACS solutions help connect PACS in multiple hospitals and integrate PACS with other hospital systems (e.g., RIS and HIS).

4.3.2 Key Technologies of Picture Archiving and Communication Systems

Hospitals generate a large amount of data through PACS daily (large medical institutions may generate over 50 GB of data each day), and the demand for accessing these data from radiologists and referring clinicians is almost constant. Therefore, PACS requires the collaboration of several key technologies to operate effectively. The key technologies for PACS involve workstation displays, networks, and storage.

4.3.2.1 Workstation Displays

With the shift from film to PACS, traditional film image viewers have been replaced by PACS workstations. Doctors view images on a computer monitor instead of using a backlit viewbox.

CRT and LCD Displays

The first computer monitors were based on cathode ray tube (CRT) technology. CRT's long history has optimized its foundational technology and minimized production costs. Liquid crystal display (LCD) technology is relatively newer and excels in many areas. CRT's main advantages are its viewing angle and initial cost, while LCDs are brighter, smaller, last longer, and offer easier quality assurance.

CRTs are priced at one-half to one-third of comparable LCDs. A comparison of LCD and CRT technologies is shown in Fig. 4.4. Doctors can view CRTs from wide angles, allowing multiple users to optimally view images simultaneously, which is significant in radiology teaching environments where attending physicians and residents need to use the same monitor for discussions. LCDs, being a type of flat-panel display, require much less desk space than CRTs, offering greater flexibility in workplace design.

Medical displays need higher brightness than household and commercial displays. Medical LCDs are generally brighter than medical CRTs, which degrade in brightness relatively quickly, requiring more frequent replacement and stricter quality assurance. Brightness is critical because radiologists can interpret images more accurately on brighter monitors.

CRT quality control is more complex than that of LCDs. Besides brightness degradation, most CRTs have curved screens that cause image distortion, and the aspect ratio may vary. If a CRT deviates from its calibration settings, images may appear too tall or too wide. LCDs, with fixed geometry, never change their aspect ratio. Some LCDs also dynamically adjust their brightness to maintain perceived brightness over the monitor's lifespan. The initial cost advantage of CRTs is offset by their shorter lifespan, making their total cost higher than that of LCDs due to more frequent replacements. The falling costs and technological improvements in LCDs have enhanced their viewing angles, making LCDs likely to fully replace CRTs for medical imaging.

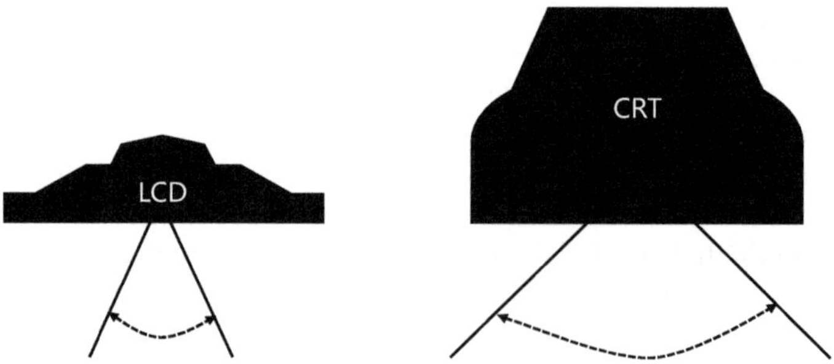

Fig. 4.4 Comparison of LCD and CRT technologies

Resolution

A monitor's resolution indicates how much data it can display at once. Each point on the screen is a pixel, and modern monitors measure pixel resolution in megapixels. Higher resolution increases costs. Additionally, very high resolution can slow monitor response time. Determining the minimum acceptable resolution for images displayed at each workstation is crucial.

Cross-sectional modes like CT, MRI, and ultrasound capture data at fixed pixel resolutions (e.g., CT images are typically 512 pixels high and 512 pixels wide). Displaying 4–6 such images on a screen requires 1–2 million pixels to accommodate the data fully. Traditional X-ray films have more pixels than most monitors, so full images on a screen must represent images without all details (downsampling). However, monitor resolutions above 2–3 million pixels do not improve speed or accuracy for traditional X-ray films. Studies suggest that a lower acceptable resolution for cross-sectional images might suffice for traditional X-ray films, although displaying on low-resolution monitors may take longer. Software allowing image zoom and pan can compensate for detail loss on low-resolution monitors.

Color and Grayscale

Color monitors seem better than grayscale-only monitors. However, the ability to display colors comes at the expense of sharpness and brightness. Each pixel in a color monitor comprises adjacent red, green, and blue elements. At normal viewing distances, this cluster blurs into a single color pixel, but these elements do not align strictly, reducing image sharpness crucial for radiology applications. Historically, color monitors lacked the brightness needed for medical imaging, making grayscale monitors more prevalent when PACS was first introduced. Nowadays, grayscale monitors are preferred because they are cheaper than color monitors of similar specifications. For most radiology applications, grayscale monitors are ideal as most medical devices capture data along a single value spectrum. Exceptions include nuclear medicine (especially PET/CT), Doppler ultrasound, and perfusion imaging, requiring color monitors, so each PACS workstation should provide color monitors.

4.3.2.2 Network

Computer networks are the infrastructure allowing data transfer from imaging devices to PACS, then to radiologists' workstations, and any additional long-term storage devices. The network distributes radiologists' diagnostic results to clinicians and enables applications like email.

Network Units

Most computers in a network can be classified as servers or clients. Servers facilitate communication between other computers and deliver information to them. Servers typically require no human intervention and respond to requests from other network computers, not directly driven by human instructions. Clients rely on servers to provide information. Radiologists typically interact only with client computers (e.g., desktop PCs). Workstations are client computers dedicated to specific purposes. Networks also include devices for data transfer between computers, such as switches, routers, and hubs.

Network Types

Local area networks (LANs) are computer networks in close proximity, usually within a single hospital. Wide area networks (WANs) connect multiple LANs across an entire healthcare system. Most networks are "wired," relying on physical connections (copper or fiber optic cables) between computers. Conversely, wireless networks use radio waves to transmit data between computers, necessitating extensive security measures due to potentially sensitive information being transmitted through the air.

Data transmission within a LAN is relatively private due to all connecting cables being within the hospital's physical boundaries. Data transmission over the internet poses greater security risks as it passes through unpredictable and unknown computer chains. Virtual private networks (VPNs) allow computers outside the LAN (e.g., a radiologist's home computer) to connect to the LAN (e.g., hospital PACS) with security levels similar to physical LAN connections. Such security measures are essential whenever identifiable patient information is transmitted.

Bandwidth

Network bandwidth is the maximum rate at which data can be transmitted between two points in a network. Bandwidth primarily depends on the transmission medium but also on the number of computers sharing the same infrastructure. The time required to send images from the PACS server to a workstation largely depends on the intermediate network's bandwidth and the number of simultaneous user requests.

When too many computers are on the same network, performance may degrade to unacceptable levels. Increasing a hospital network's bandwidth to accommodate more computers can be prohibitively expensive. During network planning, staff must recognize that PACS should have dedicated bandwidth used only by PACS workstations and servers to prevent unnecessary data transmission from disrupting departmental efficiency.

Image compression is a method to reduce the bandwidth required for rapid image transmission. By utilizing the inherent redundancy in any image, the data amount needed to define the image can be minimized. If every detail of the original image can be accurately restored, the compression scheme is called lossless compression; otherwise, it is called lossy compression. The acceptable degree of lossy compression in radiology without compromising diagnostic accuracy is highly debated, so many PACS vendors avoid this issue by using only lossless compression.

4.3.2.3 Storage

Modern radiology generates vast amounts of image data, and in a PACS environment, all relevant comparison studies must be quickly retrievable. The retrieval time, measured in seconds (s), minutes (min), or hours (h), depends on the type of digital archiving supporting PACS.

Advantages of Different Storage Media

Long-term storage of digital data offers several options: rotating disks (e.g., hard drives in personal computers), tapes (e.g., cassette tapes), optical media (e.g., CDs and DVDs), and solid-state media (e.g., USB flash drives). Most PACS use some combination of these options. Compared to other choices, optical media require more support personnel and do not scale well. Solid-state media are still too expensive for large-scale storage, but technological advancements may make them the preferred choice in the future.

Most PACS use tapes or rotating disks for long-term storage. Tapes' primary advantage is their lower cost, with the main disadvantage being longer retrieval times. Rotating disks are more expensive than tapes or optical media but have a significant advantage in retrieval times. Like data on a personal computer's hard drive, data stored on rotating disks is always immediately available, with delays only from sending data from the archive to PACS. With the continuous decline in rotating disk technology costs, this medium is becoming the preferred method for storing image data in many PACS.

Online Vs. Offline

Some data on PACS should be immediately accessible whenever radiologists request it. These data need online storage, typically including the latest images and their related comparison studies. Offline stored images are placed in harder-to-access archives and need to be restored to online status before viewing.

In a single-tier storage system, all data are always online and stored on a single medium (usually rotating disks). In a multi-tier storage system, some data are online (typically on rotating disks), and other data are offline (usually on optical media or tapes). A single-tier system with all data online offers superior performance for radiologists and clinicians but is often prohibitively expensive. Thus, a more reasonable approach is to place the most likely viewed images in online storage and downgrade unused images to offline storage.

Redundancy Techniques

Redundancy refers to storing multiple copies of imaging data. Redundancy also occurs when several computers or network components perform the same task, ensuring system operation if one component fails until the faulty component is replaced.

The redundant array of independent disks (RAID) is the most common redundancy system in PACS storage. In RAID, data are distributed across multiple hard drives so that if any drive fails, data can be rebuilt from the surviving drives.

Another form of redundancy is long-term archiving. Even when examinations are sent from imaging devices to PACS, they are copied to long-term archives when they are no longer online. A PACS with a single-tier architecture must have a backup system to archive data when primary storage fails.

Although the term redundancy is often used in data storage settings, every PACS component needs a "failover" or backup mechanism to prevent system failure from a single component failure. This reduces the probability of the entire system failing due to inevitable individual component failures.

4.4 Cutting-Edge Research in Picture Archiving and Communication Systems

4.4.1 Miniaturized and Mobile Imaging Devices and Systems

PACS was proposed to facilitate the management of various medical images generated daily. With the continuous advancement of science and technology, the sources of medical imaging have become increasingly diverse. Various miniaturized and mobile imaging devices and systems have emerged. This section briefly introduces some representative cases.

4.4.1.1 Mobile CT Scanner

CT scans utilize different X-rays to monitor diseases within the human body, characterized by relatively clear images and quick scanning times. CT equipment is generally installed in the well-protected radiology department of hospitals due to its large size, which limits its mobility. This immobility is problematic when responding to severe natural disasters or large-scale public health emergencies where timely and rapid clinical diagnosis is required. Hence, the mobile CT scanners came into being.

A mobile CT scanner, essentially a CT unit integrated with a vehicle, differs from previous attempts that simply placed a CT room on a motor vehicle. Current mobile CT scanners achieve an organic integration of the loading vehicle and the CT equipment, with the vehicle body serving as the CT room and shielding unit. This integration enhances the performance and mobility of the mobile CT scanner.

Specifically, a mobile CT scanner is a comprehensive system equipped with numerous components such as an independent examination operation room, CT equipment, power distribution system, network system, radiation protection devices, independent scanning room, air conditioning, ultraviolet air disinfection facilities, ventilation system, and dehumidifiers. It boasts high throughput of patients, rapid outdoor installation, networking capabilities, avoidance of cross-infection, and high mobility.

During the COVID-19 pandemic in 2020, CT played a significant role in screening, diagnosis, and treatment evaluation. Faced with a large number of people needing examination, the shortage of CT equipment in frontline epidemic response was severe. The mobile CT scanner, as an upgraded version of CT, proved extremely useful, providing timely and effective treatment to many patients with mild symptoms in makeshift hospitals and earning the reputation of being a "magic tool" in the fight against the pandemic.

4.4.1.2 Mobile MRI Scanner

MRI technology, based on the discovery of magnetic resonance, captures electromagnetic signals within the body and reconstructs these into images, providing detailed structural information of the human body. MRI offers high resolution for soft tissues, making it superior to CT for examining joints, muscles, and areas affected by sports injuries, such as ligaments and soft tissues around bones and the spine. Additionally, MRI involves no ionizing radiation, making it suitable for sensitive areas like the reproductive system and breasts.

Despite its advantages, MRI equipment is large, highly precise, and requires strict conditions for transport, installation, and use. Traditional MRI devices are not easily mobilized, limiting their rapid deployment in response to severe natural disasters or large-scale public health emergencies. This limitation has driven the development of mobile MRI scanners.

Due to the involvement of factors such as strong magnetic fields, low-temperature superconducting environments, and rapid switching of strong gradient fields in strong RF fields, the development of vehicle-mounted MRI systems is highly challenging. However, to date, many manufacturers have successfully developed vehicle-mounted MRI systems with different attributes. Examples include the Magnetic Resonance Diagnosis and Treatment Vehicle—Chiying A30, jointly developed by Baotou Rare Earth Medical Systems Co., Ltd. and the National Engineering Laboratory for Internet Healthcare Diagnosis and Treatment Technology, and the Magnetic Resonance Medical Vehicle independently developed by a high-tech company in Tianjin High-tech Zone and Huahai Gaosheng Investment Holding Co., Ltd. With continuous technological advancements, the functionality of vehicle-mounted MRI systems will become increasingly sophisticated, and the successively developed vehicle-mounted MRI equipment will undoubtedly meet or even exceed the rescue capabilities required for emergency disaster events.

4.4.1.3 PET

Positron emission tomography (PET) is a clinical imaging technology superior in nuclear medicine. The technique involves labeling substances needed for physiological metabolism (such as proteins, fatty acids, and glucose) with short-lived radioactive nuclides (e.g., 11C, 18F) and injecting them into the body. By observing the aggregation of these substances during metabolism, physiological metabolic activities can be visualized for diagnostic purposes.

Compared to other clinical imaging technologies, PET can display receptor and neurotransmitter activities, and biomolecular metabolism in vivo, making it widely used in diagnosing and differentiating various diseases, organ function research, disease assessment, new drug development, and treatment evaluation.

Currently, PET equipment is large and heavy, with spatial and weight constraints on placement sites. This has led to the development of Micro-PET, a miniaturized, high-resolution version of PET. Micro-PET can even scan small animals like mice, offering several advantages over other diagnostic imaging equipment:

1. Quick Imaging: The small imaging field allows for rapid imaging, providing timely dynamic reflections of physiological metabolic functions.
2. High Resolution: Achieves image resolution up to 1 mm precision.
3. High Sensitivity: Capable of reflecting molecular metabolism levels, enabling early detection of functional changes in vivo for early diagnosis.
4. Non-invasive: Minimal harm from PET imaging agents, with radiation doses from a whole-body PET scan being much lower than that of a single conventional CT scan, making it relatively safer and more reliable.

Due to these advantages, Micro-PET is frequently used in hospitals for early tumor detection, heart and brain disease identification, myocardial viability assessment, precise radiotherapy targeting, and accurate epilepsy localization. The clinical demand is substantial, with significant potential for further enhancement.

4.4.2 Image Reconstruction and 3D Printing

Image reconstruction refers to using a set of physical data related to images to create images. The input is a series of projection images, and the output is a reconstructed image. This technology has crucial clinical applications. A typical application involves using CT images collected from patients, applying mathematical principles to solve the distribution of attenuation coefficients of various tissues in a cross-section to obtain a three-dimensional reconstructed image. This 3D image can assist clinicians in diagnosis and treatment planning and can be combined with 3D printing technology for more personalized patient care.

At Tangdu Hospital of the Air Force Medical University, seven patients with skull defects or skull tumors (four males and three females, with an average defect size of (95 ± 40.4) cm^2) were scanned using a 64-slice CT between April and December 2019. Using CT image data and Mimics 19.0 software, a 3D medical model of the patients' skulls was created (as shown in Fig. 4.5). The model was used with Magics and Geomagic Wrap software to design implants. The final implants were 3D printed using polyetheretherketone (PEEK) material, and a 1:1 model was printed to perform a model surgery to help doctors verify and plan the surgery (as shown in Fig. 4.6).

Preoperative and 1-month postoperative CT images showed that the implants were stable without displacement. Preoperative trauma-induced defect areas averaged (95 ± 40.4) cm^2, and post-surgical CT images showed almost complete disappearance of defects ($P < 0.01$). Tumor-induced skull damage areas averaged (20 ± 10.4) cm^2, and postoperative CT images also showed almost complete disappearance of defects ($P < 0.01$). All seven patients had no postoperative complications; five trauma-induced bone defect patients had complete symptom resolution, and two bone tumor patients showed significant symptom relief. This demonstrated the feasibility and effectiveness of using 3D printed PEEK implants for skull defect repair in children.

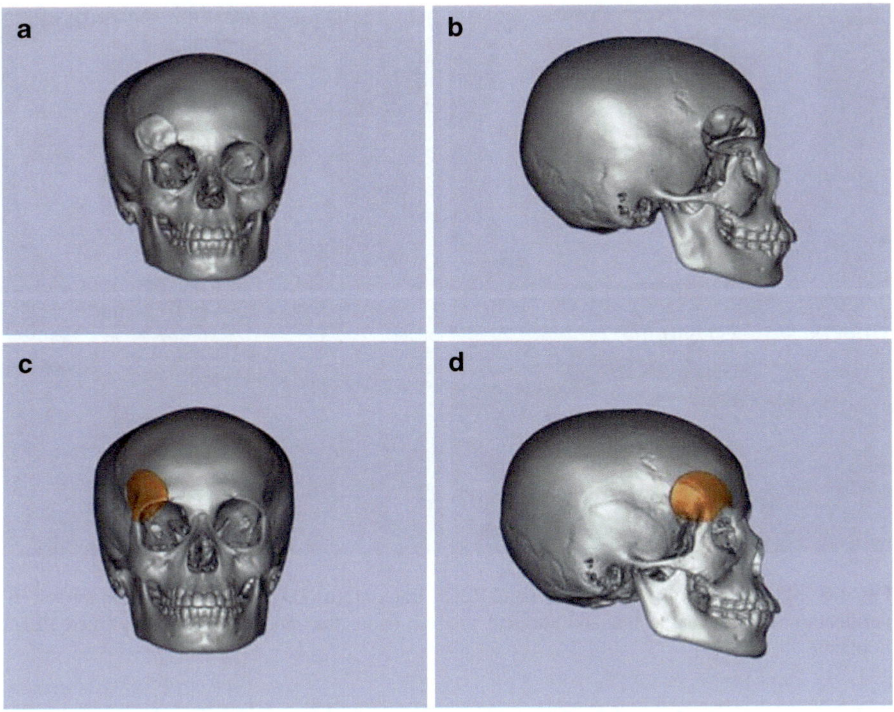

Fig. 4.5 3D model of skull defects using CAD. (**a**, **b**) 3D models of patients with tumor sections removed; (**c**, **d**) cut-out models from the complete skull model for printing

Traditional skull repair surgery varies greatly due to differences in defect size and location among patients. Preoperative CT images cannot provide accurate, intuitive skull information to the surgeon, and standardized surgical plans cannot be determined preoperatively, complicating communication with the patient's family. Using image reconstruction and 3D printing technology for auxiliary treatment can customize biomimetic implants matching the morphological characteristics of the patient's defect, thoroughly resolving the preoperative issue of spatial structure unknowns of the defect area.

4.4.3 Regional Imaging Center

A regional imaging center is led by a tertiary hospital and constructed using medical, computer, and communication technologies to build a regional remote imaging diagnosis center, involving secondary hospitals and primary healthcare institutions. Hospitals in the regional imaging center share data through a centralized data center and dedicated network, using imaging data as application objects to achieve data information sharing, adopting a hierarchical cooperation and linkage mechanism.

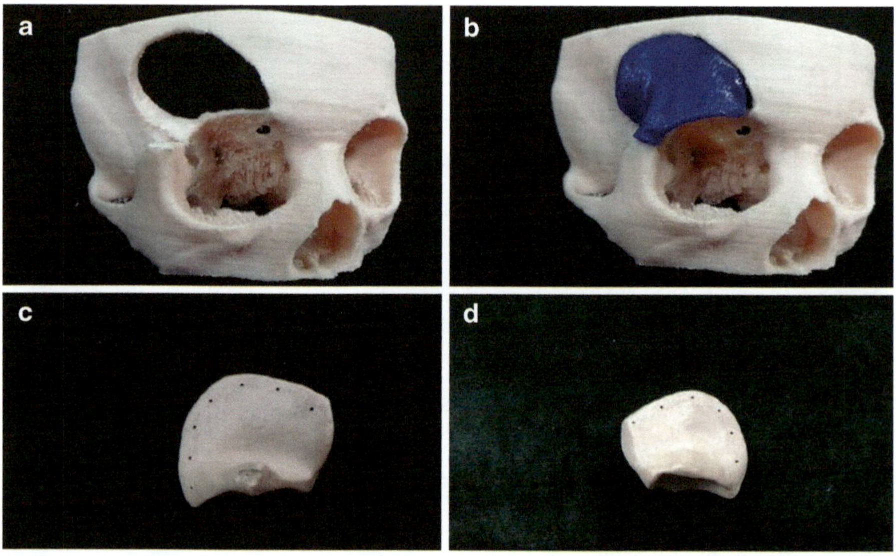

Fig. 4.6 3D printed skull defect model and PEEK implant. (**a**) 3D printed skull defect model; (**b**) verification of implant design and surgical process using the model; (**c**, **d**) 3D printed PEEK implants

4.4.3.1 Significance of Constructing Regional Imaging Centers

Regional imaging centers improve the allocation of large-scale imaging equipment resources, reduce repeated patient examinations, and realize efficient storage and management of imaging resources within imaging groups or regional medical institutions. This is crucial for accelerating medical informatization, integrating healthcare information resources, and promoting the development of medical services.

In China, medical resources are unevenly distributed between urban and rural areas and between economically developed and underdeveloped regions. Especially in remote rural areas, medical resources are scarce, and healthcare infrastructure is weak, making it difficult for local people to access medical care. Regional imaging centers can drive the development of primary healthcare institutions in the region, providing more convenient services for the public, promoting the tilt of medical resources toward grassroots people, and advancing hierarchical diagnosis and treatment development.

4.4.3.2 Principles for Constructing Regional Imaging Centers

The construction of regional imaging centers should be based on regional overall planning, implemented step-by-step, and dynamically adjusted later. The construction process should first use existing resources for infrastructure construction, then integrate the regional medical institutions' imaging sharing platform, achieving interconnection of the regional clinical information platform without changing the original PACS of the medical institutions. The entire process should follow health information exchange (HIE) standards. The design of regional imaging centers should focus on providing high-quality services to patients. Each patient should have a unique identifier for visits within the region, following principles of unification, standardization, normalization, convenience, and security to optimize patient visit processes, break information barriers, achieve mutual recognition and sharing of patient information across regions, promote integrated and homogeneous services among regional medical institutions, and establish a long-term, effective evaluation mechanism to ensure system sustainability and scalability.

4.4.3.3 Data Storage Methods in Regional Imaging Centers

Data storage methods in regional imaging centers are divided into three types: centralized, distributed, and hybrid storage.

Centralized Storage

Requires establishing a regional imaging storage center. Secondary hospitals and primary healthcare institutions must upload imaging and report data to the storage center, and images need to be retrieved through the regional imaging center. This method requires high bandwidth data upload and retrieval but offers easy management.

Distributed Storage

Imaging data are stored within each medical institution, without establishing a physical imaging storage center, only an imaging index information center. Secondary hospitals or primary healthcare institutions retrieve images through the regional imaging center's index information, accessing the specified storage location. This method requires no data upload and has low bandwidth requirements but slower retrieval speeds.

Hybrid Storage

Combines the advantages of the above methods for flexible storage. It establishes a regional imaging storage center, using centralized storage for smaller primary healthcare institutions and distributed storage for larger secondary hospitals, with the storage center retaining only imaging index information.

4.4.3.4 Case Studies of Regional Imaging Center Construction

Shanghai Hongkou Regional Clinical Imaging Center

The Hongkou Regional Clinical Imaging Center (HKMIDC) was built on the framework of an existing regional public health information platform. The project achieved the construction of a shared imaging information data platform in Hongkou and PACS/RIS systems in eight community health service centers. Imaging data from community health service centers are centrally stored on the center's cloud platform, while secondary hospitals have independent PACS and use distributed storage. The Hongkou District Health Bureau designated the North Campus of the First People's Hospital to handle center diagnostics and provide consultation services for difficult cases in secondary hospitals.

To address the unique patient identification issue, the regional imaging center uses an IHE PIX-based patient ID cross-referencing mechanism to interface with the regional public health information platform for patient identification. The system also enables the interoperability between PACS/RIS and other clinical information systems. This means that PACS at the municipal diagnostic center and community level can access corresponding patient personal health records and other clinical data from the public health information platform. Additionally, the hospital's HIS can access imaging results and diagnostic reports provided by the medical imaging center.

Maine Integrated Imaging Project

The Maine Department of Health, Maine Medical Center (MMC), and other healthcare providers developed the Consolidated Imaging Initiative (CIPACS), exploring ways for multiple organizations to store radiological images in MMC's PACS and retrieve and display these images within each organization's clinical systems. CIPACS initially implemented a shared system with two rural hospitals. Participating rural hospitals can save on PACS construction costs, improve care quality, and enhance access to radiologists. MMC benefits from cost-sharing among multiple organizations. Through this shared system, each hospital can access radiological information from other hospitals, improving diagnostic accuracy.

Through CIPACS, all images taken at the two rural hospitals are stored on MMC's servers. By storing images on a single server, hospitals can access their and others' images via a wide area network (WAN) connection with MMC, eliminating the need for each hospital to maintain its server. MMC checks and maintains each PACS device, providing IT support and installation upgrades, while rural hospitals only pay for new radiological equipment, network connections, and data transmission costs.

These case studies highlight the practical benefits and implementation strategies of regional imaging centers, showcasing how centralized and distributed data storage methods can be effectively employed to enhance healthcare delivery and resource management.

4.5 Summary

At the beginning of the twenty-first century, with the widespread adoption of PACS, radiology departments gradually transitioned from film-based operations to digital-based operations. The advent of PACS transformed the landscape of radiology, accelerating the shift toward digital image acquisition, centralizing image storage, integrating regional systems, and paving the way for tele-radiology [1].

Despite these advantages, the implementation of PACS still faces many challenges, such as the difficulty in integrating PACS systems across multiple hospitals, limited storage capacity, backup and recovery solutions, and data migration issues. Cloud-based PACS may offer a promising solution to these problems. Overall, the research and development of PACS must continue to meet the needs and demands of a broader range of PACS users [1].

Reference

1. Loux S, Coleman R, Ralston M, et al. Consolidated imaging: implementing a regional health information exchange system for radiology in Southern Main. In: Advances in patient safety: new directions and alternative approaches. vol. 4. Technology and medication safety. Rockville: Agency for Healthcare Research and Quality; 2008.

Clinical Decision Support Systems

5

Contents

5.1 Overview of Clinical Decision Support Systems 130
5.1.1 Introduction to Clinical Decision Support Systems 130
5.1.1.1 Right Channel 131
5.1.1.2 Right Time 131
5.1.1.3 Right Intervention Format 131
5.1.1.4 Right Person 131
5.1.1.5 Right Information 132
5.1.2 Classification of Clinical Decision Support Systems 133
5.1.2.1 Knowledge-Based CDSS 133
5.1.2.2 Non-knowledge-Based CDSS 135
5.1.3 Development History of Clinical Decision Support Systems 135
5.2 Construction Methods and Inference Algorithms of Clinical Decision Support Systems 138
5.2.1 Construction Methods of Clinical Decision Support Systems 138
5.2.1.1 Problem Definition 138
5.2.1.2 Feasibility Analysis 138
5.2.1.3 Requirements Analysis 139
5.2.1.4 Software Design 140
5.2.1.5 Coding 140
5.2.1.6 Testing 141
5.2.1.7 Maintenance 142
5.2.2 Inference Algorithms of Clinical Decision Support Systems 142
5.2.2.1 Rule-Based Inference 142
5.2.2.2 Probability Reasoning 144
5.2.2.3 Case-Based Reasoning 146
5.2.2.4 Deductive Reasoning and Inductive Reasoning 149
5.3 Case Studies of Clinical Decision Support Systems 150
5.3.1 MYCIN 150
5.3.2 Dxplain 152
5.3.3 SimuConsult 152
5.3.4 CADUCEUS 152
5.3.5 ISABEL 153
5.4 Frontier Research in Clinical Decision Support Systems 153
5.4.1 Multimodal Fusion Assisted Diagnosis 153

J. Li et al., *Healthcare Information Systems*, Innovative Medical Devices,
https://doi.org/10.1007/978-981-97-9551-2_5

5.4.1.1 Fusion of Clinical Data and Imaging Data 154
5.4.1.2 Fusion of Different Types of Imaging Data 154
5.4.1.3 Fusion of Physiological Signals with Other Data 155
5.4.1.4 Fusion of Facial Expressions with Other Data 155
5.4.2 Disease Prognosis Prediction and Risk Factor Warning 156
5.4.3 Shared Decision-Making and Health Management 158
5.4.4 Assisted Precision Screening for Rare and Genetic Diseases 159
5.5 Summary 161
References 161

Clinical decision support systems (CDSS) are a cutting-edge development in today's healthcare information systems. They primarily utilize advanced computer algorithms and comprehensive medical knowledge bases to improve the accuracy and completeness of decisions made by medical personnel when treating patients. This, in turn, reduces the incidence of medical errors, enhances the quality of healthcare, and lowers medical costs. With the rapid advancement of medical equipment and information technology, increasingly complex clinical situations and the explosive growth of clinical data have placed higher demands on CDSS. One common issue, "alert fatigue," has drawn considerable attention from researchers. Consequently, developing a CDSS that is comprehensive across the entire diagnostic and treatment process, safe, efficient, and user-friendly in terms of human-computer interaction has become a major focus of current research.

5.1 Overview of Clinical Decision Support Systems

5.1.1 Introduction to Clinical Decision Support Systems

A Clinical Decision Support System (CDSS) is an interactive computer system designed to assist healthcare workers, patients, and other potential users in intelligently acquiring or filtering clinical symptom data and knowledge, aiding in the judgment of specific issues, improving medical services, and enhancing healthcare quality. CDSS applications are widespread and often integrated with electronic health record (EHR) systems to capture real-time patient data. It is involved in all aspects of the diagnostic and treatment process, including triage, diagnosis, treatment, nursing, billing, and prescription, providing patients with accurate, personalized treatment plans. Scholars have proposed that "the ultimate goal of electronic health records is CDSS."

To ensure that CDSS can effectively improve medical standards, Osheroff proposed the "Five Rights of Clinical Decision Support" framework: providing the right information to the right person through the right channel, in the right intervention format, at the right time within the workflow. Currently, many top-tier hospitals in China, including Peking University Third Hospital, follow this framework to build CDSS, and it is recommended by the Centers for Medicare & Medicaid Services as a best practice for improving quality. Below is a brief introduction to the specific content of these "Five Rights."

5.1.1.1 Right Channel

Clinical Decision Support (CDS) can be delivered to patients through EHR, wearable devices, smartphone apps, etc. The practical operation requires consideration of user scenarios. For example, for outpatient doctors, EHR is the best platform for delivering decision support as it is their primary work platform. For patients receiving home care, the best platform might be a smartphone app.

5.1.1.2 Right Time

Effective information often gets delivered at the wrong time in medical information systems, or it may be invalid when sent. For example, a CDSS might capture the keyword "sulfonylurea" when a doctor prescribes a drug containing this compound to a patient taking aspirin, and warn about potential adverse reactions. Clearly, this warning comes at the wrong time—the optimal time would be at the start of the prescription process. Additionally, some alerts are triggered during the patient's examination process, requiring the doctor to click on the alert window to continue with the examination. This obviously disrupts the doctor's current examination flow. The best timing would be to issue the warnings after the examination is completed.

5.1.1.3 Right Intervention Format

CDS intervention formats vary, including alerts, orders, protocols, and buttons. Decision recipients need to determine their issues and choose the best format to address them. Designers must identify the clinical workflows requiring CDS and determine the appropriate intervention formats during CDSS development. For example, when a doctor is prescribing medication for a patient, the CDSS needs to assess whether the current prescription might cause an adverse drug reaction based on the patient's medication history, allergy history, and medical history. The most effective approach is to pre-emptively remind the doctor of the drugs that are unsuitable for the patient on the EHR system before the prescription is entered, and to provide the basis for the decision.

5.1.1.4 Right Person

The current medical model involves a team including doctors, pharmacists, nurses, and therapists. Thus, CDSS needs to deliver the correct information to the appropriate person. For instance, if a patient resists a doctor's recommendation, it can be communicated to the patient's relatives to help improve compliance and treatment quality.

5.1.1.5 Right Information

The information provided must adhere to evidence-based medicine principles, derived from a set of recognized guidelines, such as various clinical guidelines issued by the National Health Commission. For instance, for patients with abnormal kidney structure or function lasting more than 3 months, it should be considered that they might have chronic kidney disease (CKD). This diagnostic criterion was established by the Kidney Disease: Improving Global Outcomes (KDIGO) based on years of medical data from numerous patients and with the participation of kidney experts from around the world.

With the rapid development of medicine and computer technology, medical knowledge is growing explosively. Long hours and high-intensity work make it difficult for doctors to stay updated, and incomplete knowledge can lead to missed or incorrect diagnoses. CDSS, storing extensive multidisciplinary knowledge, compensates for this, allowing doctors to focus more on patient communication and make more accurate, comprehensive decisions. In summary, CDSS has the following clinical significance:

1. Reducing the incidence of medication/prescription errors and adverse events to improve clinical outcomes. According to statistics, the number of adverse drug reaction (ADR) events in the United States exceeds 2 million annually, resulting in 1 million deaths. CDSS can promptly remind physicians of contraindications for the combined use of different medications, conflicts between drugs and the patient's past medical history, and potential nephrotoxicity and hepatotoxicity when prescribing. Evans and others reported that Yancheng LDS Hospital developed a CDSS for rational drug use recommendations for antimicrobial drugs. A prospective study was conducted on 12 intensive care unit (ICU) patients for 1 year, and it was found that the use of the system led to a one-third reduction in the use of antimicrobial drugs in ICU patients, with an average reduction of 6.7 days in hospital stay [1].
2. Improving adherence to clinical guidelines. Traditional clinical guidelines and care pathways are often difficult to implement due to low adherence by doctors. CDSS digitalizes these pathways and guidelines, constantly reminding doctors during routine consultations.
3. Controlling hospital medical costs and reducing expenses. CDSS can help doctors reduce redundant lab tests and use more cost-effective drugs and treatment plans. For example, in 2012, the total cost of diabetes-related treatments in the USA was about $245 billion, but using CDSS in diabetes care saved 14% in treatment costs.
4. Supporting clinical and diagnostic coding, and patient classification. Doctors can choose appropriate diagnostic codes from a list on the CDSS interface, improving clinical documentation quality and facilitating the implementation of clinical plans. For example, a study found that 71% of splenectomy patients did not have this procedure recorded in their problem list in EHRs, leading to missed vaccinations. Implementing CDSS improved this situation.

5. Aiding clinical decision-making and enhancing doctor efficiency. The primary purpose of CDSS is to assist doctors in making quick, accurate decisions, compensating for their lack of experience in diagnosing certain diseases. For example, CDSS can help radiologists select the most appropriate tests, remind them of best practice guidelines, or warn about contraindicated contrast agents. A study at Virginia Mason Medical Center showed that CDSS significantly reduced inappropriate MRI and CT use.
6. Better data retrieval and presentation, improving medical efficiency. CDSS can filter important patient features and relevant medical literature through its inference engine, presenting them to doctors and reducing the time spent on paperwork.

It is important to note that despite the significant role of CDSS in clinical practice, it also brings some negative issues. One common problem is "alert fatigue," where excessive and unimportant warnings desensitize doctors, leading them to miss critical warnings and causing serious patient safety issues. Additionally, over-reliance on CDSS can reduce doctors' skill levels. CDSS's role in the healthcare system is to assist and support; the doctor remains the true decision-maker in clinical decisions. Some medical experts believe that CDSS disrupts existing clinical workflows, and these issues require solutions from medical informatics experts.

5.1.2 Classification of Clinical Decision Support Systems

Currently, there are various ways to classify CDSS. According to the timing of intervention, CDSS can be divided into pre-diagnostic, intra-diagnostic, and post-diagnostic systems. According to whether they actively provide decision support, CDSS can be categorized as active or passive. The most widely accepted classification divides CDSS into knowledge-based and non-knowledge-based systems. Knowledge-based CDSS primarily follows "IF-THEN" rules to retrieve data and output results, while non-knowledge-based CDSS relies mainly on various machine learning and deep learning algorithms. Although the use of non-knowledge-based CDSS in medicine has rapidly developed, many challenges remain. The common framework of CDSS is shown in Fig. 5.1. The following sections will detail the two types of CDSS.

5.1.2.1 Knowledge-Based CDSS

Knowledge-based CDSS originated from early expert systems. Researchers aimed to develop a computer program that could simulate human thinking and replace clinical experts, becoming a "doctor." As research progressed, the goal shifted from simulating expert decisions to assisting clinical experts in decision-making. Instead of just providing "answers," these systems now also provide the rationale behind the answers. Users have also transitioned from passive recipients to actively interacting with CDSS, collaboratively guiding optimal clinical decisions.

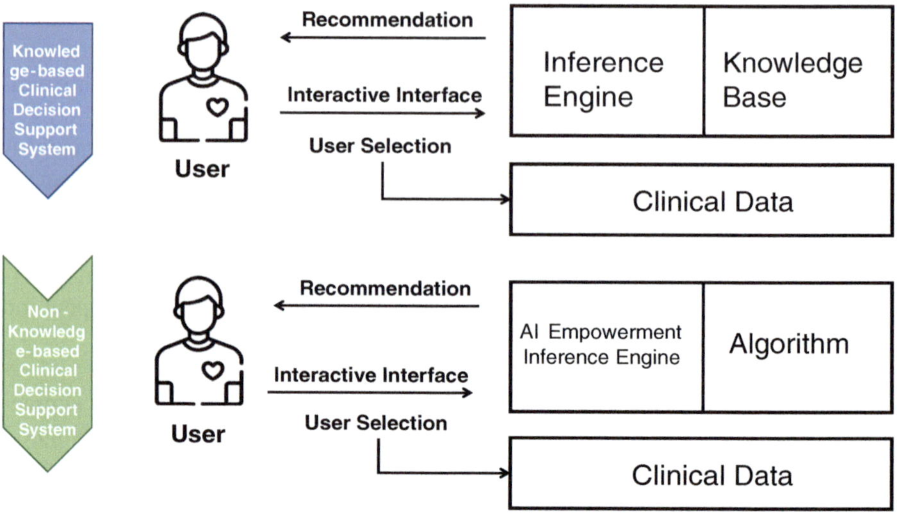

Fig. 5.1 Common framework of CDSS

Knowledge-based CDSS mainly comprises three parts: the knowledge base, the inference engine, and the communication interface. The knowledge base is the foundation of CDSS, composed of compiled information, typically represented in "IF-THEN" rules. For example, "IF" the system detects that a doctor is prescribing medication for a diabetes patient who is in stage 4 chronic kidney disease, "THEN" it will alert the doctor to reduce the dosage of sulfonylureas, insulin, and metformin by half, providing the rationale that patients with severe renal impairment have altered drug metabolism, increasing the risk of hypoglycemia.

In addition to the relationship between drugs and diseases, the knowledge base can include the probability relationships between signs/symptoms and diagnoses, drug–drug adverse reactions, recommended relationships between diseases and lab tests, and causal relationships between test results and diseases. The rules can be sourced from literature and clinical guidelines or clinical experts' practical evidence. Generally, the construction of the knowledge base uses literature knowledge as the foundation and supplements it with practical evidence. The knowledge base is usually organized using ontology.

The inference engine is the core of CDSS, primarily combining the rules from the knowledge base with actual data to derive conclusions. For example, when a doctor orders an "MRI enhanced scan" for a patient, the inference engine analyzes the knowledge base as follows:

(1) What are the contrast agents for MRI enhanced scans?
(2) Which contrast agents could adversely affect the patient's existing conditions? What is the rationale?
(3) Are there any alternative tests to the MRI enhanced scan? What is the rationale?
(4) ...

Finally, these comprehensive inference results are fed back to the end user through the human–computer interaction mechanism.

The human–computer interaction mechanism can be a website, application, or interface within an EHR. It is mainly divided into user interface (UI)-based interfaces and service-based interfaces. The UI directly presents knowledge inferred from the knowledge base via a website, while the service interface transmits knowledge and data based on the HL7 health information exchange standard. The technology related to CDSS human–computer interaction is developing rapidly. For example, InfoButton technology can provide necessary decision-related information to doctors without interrupting their workflow.

Knowledge-based CDSS generally responds quickly and provides a rationale for each decision, offering strong interpretability. The technology is relatively mature, but the reliability of CDSS heavily depends on the quality of the knowledge base and the accuracy of its rules. Given the rapid updating of medical knowledge, maintaining and updating the knowledge base requires significant effort and manpower.

5.1.2.2 Non-knowledge-Based CDSS

As shown in Fig. 5.1, the structure of non-knowledge-based CDSS is roughly similar to that of knowledge-based CDSS. The primary difference is that non-knowledge-based CDSS typically utilize artificial intelligence, such as machine learning algorithms, to learn rules from past experiences or discover patterns from clinical data, rather than relying on an existing knowledge base. Therefore, it usually requires a sufficient amount of preliminary data to train the algorithms to ensure the reliability of the derived rules and patterns. Common algorithms include artificial neural networks (ANN), genetic algorithms (GA), and pattern recognition algorithms (PRA). Although research on non-knowledge-based CDSS is very popular, few have been successfully implemented in practice. Only a few CDSS have been applied, such as the AI product IDx-DR, which was approved by the FDA in 2018 to detect mild diabetic retinopathy. This product is mainly used for screening during physical examinations. The primary reason for the limited application of non-knowledge-based CDSS is its poor interpretability. The entire reasoning process is hidden in a "black box," making it difficult to provide doctors with clear diagnostic rationales. Despite potentially superior predictive performance compared to knowledge-based CDSS, doctors remain skeptical and cautious about its use. Therefore, many researchers are now considering combining knowledge-based and non-knowledge-based CDSS to leverage the strengths of both approaches. This hybrid method aims to improve predictive performance while providing a certain level of interpretability.

5.1.3 Development History of Clinical Decision Support Systems

The development history of CDSS is illustrated in Fig. 5.2. The origins of clinical decision support systems date back to the late 1950s when scholars like Ledley and Lusted published articles in the journal Science discussing the principles and

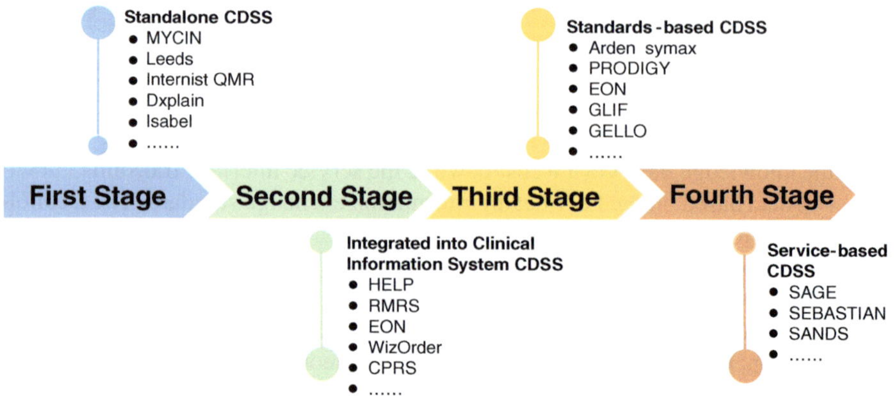

Fig. 5.2 Development history of CDSS

feasibility of using symbolic logic and probability to aid physicians in decision-making. This marked the beginning of CDSS research [2]. The initial CDSS, also known as expert systems, primarily compiled the experience and knowledge of medical experts into a knowledge base and used logical reasoning to make decisions. These early CDSS were often standalone systems with poor integration and low efficiency, requiring manual data input and serving mostly single departments or specific steps in the diagnostic process. Doctors could only passively accept decision recommendations without interacting with the system. A typical example is AAPHelp, developed in 1971, which used the Naive Bayesian method to predict acute abdomen based on patient symptoms. Despite its excellent diagnostic performance, comparable to clinical experts, it was highly controversial and not widely adopted due to skepticism about using computers for clinical decision-making at the time. In 1976, the Shortliff team at Stanford University developed MYCIN, which provided decision support for diagnosing bacteremia based on rule-based reasoning and was later expanded to diagnose other infectious diseases. In 1982, the University of Pittsburgh developed Internist, which used heuristic rules and decision tree logic to assist internists in prescribing medication. Although these systems achieved good testing performance, they were not widely adopted in clinical practice.

Due to these issues, researchers began developing the second generation of CDSS. These systems were integrated into EHR systems, computerized physician order entry (CPOE) systems, and clinical information systems (CIS), allowing CDSS to access data from electronic health records in real-time for proactive response. A representative example from this period is the HELP (Health Evaluation through Logical Processing) system developed by the University of Utah in 1967. This system integrated CDSS with the hospital information system (HIS), interacting with billing, laboratory, electronic medical record, and imaging systems through a local area network (LAN). It included an integrated clinical database, CDSS, programs supporting hospital clinical and administrative functions, and software tools for maintaining and expanding these components. It was installed in 20 hospitals operated by Intermountain Healthcare. Other notable examples include the Regenstrief Medical Record System (RMRS) developed by the Regenstrief Institute in Indiana and the Brigham Integrated Computing System (BICS) developed by Brigham and Women's Hospital, an affiliate of Harvard Medical School. These systems achieved CDSS integration with other hospital systems and were applied in academic medical centers. However, the second generation of CDSS faced challenges such as poor system interoperability and complex knowledge management.

To address knowledge management issues, researchers developed the third generation of CDSS. A typical representative is the Arden Syntax, designed for representing and sharing knowledge. The Arden Syntax uses Medical Logic Modules (MLMs) as its representation units. MLMs consist of maintenance, library, knowledge, and resources sections, containing the logic to make a single medical decision. CDSS can use MLMs to represent medical conditions and recommendations, sharing medical knowledge within hospital systems. The Arden Syntax has become part of the HL7 standard. Systems like RMRS widely adopted this syntax for knowledge management. However, it has limitations: constructing specific compilers for the Arden Syntax is challenging, and encoding standards restrict the content users can code.

Thus, the fourth generation of CDSS emerged. Unlike the integrated model of the second and third generations, CDSS returned to being a standalone component, providing APIs to healthcare information systems in a service-oriented manner. Heterogeneous medical information systems can reuse these components by calling the APIs. A typical example is the Standard-based Sharable Active Guideline Environment (SAGE), developed collaboratively by IDX System Corporation, IHC, and the Stanford Medical Informatics Center. SAGE includes a model and services supporting guideline modeling and execution, accessing EHR terminology through the Virtual Medical Record (VMR) method, and providing appropriate mappings across different medical system terminologies. It is compatible with service-oriented architecture (SOA). Other examples include SEBASTIAN, a clinical decision support web service developed by Duke University, which serves as the basis for the HL7 decision support service draft standard. The fourth generation of CDSS is currently being applied in several countries.

The development history of CDSS reveals many limitations in its clinical use. Although technological advancements have addressed some issues, many challenges remain. For instance, as CDSS becomes increasingly complex, it imposes higher demands on both users and maintenance staff. Furthermore, in reality, medical information systems within different medical institutions and even within the same medical organization are highly diverse, with various developers. How to extract and interact with information across these heterogeneous systems is a challenging issue that plagues today's medical information specialists.

5.2 Construction Methods and Inference Algorithms of Clinical Decision Support Systems

5.2.1 Construction Methods of Clinical Decision Support Systems

As mentioned earlier, CDSS primarily consists of three parts: a knowledge base/intelligent algorithms, an inference engine, and a human–computer interaction mechanism. To ensure the effectiveness of CDSS applications, CDSS needs to be developed and constructed following standardized procedures. The construction method for a knowledge-based CDSS is as follows.

5.2.1.1 Problem Definition

Firstly, it is essential to clarify the purpose of developing the CDSS, identify the clinical problems it needs to solve, determine the decision support required in various diagnostic and treatment processes, and specify which hospital information systems it needs to interact with. It is also necessary to identify the medical personnel who will participate in the decision support process, their functions, and decision-making scenarios. Developers need to describe these issues in detail, create corresponding specification documents, and discuss them with relevant clinical experts. For example, the basic description for a CDSS aimed at the rational use of antimicrobial drugs would include strict adherence to the graded management of antimicrobial drugs, monitoring physicians' authority to prescribe these drugs, and requiring approval from senior physicians for drugs beyond their authority. The system would also collect real-time information on patients' vital signs, personal information, medical history, and previous tests and examinations to provide recommended antimicrobial treatment plans. Additionally, it would periodically collect, analyze, and compare the usage statistics of antimicrobial drugs for outpatient and inpatient populations, and send the generated reports to the appropriate hospital management personnel.

5.2.1.2 Feasibility Analysis

Feasibility analysis examines whether the above system description can be developed and implemented. It mainly includes the following aspects:

1. Theoretical feasibility: This involves evaluating whether the existing standard model frameworks and knowledge bases can support the functions of the CDSS and whether there are similar CDSS cases that have been successfully implemented in the past.
2. Technical feasibility: This includes assessing whether the current methods for constructing knowledge bases, knowledge representation methods, decision support algorithms, and human–computer interaction technologies can support the functionalities and interfaces of the CDSS, ensuring its proper operation. It also involves checking if the existing hospital information systems provide the necessary interfaces to interact with the CDSS.

3. Economic feasibility: This considers the cost and benefit issues of implementing the CDSS, ensuring that the construction of the CDSS will not exceed the budget significantly and that the benefits of implementing the CDSS outweigh the costs.
4. Social feasibility: This focuses on how to train medical staff to use the CDSS after deployment, ensuring its practical implementation. It also includes clarifying the responsibilities and methods for subsequent maintenance, updates, and handling potential infringement issues.

For a CDSS aimed at the rational use of antimicrobial drugs, the considerations include developing the system based on the existing literature and expert experience, and using mature algorithms on the current instruments and equipment to ensure theoretical feasibility. The electronic health records must be compatible with the developed CDSS, and the existing network must support real-time information retrieval and interaction, ensuring technical feasibility. The costs of constructing the CDSS mainly involve the labor fees for developers and the purchase of some knowledge sources. Once successfully deployed, the system can reduce the number of skin tests, lower the readmission rates caused by improper use of antimicrobial drugs, and improve the efficiency of medical staff. Over time, these benefits can offset the costs, ensuring economic feasibility. The CDSS should have a user-friendly interface, allowing medical staff to use it with minimal training, and it should not disrupt existing clinical workflows, ensuring social feasibility.

5.2.1.3 Requirements Analysis

Requirements analysis is the process of clarifying the specific functions and requirements of the software, serving as the foundation for constructing the CDSS. This process involves collaborative discussions between developers and medical staff, utilizing methods such as questionnaires, face-to-face interactions, and process observations to determine the functionalities, performance, and interfaces with other hospital information systems for the CDSS. After completing the investigation, developers construct data models, functional models, and behavioral models based on the requirements and finally provide the CDSS requirements specification.

1. Functional requirements for rational use of antimicrobial drugs CDSS
   (a) Real-time monitoring of patient medication behavior.
   (b) Hierarchical management of antimicrobial drugs.
   (c) Real-time monitoring of physicians' prescription authority for antimicrobial drugs.
   (d) Generating recommended antimicrobial prescriptions based on patient vital signs, diagnoses, and examination data.
   (e) Conducting consultations for emergency and special use of antimicrobial drugs.
   (f) Regularly compiling statistics on hospital antimicrobial drug usage and generating statistical reports.
2. Performance requirements for rational use of antimicrobial drugs CDSS

(a) The system must have fast inference and response speeds to achieve real-time alerts and recommendations, with system response times less than 5 s.
(b) The knowledge base must cover all antimicrobial drugs listed in the "Classification management directory of clinical application of antimicrobial drugs" and at least 95% of the diseases in ICD-10, with a minimum of 1000 related literature sources in the knowledge base.
(c) The CDSS should support at least 500 concurrent users.
(d) The CDSS must ensure data security, allowing only authorized medical personnel to access patient data.
(e) The network must be stable and reliable during CDSS operation.
(f) The CDSS interface must be simple to operate and user-friendly.

In the requirements analysis process, a data flow diagram (DFD) can be used to construct the CDSS requirements model, and relevant data dictionaries, decision tables, and other information can be refined layer by layer.

5.2.1.4 Software Design

Software design mainly involves converting the requirements analysis of CDSS into computer models, consisting of two stages: high-level design and detailed design. High-level design involves defining the various functional modules within the CDSS, the relationships and interactions between these modules, the hierarchical structure, data structures, and database architecture. Detailed design provides comprehensive descriptions of each part outlined in the high-level design, translating each functional module's description into specific, precise procedural descriptions that can be implemented in the next stage using programming languages. Flowcharts, NS diagrams, problem analysis diagrams (PAD), and pseudocode can be used to describe software design. It is important to ensure that the CDSS software design does not disrupt existing diagnostic and treatment workflows to avoid interfering with doctors' consultations and reducing their efficiency. The high-level design flowchart for the CDSS for rational use of antimicrobial drugs is shown in Fig. 5.3.

5.2.1.5 Coding

The coding stage involves implementing the high-level and detailed design of the CDSS using programming languages. During coding, it is essential to ensure that the program structure is clear, readable, and easily maintainable. The software must meet the functional and performance requirements specified in the requirements analysis, and the different CDSS modules must interact according to the software design. Attention should be paid to setting alert thresholds to address common issues like "alert fatigue." Given the busy schedules of doctors, the interface design must be simple and clear to balance functionality with efficiency. The knowledge base can be constructed using ontology, which provides a formalized specification of a shared conceptual model. Ontologies capture common knowledge and understanding within a domain and serve as a common language for exchanging information between different knowledge systems. Ontology modeling elements (classes, relationships, functions, axioms, and instances) can explicitly define medical

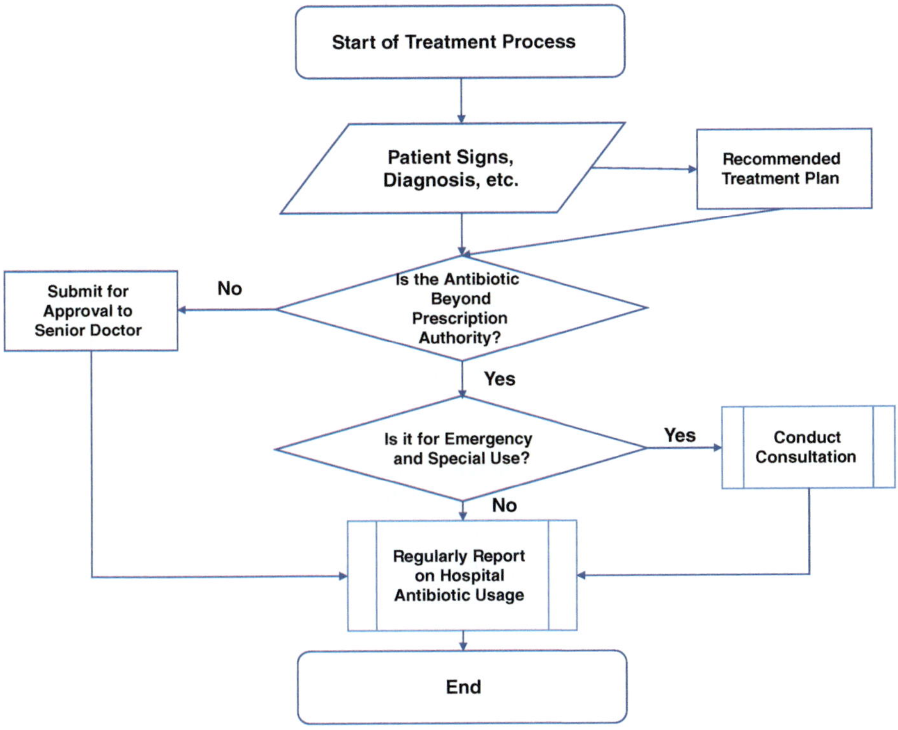

Fig. 5.3 Outline design flowchart for the rational use of antibiotics CDSS

concepts and their relationships, making it a common method for constructing medical knowledge bases. The inference engine's algorithms can be implemented using programming languages like Java or Python. Java is an object-oriented programming language known for its powerful features, multi-threading, distributed nature, and high security, making it a mainstream programming language. Python supports multiple programming paradigms, is simple and efficient, easily extensible, and portable, and has a rich standard library, gaining popularity in recent years. The human-computer interaction interface should ensure compatibility with the hospital's existing CDSS, particularly interface compatibility, and emphasize patient safety with robust privacy protection mechanisms and well-designed interfaces to minimize medical errors.

5.2.1.6 Testing

Testing involves running the coded CDSS to identify and address any issues based on the problem definition and requirements analysis. The testing process can use simulated data from real patient diagnostic and treatment processes, with relevant medical staff simulating a real clinical environment. It is important to note that, in principle, the more tests conducted, the more issues can be identified. However, in the real world, the number of tests is limited, so a balance between the number of tests and testing costs must be considered. Testing methods include static analysis and dynamic analysis: static analysis involves manually testing step-by-step, while dynamic analysis involves designing different clinical scenarios in advance, determining system functions within those scenarios, and comparing the results with expected outcomes.

Testing the CDSS for rational use of antimicrobial drugs includes program testing, functional testing, performance testing, and interface testing. Functional and performance testing should meet the requirements specified in the requirements analysis. Program testing involves checking for syntax errors, redundant code, and ensuring every step produces an output. Interface testing includes self-validation and prompts for erroneous or invalid clinical data inputs and ensuring the interface adapts to different browsers and screen sizes.

5.2.1.7 Maintenance

Given the rapid growth of medical knowledge and the continuous updates to clinical guidelines, it is inevitable that new issues will be discovered during the usage of CDSS, even after thorough testing. Since CDSS influences doctors' decisions and, consequently, patient health management, maintenance personnel must regularly maintain the CDSS to ensure its ongoing proper functioning within the hospital.

5.2.2 Inference Algorithms of Clinical Decision Support Systems

As previously mentioned, the inference engine is the core of CDSS, and inference algorithms are the core of the inference engine. A good inference algorithm can help doctors understand and extract more information about patients, compensate for gaps in knowledge and clinical testing, reduce unnecessary clinical expenses for patients, and improve patient health management. Currently, common inference algorithms include rule-based inference, probabilistic inference, case-based reasoning, deductive reasoning, and inductive reasoning. The specifics are as follows.

5.2.2.1 Rule-Based Inference

Rule-based inference was the first inference algorithm to appear in CDSS. Its architecture mainly consists of two parts: a knowledge base represented by "IF-THEN" rules and an inference engine using forward or backward chaining. The rule-based inference works as follows: for a given input problem, the system first uses a rule matching algorithm to find suitable rules, then generates intermediate results based on forward or backward chaining mechanisms, repeating this process until the desired result is obtained. "IF-THEN" denotes that if the condition is true, then execute scheme A. A common variation is "IF-THEN-ELSE," meaning if the condition is true, execute scheme A; if false, execute scheme B.

Conventional "IF-THEN" rule matching requires strict Boolean expression matching for conditions and conclusions. However, many clinical descriptions are vague, uncertain, or partially matched. For example, terms like "suspected," "possible," and "cannot be ruled out" often appear in patient records, indicating that certain symptoms or test results suggest a disease but are not definitive for diagnosis. In such cases, the CDSS needs to infer the most likely diagnosis or suggest further tests to confirm the diagnosis. Researchers have thus proposed fuzzy "IF-THEN" rules. These use fuzzy propositions like "a is A" for the premise, where A is a fuzzy set. For example, "high blood pressure" is a fuzzy proposition, with "high" being a fuzzy concept. Fuzzy propositions can be linked through operations like complement, union, and intersection. Fuzzy rules are widely used in diagnostic assistance, medical behavior analysis, and treatment support.

Forward Chaining

Forward chaining (or forward chained reasoning) involves starting from existing data and using inference rules to obtain more data until the final result is reached. It is a top-down reasoning approach. For instance, using "IF-THEN" rules, a forward reasoning inference engine continuously searches for rules that match the known conditions and then infers conclusions based on those rules, adding the conclusions to the data. This process is repeated until the desired result is found. For example, if the goal is to determine the recommended dose of metoprolol for a patient with an estimated glomerular filtration rate (eGFR) of less than (30 mL/min)/1.73 m^2, the knowledge base might contain the following rules.

(1) If a patient starts or is taking metoprolol, regular monitoring of blood count, blood pressure, heart function, liver function, and kidney function is required to avoid adverse drug reactions.
(2) If the patient's eGFR <(30 mL/min)/1.73 m^2, it indicates severe renal impairment.
(3) If the patient has severe renal impairment, the dose of beta-adrenergic receptor blockers should be halved.
(4) Metoprolol is a beta-adrenergic receptor blocker.

Based on these rules, (4) is axiomatic knowledge. From knowledge (4), we know that metoprolol is a beta-adrenergic receptor blocker. According to rule (2), we determine that the patient has severe renal impairment and add this information to the patient's data. According to rule (3), the metoprolol dose for this patient should be halved. Rule (1) suggests that the doctor should regularly check the patient's blood count, blood pressure, heart function, liver function, and kidney function to avoid adverse reactions. Finally, the recommendation to reduce the dose and monitor the patient regularly will be presented to the doctor. The inference engine continuously searches for rules that match the conditions and outputs conclusions, hence it is also called data-driven reasoning. A representative example of forward chaining is the Germwatcher system at Barnes-Jewish Hospital in St. Louis, which uses forward chaining for hospital infection monitoring.

Backward chaining (or backward chained reasoning) is the opposite of forward chaining. It starts from known conclusions and works backward to find conditions that support the conclusions. Unlike forward chaining, where true conditions lead to true conclusions, backward chaining cannot deduce that conditions are true solely based on true conclusions because the rules in the rule base do not always meet the necessary and sufficient conditions.

Using the same knowledge base for forward chaining, backward chaining first looks for information about metoprolol, deducing that it is a beta-adrenergic receptor blocker and adding this information to the data. The inference engine then looks for rules regarding the dosage of metoprolol and beta-adrenergic receptor blockers, i.e., rule (3), and searches for information about impaired renal function. According to rule (2), the patient has impaired renal function, leading to the conclusion that the metoprolol dose should be halved. Backward chaining is highly goal-oriented and is also known as goal-driven reasoning.

The example illustrates the differences between the two reasoning methods. Backward chaining is suitable for scenarios with few ultimate answers, such as the MYCIN system, which uses backward reasoning to identify microorganisms causing bacteremia or meningitis because the number of possible microorganisms is limited. Forward chaining is more appropriate for scenarios with many possible answers to avoid combinatorial explosion, making it difficult to test. Therefore, it is crucial to clarify the appropriate reasoning method when developing a CDSS. Typically, simple diagnostic support functions use backward chaining, while medical plan management, equipment management, and test result interpretation often use forward chaining. Some CDSSs support both methods for comprehensive reasoning, such as those used for clinical explanations.

Advantages and Disadvantages of Rule-Based Inference

From the above introduction, it can be seen that the advantages of rule-based reasoning include: (1) It aligns with the way doctors think, with strong interpretability; (2) The reasoning process is simple and rigorous.

However, its disadvantages are also quite evident, including: (1) Regular maintenance and updates of the system are required; (2) The construction of the rule base is complex; (3) It cannot generate new knowledge; (4) It has high requirements for the knowledge base, but in reality, it is difficult for the knowledge base to encompass all the necessary knowledge.

5.2.2.2 Probability Reasoning

Probability reasoning is a common form of reasoning in clinical practice. As mentioned earlier, clinical tests are filled with descriptions of uncertainty and incompleteness. While some medical personnel do not include quantitative descriptions, computers need to use specific numerical representations to convert these uncertain descriptions into definite conclusions for reasoning. Probability is the quantification of these uncertain descriptions, usually ranging from 0 to 1, where a probability of 0 indicates the conclusion is false, and a probability of 1 indicates the conclusion is true. Typically, most probabilities in clinical descriptions are greater than 0 and less than 1.

In clinical testing, ideal results are clearly delineated. However, in reality, due to factors such as operational procedures, test results among large populations may overlap. Therefore, terms like true positive (TP), false positive (FP), true negative

(TN), and false negative (FN) are used to describe test outcomes. Based on these four scenarios, the following metrics or curves are generated to measure the effectiveness of tests or decisions:

1. Precision = TP/(TP + FP)
2. Sensitivity (or true positive rate, recall) = TP/(TP + FN)
3. Specificity (or true negative rate, selectivity) = TN/(TN + FN)
4. Negative Predictive Value (NPV) = TN/(TN + FN)
5. The receiver operating characteristic (ROC) Curve, also known as the receiver operating characteristic curve, with the area under the ROC curve (AUC) used to measure the effectiveness of model classification and prediction, as shown in Fig. 5.4.

Common probability reasoning methods include Bayes' theorem, decision trees, Markov chains, and others. Bayes' theorem can assist doctors in reducing uncertainty and adjusting prior probabilities based on a patient's current condition to derive posterior probabilities, aiding in decision-making. For random events A and B, where the probability of event B occurring is non-zero, the probability of event A occurring given that event B has occurred is:

$$P(AB) = \frac{P(A)P(BA)}{P(B)}$$

In this formula: P(A|B) represents the conditional probability of A occurring given that B has occurred, also known as the posterior probability of A. P(A)

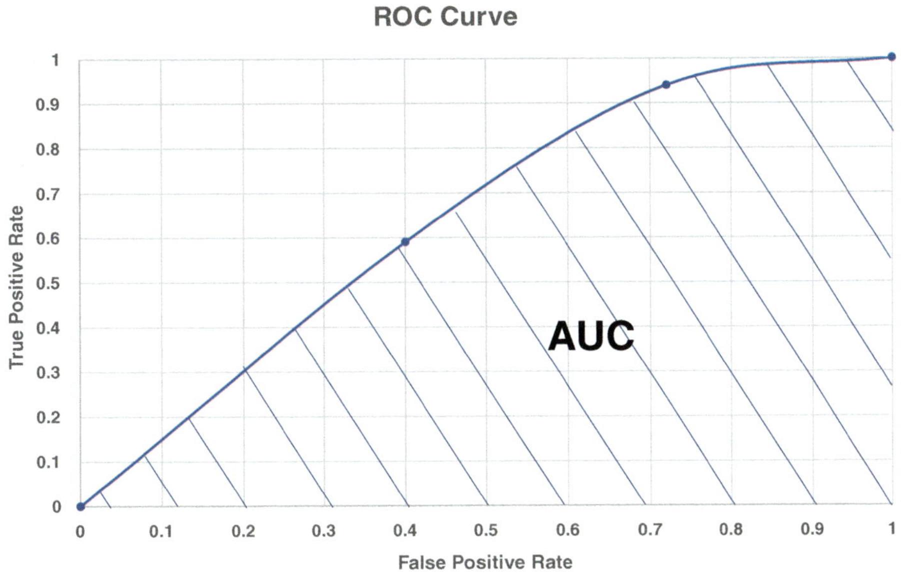

Fig. 5.4 ROC curve

represents the occurrence rate of A, also known as the prior probability of A. P(B|A) represents the conditional probability of B occurring given that A has occurred, also known as the posterior probability of B. P(B) represents the occurrence rate of B, also known as the prior probability of B.

Bayes' theorem is widely used in clinical settings and has spawned many versions. For example, the Naive Bayesian Model (NBM) applies Bayes' theorem under the condition of strong independence of features to simply classify diseases. It has played a significant role in disease diagnosis and prediction.

A decision tree is a structure similar to a flowchart, where each chance node (usually represented by a circle) represents a test of an attribute (such as high blood pressure or low blood pressure), and each decision node (usually represented by a rectangle) represents the result of a branch test. The terminal node (usually represented by a triangle) indicates the end of the branch where no further splitting occurs. Decision tree analysis typically includes three steps: feature selection, decision tree generation, and decision tree pruning. Common decision tree algorithms include the ID3 algorithm, C4.5 algorithm, and Classification and Regression Tree (CART), which use information gain, information gain ratio, and Gini coefficient, respectively, for feature selection. Due to the potential for overfitting, where the decision tree classifies unknown data inaccurately, pruning is necessary to remove some nodes and reduce the complexity of the decision tree. To enhance classification effectiveness, researchers have combined multiple decision trees in a classifier, known as the Random Forest method. This approach has been widely studied and applied in medical imaging classification, tumor diagnosis, and other fields.

A Markov chain is a stochastic model that describes a sequence of possible events. Its most important property is that the probability of a given current state depends only on the previous state and is independent of other states, known as the Markov property.

When Clinical Decision Support (CDS) involves risks that change continuously over time, such as during treatment when a patient's health status is continuously changing, a Markov chain can be constructed. This model assumes that a patient is always in one of a finite number of health states, allowing the study of state changes and the factors influencing these changes.

Compared to rule-based reasoning, probability reasoning can handle incomplete and imprecise data from a probabilistic perspective, providing a more objective reference for doctors in decision support and offering strong interpretability. However, when the data volume is large, probability calculations become complex, reducing inference efficiency. Additionally, some events rely on subjective probabilities, which can decrease the accuracy of probability reasoning.

5.2.2.3 Case-Based Reasoning

Case-based reasoning (CBR) is the process of solving new problems based on the solutions to similar past problems. This approach closely mirrors the actual decision-making process of doctors, who often rely on the experience of previous cases to address current patient issues.

The steps in case-based reasoning are as follows:

Retrieval

For a given target problem, search for cases related to that problem. These cases include the problem itself, the solution, and the way the solution was implemented. For example, when a doctor faces a patient with secondary hypertension, they will actively recall past cases, determine that the condition can be controlled, and remember the methods used for control.

Reuse

When mapping the decision process from past cases to the current case, it is usually impossible to directly apply previous experiences without modifications. Adjustments must be made based on the current patient's situation. For example, in patients with secondary hypertension, the underlying chronic conditions may differ, requiring the doctor to adapt their decision-making process accordingly.

Revision

After mapping the old case, it is necessary to simulate the new solution in the real world and make modifications as needed. For instance, a doctor prescribes metoprolol to a patient with secondary hypertension and chronic kidney disease, advising them to take the medication for two weeks and then return for a kidney function test. If, after 2 weeks, the patient's eGFR slightly decreases and no other significant changes in diet or habits are observed except for the medication, the doctor might suspect that metoprolol is affecting kidney function. Therefore, the doctor must revise the patient's treatment plan, either by reducing the metoprolol dosage or selecting an alternative antihypertensive drug.

Maintenance

Once the current solution has been successfully adapted to the case, the decision-making experience gained is stored as new knowledge in the brain. For example, in the case mentioned above, after adjusting the dosage, the patient's blood pressure was effectively controlled, and eGFR returned to normal. Therefore, the doctor records this case to prepare for decision-making with future similar patients. Table 5.1 provides an example of case-based reasoning from a study.

These three cases have many similarities, with only some attribute values differing slightly. Therefore, medical experts rated the similarity of each symptom feature between each pair of cases, with similarity values ranging from 0 to 1, where 0 indicates completely dissimilar and 1 indicates completely similar. The higher the value, the greater the similarity, as shown in Table 5.2.

The global case similarity is calculated using Euclidean distance, resulting in the following similarities: sim (Case 1, Case 2) = 0.84, sim (Case 1, Case 3) = 0.67, sim (Case 2, Case 3) = 0.70. In real situations, the importance of different attributes may vary. Therefore, attribute weights can be introduced when calculating similarity.

The main advantage of case-based reasoning is that it references a large number of real cases. In clinical practice, disease cases are relatively easy to obtain, making it relatively simple to build a relevant knowledge base. However, the quality of case-based reasoning is influenced by the quality of the case knowledge base. If previous

Table 5.1 Example of case-based reasoning in hypertension diagnosis and treatment

Attribute	Case 1	Case 2	Case 3
Hypertension grade	3rd degree	3rd degree	3rd degree
Gender	Male	Male	Female
Age	50	53	52
Smoking	No	No	Yes
Hemoglobin	141 g/L	110 g/L	119 g/L
Red blood cell count	None	None	None
Family history of CVD	None	Yes	Yes
Abdominal obesity	None	Yes	Yes
Proteinuria	None	None	+
Glucosuria	+	+	+
Serum iron	50 μg/dL	45 μg/dL	48 μg/dL
Serum ferritin	6 μg/L	5 μg/L	6 μg/L
History of stroke	Ischemic stroke	Cerebral hemorrhage	None
History of heart disease	Angina	Coronary artery bypass	None
Diabetic nephropathy	None	Yes	None
Renal impairment	None	None	None
Fasting blood glucose	9.6 mmol/L	8.6 mmol/L	8.8 mmol/L

Table 5.2 Similarity between patient records

Attribute	Case 1 vs. case 2	Case 1 vs. case 3	Case 2 vs. case 3
Hypertension grade	1.00	0.75	0.75
Gender	1	0	0
Age	1	2/3	1/3
Smoking	0	0	1
Hemoglobin	1	0.7	0.3
Red blood cell count	1	5/6	1/6
Family history of CVD	1	1	1
Abdominal obesity	0	0	1
Proteinuria	1	0	0
Glucosuria	0.8	0.8	1
Serum iron	1	0.4	0.6
Serum ferritin	1	0	1
History of stroke	0.75	0.5	0.75
History of heart disease	0.8	0.4	0.6
Diabetic nephropathy	0	1	0
Renal impairment	1	1	1
Fasting blood glucose	1.0	0.8	0.2

cases contain errors, it will directly affect the accuracy of the reasoning. Additionally, the sparsity of cases can also impact the accuracy of the reasoning.

5.2.2.4 Deductive Reasoning and Inductive Reasoning

Deductive reasoning and inductive reasoning are two common modes of reasoning in medicine. In fact, most reasoning modes can be classified into these two types. Deductive reasoning is the process of deriving a conclusion from one or more premises, moving from the general to the specific. This method is similar to forward reasoning, using a top-down approach where the conditions are clear and, if the premises are true, the conclusion is guaranteed to be correct. Inductive reasoning, on the other hand, extends views formed from individual instances to a broader range, moving from the specific to the general. This bottom-up approach draws conclusions based on given evidence, but the correctness of these conclusions depends on factors like sample size and representativeness.

Representative forms of deductive reasoning include syllogism, hypothetical reasoning, and relational inference. A syllogism derives a conclusion based on one condition's hypothesis and another's conclusion, typically in the following form:

(1) Assume $P \rightarrow Q$.
(2) Given $Q \rightarrow R$.
(3) Therefore, $P \rightarrow R$.

Hypothetical reasoning involves reasoning based on the logical nature of hypothetical propositions, which are "IF A THEN B" statements where A is the antecedent and B is the consequent. This can be categorized into sufficient condition, necessary condition, and sufficient and necessary condition reasoning. Relational inference involves using relational judgments as premises and conclusions in deductive reasoning. It can be categorized into direct and indirect relational inference, depending on whether it involves one premise or more. Direct relational inference includes symmetric and antisymmetric relational reasoning, while indirect relational inference includes transitive and anti-transitive relational reasoning. In actual clinical practice, doctors often use deductive reasoning. They propose hypotheses based on general knowledge and experience, design lab tests based on these hypotheses, eliminate hypotheses, and arrive at a final diagnosis. For example, the Guangzhou Women and Children's Medical Center designed a pediatric diagnostic CDSS based on deductive hypotheses, achieving high accuracy and F1 scores in predicting various pediatric organ diseases and generalized systemic diseases.

Deductive reasoning has its limitations. Firstly, it is based on prior knowledge and cannot uncover new knowledge. Additionally, within the scope of deduction, it cannot guarantee the accuracy of the premises.

Inductive reasoning includes forms such as complete induction and incomplete induction. Complete induction involves deriving that all objects in a category possess (or do not possess) a certain attribute by observing that every individual object in that category has (or lacks) that attribute. For example, if the premise is "All of Zhang's elders are diabetic," complete induction would infer that "Zhang's grandfather is a diabetic." However, complete induction is difficult to achieve in the real world. Therefore, researchers have developed incomplete induction.

Incomplete induction involves inferring that all objects in a category possess (or do not possess) a certain attribute based on a representative sample of that category. For instance, before a drug is marketed, it must undergo clinical trials to verify its efficacy against a particular disease. Because the number of patients treated after the drug's release may be countless, ideally, as many subjects as possible should be included in the trial. However, in reality, it is challenging to find such a large number of subjects. Therefore, clinical trials typically select a certain number of subjects, and if the drug shows efficacy and no major adverse reactions in this group, it is considered effective for the disease and can be considered for marketing.

Compared to deductive reasoning, inductive reasoning is more likely to discover new knowledge. However, the process of inductive reasoning has high requirements. If the sample chosen is not representative or the sample size is too small, the accuracy and adequacy of the conclusion cannot be guaranteed.

5.3 Case Studies of Clinical Decision Support Systems

5.3.1 MYCIN

MYCIN is a backward reasoning Clinical Decision Support System (CDSS) developed by Edward Shortliffe at Stanford University in the early 1970s. AI pioneer Allen Newell referred to it as a "pioneer in the field of expert systems." The system utilizes rule-based reasoning to diagnose bacteria causing severe infections (such as bacteremia and meningitis) based on patient symptoms and laboratory results and recommends antibiotics based on the patient's weight and condition. The structure of MYCIN is shown in Fig. 5.5. MYCIN comprises two databases: a static database storing approximately 600 reasoning rules, and a dynamic database storing patient data. The system consists of three main modules: (1) Consultation System: The core system of MYCIN, mainly interacting with doctors to gather patient information. (2) Explanation System: Provides relevant knowledge on infectious disease treatment and justifies its recommendations. (3) Knowledge Acquisition System: Allows experts in infectious diseases to provide decision rules they deem useful for clinical decisions and update the knowledge base [3].

MYCIN employs backward reasoning. Its typical rule format is shown below, primarily written in INTERLISP. The term "CNTXT" is a MYCIN variable used to bind context. "$AND" is a Boolean function that minimizes certainty factors (numbers between −1 and 1, representing the confidence in the conclusion). When combining multiple statements with AND functionality into a single composite statement in MYCIN, the smallest certainty factor among all statements is used as the certainty factor for the composite statement. The body of the rule is executable LISP code. The highly programmatic, modular, and structured nature of MYCIN rules allows the system to flexibly check and manipulate them, which inspired a series of subsequent CDSSs.

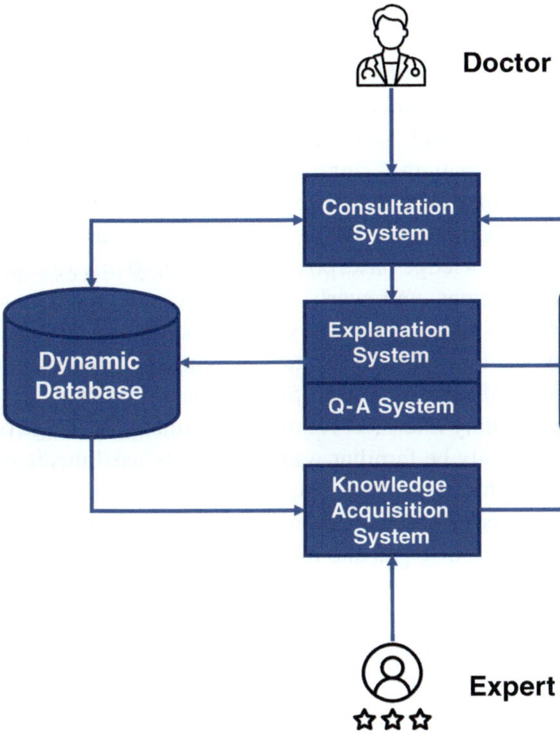

Fig. 5.5 MYCIN framework diagram

```
PREMISE: $AND (SAME CNTXT GRAM GRAMNEG)
              (SAME CNTXT MORPH ROD)
              (SAME CNTXT AIR ANAEROBIC)
ACTION: (CONCLUDE CNTXT IDENTITY BACTEROIDES TALLY .6)
```

If

1. The gram stain of the organism is gamneg,
2. The morphology of the organism is rod, and
3. The aerobicity of the organism is anaerobic

Then: There is suggestive evidence (.6) that the identity of the organism is bacteroides.

Unfortunately, despite MYCIN's excellent performance in internal tests, it was never implemented in clinical practice. This was due to ethical and legal issues related to using computer-assisted diagnosis in medicine at the time, the need for doctors to manually input patient information into MYCIN, and its requirement to run on large computer systems.

5.3.2 Dxplain

Dxplain is a Clinical Decision Support System (CDSS) designed and developed in 1984 by the Computer Science Laboratory at Massachusetts General Hospital, with the support of the American Medical Association (AMA). The system generates differential diagnoses based on patients' signs, symptoms, laboratory results, and other clinical findings. It provides evidence for each differential diagnosis and follow-up suggestions to help doctors make more accurate diagnoses. Additionally, Dxplain serves as a medical knowledge base, covering over 2000 diseases, approximately 4700 clinical manifestations, and nearly 65,000 disease-clinical manifestation relationships, each with a simple explanatory note. Doctors can search for and consult disease-related knowledge within the system, making it an important educational tool in American medical schools. By 2005, it had over 33,189 users.

Dxplain features a user-friendly interface, requiring minimal knowledge of computer technology; users need only be familiar with commonly used medical terminology. It also offers an "online help" function to assist users in understanding system commands. The knowledge base is comprehensive, providing the frequency of each clinical finding in various diseases and the strength of evidence for diagnosing a specific disease based on that finding. Another key factor in Dxplain's successful development is its collaboration with doctors, incorporating their feedback to continuously update and improve the knowledge base, thereby gaining increasing recognition from the medical community.

5.3.3 SimuConsult

SimuConsult is a Clinical Decision Support System (CDSS) designed by doctors for doctors, primarily utilizing Bayes' theorem for probabilistic reasoning. Its main functions include differential diagnosis, diagnostic recommendations, and disease assessment. Doctors need only input the patient's clinical signs and test results, and the system will provide a relevant diagnostic list along with the probable likelihood of each disease. The system also reviews the patient's symptoms and suggests additional tests to help clarify the diagnosis. Moreover, it compares the patient's symptoms with known disease symptoms to assess the accuracy of the preliminary diagnosis. In addition to clinical information, SimuConsult can incorporate genetic information for decision-making, allowing doctors to import a table of genomic variants to identify genes related to the patient's current signs.

5.3.4 CADUCEUS

CADUCEUS is a CDSS developed in the mid-1980s by scholars at the University of Pittsburgh. Their goal was to improve upon MYCIN by enabling the discovery of diseases with finer granularity and expanding the knowledge base to include all internal medicine drugs. CADUCEUS introduced many improvements over

MYCIN, integrating both rule-based and inductive reasoning. It can handle data dilution issues and assist in diagnosing patients with multiple underlying conditions. Currently, the system supports the diagnosis of 1000 different diseases.

5.3.5 ISABEL

ISABEL is a Clinical Decision Support System (CDSS) for pediatric disease differential diagnosis, developed in 2002 by the UK-based Isabel Medical Charity. The system was inspired by the misdiagnosis of a three-year-old girl named Isabel, who suffered from necrotizing fasciitis complicated by chickenpox. Her parents felt the need to develop a pediatric-focused CDSS to prevent similar incidents [4].

ISABEL consists of the Isabel Diagnosis Checklist System (IDCS) and a knowledge component. The IDCS is a database containing over 11,000 diagnoses and 4000 drugs. Doctors can manually input patient symptoms and clinical signs or import them from integrated Electronic Health Records (EHR). ISABEL then checks these inputs against its database and uses its built-in natural language processing tools to search medical textbooks and literature databases, providing a list of potential diagnoses or drugs that could explain the patient's symptoms.

ISABEL's functionalities are very powerful, currently including three components: the Isabel Pro DDX Generator, the Isabel Symptom Checker, and the Isabel Clinical Educator. The Isabel Pro DDX Generator is primarily aimed at healthcare professionals. According to clinical trials, 96% of cases require only the initial clinical features to be provided, and the generated disease list already includes the patient's actual disease. The Isabel Symptom Checker is mainly for patients themselves; they only need to input their conditions, and the system will provide a list of relevant diagnoses. The Isabel Clinical Educator is aimed at medical students, allowing them to measure and refine their clinical reasoning skills.

ISABEL is user-friendly and easy to operate. Doctors need only input the patient's gender, age, nationality, and relevant symptoms, and the system will generate a corresponding diagnosis list and clinical evidence within seconds. With ISABEL's robust knowledge base, doctors can reduce medical errors caused by cognitive mistakes. Clinical trials have shown that ISABEL can help doctors improve their diagnostic accuracy by 33%.

5.4 Frontier Research in Clinical Decision Support Systems

5.4.1 Multimodal Fusion Assisted Diagnosis

With the rapid advancement of medical informatics and medical equipment, the structure of medical data has become increasingly diverse. Common data types include text data, imaging data, omics data, and pathological data. The development of reasoning algorithms and data analysis techniques has also promoted the emergence of multimodal fusion. A modality refers to a type of information or a representation format for storing information. Common modalities include natural language (both written and spoken), visual (images or videos), auditory (including sounds, music, etc.), tactile, gustatory, and physiological signals.

Multimodal fusion, also known as multi-source information fusion, refers to the process of handling data from different modalities in analysis and recognition tasks. Multimodal fusion for assisted diagnosis integrates data from various modalities of a patient, enabling complementary diagnostic information. Additionally, multimodal fusion can generate new combined features, further improving diagnostic accuracy.

Currently, multimodal fusion for assisted diagnosis is widely used in clinical practice. Common types of multimodal fusion in clinical settings include:

5.4.1.1 Fusion of Clinical Data and Imaging Data

In actual diagnostic processes, doctors often use imaging data from Electronic Health Records (EHR) to provide background information for image diagnosis and supplement patient diagnosis based on image diagnosis results. Studies have shown that the absence of relevant clinical data during imaging can affect the accuracy of image diagnosis. Therefore, how to integrate EHR data with imaging data to improve diagnostic accuracy has become a leading development direction.

Some researchers have already explored this area. Researchers from Stanford University have integrated CT pixel data with demographic data, sign data, and laboratory test data from patients' EHRs to automatically classify cases of pulmonary embolism (PE). They found that the fusion model's AUC was superior to that of unimodal models relying solely on imaging data or EHR data. Researchers from the University of Toronto in Canada have used MRI images, clinical assessment scores from the Alzheimer's Disease Assessment Scale-Cognitive (ADAS13), genetic data, and demographic data to model symptom trajectories in Alzheimer's disease (AD) patients. They found that using longitudinal multimodal data could effectively predict the decline trajectory categories in AD, which could be used for early detection of AD patients at risk of clinical decline. Additionally, other scholars have integrated demographic information with dermoscopy images for skin cancer diagnosis, improving model performance compared to unimodal data models. Other studies, such as those on small cell cytoreduction diagnosis and glaucoma classification, have also used the fusion of clinical data and imaging data for assisted decision-making.

5.4.1.2 Fusion of Different Types of Imaging Data

Different imaging modalities have their own advantages and disadvantages. Common imaging techniques include CT, MRI, ultrasound, PET, and single-photon emission computed tomography (SPECT). CT is moderately priced with high image resolution and clear bone imaging, but its performance is poor for muscles and fat. MRI is more expensive but also offers high image resolution, performing well for fat, spinal cord, and muscle imaging, and is especially suitable for brain imaging, though it is less sensitive to bone tissue compared to CT. PET/SPECT is expensive and has low image resolution but is highly sensitive for tumor diagnosis and molecular metabolic activity. Ultrasound is low-cost and has low image resolution but is very safe and suitable for blood flow-related examinations. Researchers have explored the fusion of different imaging modalities based on their characteristics.

Indian researchers used discrete wavelet transformation to fuse MRI and PET images, finding that compared to unimodal images, the fusion provided more detailed anatomical and hyperspectral information for radiologists in cases such as Alzheimer's disease. German researchers fused CT images with PET images of prostate-specific membrane antigen ligands, developing new multimodal quantitative imaging indicators for assessing skeletal tumor burden in prostate cancer. Norwegian researchers combined ultrasound and MRI images, discovering that ultrasound-guided neurosurgery helped evaluate anatomical changes, potentially improving surgical quality. Other examples of imaging data fusion include CT and ultrasound fusion, as well as PET and CT image fusion.

5.4.1.3 Fusion of Physiological Signals with Other Data

Physiological signal measurement plays a crucial role in clinical practice. Common physiological signals include electrocardiogram (ECG), electromyogram (EMG), partial pressure of oxygen (PO_2), blood pressure (BP), and urine pH. These measurements are usually supplementary and need to be combined with other clinical data to confirm specific diagnoses.

For example, ECG signals alone cannot accurately locate and characterize most arrhythmias. Therefore, French researchers fused ECG information with body surface mapping based on delayed enhancement MRI to study patients with Wolff-Parkinson-White syndrome, ventricular tachycardia, and atrial fibrillation. They found that the multimodal model could achieve comprehensive non-invasive evaluation of arrhythmias, showing potential diagnostic applications. Additionally, in identity recognition and verification, many researchers have combined ECG signals with fingerprints and voice signals for multimodal fusion to verify patient identity, yielding positive results.

5.4.1.4 Fusion of Facial Expressions with Other Data

Early stages of mental disorders often manifest as abnormalities in facial expressions and vocal expressions. Therefore, integrating modalities such as facial expressions and vocal expressions for emotion analysis to aid in the early diagnosis of mental disorders is currently a research hotspot. This type of research is also known as multimodal emotion analysis. Additionally, multimodal emotion analysis can be used to detect whether patients are withholding or misreporting information during consultations.

Depression is one of the most common mental disorders, affecting 350 million people worldwide according to WHO statistics. Despite its prevalence, its varied manifestations can lead to misdiagnosis, and self-assessment diagnostic methods can be subject to subjective bias. Researchers have used statistical features from speech behavior, eye movements, and head posture to distinguish between patients with major depressive disorder and healthy individuals, finding that the classification level of the model is significantly higher than chance, and that a model integrating all modalities performs significantly better than single-modality models. Other researchers have extracted multimodal features such as audio, video, and text to analyze patients' voices and facial expressions, predicting the severity of depression. These models outperformed single-modality prediction models.

Although multimodal fusion for assisted diagnosis has achieved some clinical success, many results are still in the research stage and have not yet been formally implemented in clinical practice. Several problems and challenges remain in multimodal fusion for assisted diagnosis:

1. Feature representation: Integrating features from different modalities can lead to the curse of dimensionality. A major challenge is learning complementary information from different modality features while eliminating redundancy to reduce unnecessary feature dimensions.
2. Feature alignment: There may be relationships between different modality features that need to be aligned during data processing. Resolving conflicts between different modality features and achieving feature alignment is a current research focus in multimodal learning.
3. Feature fusion: After feature alignment, information from two or more modalities needs to be integrated to perform prediction tasks. Balancing different modalities and their feature scales to achieve complementary strengths and eliminate redundancy is a significant challenge.
4. Feature transformation: Converting features between different formats without losing original information is a severe challenge, especially in the medical field where many modalities are used and there are substantial differences between them. Careful selection of transformation methods is required based on the specific problem.
5. Co-learning: Learning knowledge from different modality features to obtain superior diagnostic features compared to single-modality features is a core challenge in multimodal assisted diagnosis.

5.4.2 Disease Prognosis Prediction and Risk Factor Warning

With the development of modern medicine and significant improvements in living standards, doctors are now concerned not only with the cure rates of diseases but also with the quality of life of patients under a given treatment plan. The WHO has included quality of life as a new standard of health, representing the ultimate goal of all health interventions. Disease prognosis prediction and risk factor warning are essential means to improve quality of life. Disease prognosis prediction refers to predicting the likelihood of disease recurrence, death, disability, or complications over a future period based on the current disease state. Risk factor warning indicates that a current factor in the patient increases their risk of developing a particular disease.

Disease prognosis prediction and risk factor warning are among the hottest topics in current research. For example, from January 2015 to January 2019, more than

4500 related papers were published on patient readmission. Predicting disease-related risk factors, reducing adverse prognostic events, and decreasing readmission rates can significantly lower hospital operating costs and improve patient care quality. In 2017, the Centers for Medicare & Medicaid Services in the United States reported to Congress, requiring hospitals to disclose readmission rates. In 2010, the United States established the Hospital Readmissions Reduction Program (HRRP), imposing financial penalties on hospital systems with higher than expected readmission rates. This program was officially implemented in 2013 and has promoted research in disease prognosis prediction and risk factor warning to some extent.

Commonly used data for this research includes demographic data, symptoms, signs, and laboratory test results from Electronic Medical Records (EMR). Shuai Zhang et al. used demographic, sign, radiological, laboratory test, and mortality data from over 800 patients infected with COVID-19. Using multivariate Cox regression, they identified five independent risk factors and developed a nomogram scoring system to predict the 14-day and 28-day survival rates of COVID-19 patients based on these factors. This system demonstrated strong discrimination and calibration in external validation cohorts[5]. Chen et al. from Stanford University developed a CDSS named OrderRex, which can automatically mine decision support orders, diagnoses, and laboratory test data from EMRs. Using a series of Bayesian methods, it evaluates the patient's initial course of disease. The study found that this system could provide personalized treatment recommendations and accurately predict clinical outcomes such as ICU life support, discharge, and readmission [6]. Hao et al. used data from all patients within the Maine Health Information Exchange system, using 2012 data for retrospective development and 2013 data as prospective data. They extracted demographic, diagnostic, laboratory test, and medical history data from the EMR and used an unsupervised clustering algorithm to classify the risk of readmission within 30 days for hospitalized patients, providing a daily risk score [7]. Park et al. used laboratory tests, surgery, medication, and radiotherapy data from over 5000 prostate patients to construct a CDSS. This system was used for prognosis management after radical prostatectomy and for extracting and visualizing important disease risk factors in prostate cancer decision-making [8].

Despite the numerous studies on prognosis prediction and risk factor warning, several issues remain. Many studies have only utilized clinical signs and laboratory data, with a low utilization rate of patients' social data (e.g., occupation, salary). Some studies have shown that incorporating relevant psychosocial characteristics into readmission prediction models can significantly improve their predictive performance. Additionally, there is still much debate about whether CDSS provides significant clinical benefits for disease risk factor management. Some researchers evaluated the impact of CDSS on cardiovascular risk factor management and found no significant clinical benefits. However, they noted that this might be due to a lack of long-term evidence and sufficient sample sizes. They also found that the type of prompts and messages could affect the CDSS's effectiveness in improving cardiovascular risk factors. This highlights the need to fully consider human-computer interaction mechanisms when developing models to ensure user-friendly and straightforward operation.

5.4.3 Shared Decision-Making and Health Management

Shared Decision-Making (SDM) is a new model of medical decision-making that centers on the patient. Unlike the previous paternalistic approach where the doctor was the authority and the patient was passive, SDM establishes an equal partnership between the doctor and the patient. Both parties jointly discuss and participate in every step of the decision-making process to develop the most suitable individualized clinical decisions for the patient. This model allows doctors to better understand the patient's values and preferences, make appropriate decisions, enhance patient trust in the doctor, and increase patient adherence to treatment plans. It also promotes better health management by the patient outside of the hospital.

This decision-making method was first proposed in the early 1970s in Reimann's publication "Shared Decision Making and Shared Responsibility: The Dilemmas of Modern Educational Institutions." In 1970, Ketter introduced SDM into the medical field in "Shared Decision Making in the Hospital Ward." Initially, SDM involved placing disease-related posters and pamphlets in hospitals to help patients understand the background and standard treatments for their conditions, and then doctors began interactive decision-making with patients. Today, an increasing number of decision support tools have emerged to facilitate the SDM process.

The medical community currently places great importance on the SDM model. In 2001 and 2003, the first International Shared Decision Making Conference and the International Patient Decision Aid Standards (IPDAS) collaboration were established to promote the development of shared decision-making.

A typical example of an SDM support tool is the Patient Decision Aids (PDA) launched by the Ottawa Hospital Research Institute in Canada. This tool provides information about the decisions that need to be made, the options available, and the outcomes of those options, clarifying personal values to help individuals participate in decision-making. The implementation steps of PDA for patient decision support and decision-making assistance are divided into the following five steps.

1. Determining the decision

   Identify which aspects of the diagnostic and treatment process require patient decisions and what the decision difficulties are. For example, parents of children with short stature often hesitate about whether to use growth hormone therapy. This process can use the key issues workbook from the Ottawa Decision Support Framework (ODSF) to determine the views of patients and healthcare providers on the decision-making needs.
2. Finding patient decision aids

   Search for and review decision aids to find the most suitable and high-quality tools. PDA offers decision aids for over 200 health issues, helping patients and physicians make specific and well-considered interventions.
3. Identifying and addressing barriers to SDM implementation

   Identify potential barriers to using PDA, such as patients' limited education, inability to operate a computer, poor attitudes, or doctors' lack of confidence in

PDA. Surveys of patients and healthcare providers can determine their attitudes and willingness to use PDA.

4. Implementing decision support and providing training

   Assign responsibility for PDA, provide user training, input patient information into the decision aid tool, or integrate it with EHR to obtain patient information.

5. Monitoring and evaluating usage and effectiveness

   Use decision support analysis tools (like DAST10), decision regret scales, decision preparation scales, and decision conflict scales to analyze patient-provider interactions. Assess the level of regret patients feel post-decision, their views on decision preparation, and their perception of decision uncertainty to gage the quality of decision support and patient outcomes.

Additional common SDM decision support tools include Decision Points by Healthwise, Consumer Summary by the Agency for Healthcare Research and Quality (AHRQ), and Decision Aid by the National Institute for Health and Care Excellence (NICE). The concept of SDM was introduced to China in 1998, leading to extensive research and theoretical contributions by many scholars. From 2016 to 2018, the International Traditional Chinese Medicine Anti-Cancer Forum and the Doctor-Patient Shared Decision Making and Communication Forum were held to discuss the development and implementation of SDM in China.

There are many issues to address in promoting SDM, such as patients' difficulty in quickly understanding their health conditions and the potential for SDM to increase doctors' workload, thereby reducing their enthusiasm for its use. Tailoring SDM to individual patient differences remains a significant challenge.

5.4.4 Assisted Precision Screening for Rare and Genetic Diseases

The definition of rare diseases (or orphan diseases) varies by region, generally referring to diseases with an incidence of 1/200,000 to 1/1000. Genetic disorders are diseases caused by abnormalities in one or more genes in the genome. In this context, the term refers to diseases with a single genetic cause involving a gene or chromosome, rather than common polygenic diseases. Although the prevalence of rare diseases is low, data from the American organization Global Genes in 2016 showed that 350 million people worldwide suffer from over 7000 rare diseases. Additionally, there are over 6000 known genetic disorders, with 1 in 50 people having a known monogenic disease and 1 in 263 having a chromosomal disease. Most rare diseases are genetic disorders, and most genetic disorders are considered rare diseases.

Rare and most genetic diseases are uncommon, and some have subtle early symptoms. Therefore, some doctors lack the experience and knowledge to diagnose these diseases accurately, leading to frequent misdiagnoses and missed diagnoses. Statistics show that rare diseases affect over 30 million Americans, with 40% of patients being misdiagnosed or undiagnosed. CDSS can address this knowledge gap. Based on existing knowledge bases and reasoning algorithms, CDSS can alert clinical experts to the risk and diagnostic basis of a rare or genetic disease in a current patient, helping them take further targeted screening strategies for precise diagnosis.

Rare and genetic diseases typically involve changes in genes and proteins. Therefore, CDSS for rare and genetic diseases includes not only clinical signs, symptoms, demographic characteristics, and laboratory tests but also genetic and phenotypic data. Köhler et al. used semantic similarity metrics and the human phenotype ontology (HPO) to measure the similarity between current disease characteristics and genetic diseases, achieving differential diagnosis of monogenic diseases [9]. Koile et al. developed a tool called GenIO, which utilizes genomic and clinical data provided by doctors to analyze symptoms and suspected diseases. This tool classifies and filters diseases to aid in the screening of rare genetic diseases [10]. Shen et al. incorporated phenotypic data and knowledge from the MEDLINE database, designing data fusion strategies to expedite the diagnosis of rare diseases using a collaborative filtering model [11].

Common screening methods for rare and genetic diseases, besides the aforementioned semantic similarity metrics and collaborative filtering algorithms, also include machine learning algorithms and information retrieval methods. Sidiropoulos et al. used a probabilistic neural network (PNN) as a classifier to categorize rare brain cancers based on brain morphology and texture features. They validated the classifier using ten-fold cross-validation, demonstrating high classification accuracy [12]. Rother et al. utilized a classifier ensemble combining eight machine learning algorithms, including support vector machines (SVM), artificial neural networks (ANN), and random forests. They based their analysis on questionnaire data from children and their parents to diagnose rare pediatric lung diseases. The tenfold cross-validation showed that the ensemble classifier had high sensitivity and accuracy, aiding general practitioners in screening and diagnosing rare pediatric lung diseases [13]. Information retrieval involves searching for case reports of rare disease patients, comparing, and identifying similar features among patients to determine if a patient has a rare disease. The FindZebra diagnostic support tool's knowledge base includes more than ten sources, such as the Online Mendelian Inheritance in Man (OMIM) and the Genetic and Rare Diseases Information Center (GARD). Users can input symptoms and phenotypic data to receive potential diseases and related genes, assisting clinicians in diagnosing rare monogenic diseases. This tool is currently available for free online access and use [14].

Despite advances in genetic testing, prenatal screening, pre-pregnancy screening, and newborn screening, which enable the detection of some rare and genetic diseases before or shortly after birth, many conditions (such as Huntington's disease) cannot be detected early. These diseases often manifest only in adulthood. Additionally, some rare diseases are not genetic but are caused by environmental factors and lifestyle choices. Therefore, computer-assisted precision screening for rare and genetic diseases still holds significant application value.

5.5 Summary

After more than 70 years of development, Clinical Decision Support Systems (CDSS) have been widely applied in clinical practice. They help doctors improve diagnosis and treatment quality, enhance patient care, and clinical outcomes, and reduce hospital operating costs, ultimately achieving a win-win situation for doctors, patients, and hospitals. This chapter provides an overview of the basic concepts, significance, development history, and framework of CDSS, focusing on decision reasoning methods, practical cases, and cutting-edge research in CDSS.

Despite many achievements, CDSS still has several areas needing improvement, such as system interface optimization, integration with current clinical workflows, and addressing alert fatigue. It is believed that with the future development of medical and information technology, more CDSS with various functionalities will be integrated into clinical practice and see extensive application.

References

1. Evans RS, Pestotnik SL, Classen DC, et al. A computer assisted management program for antibiotics and other antiinfective agents. N Engl J Med. 1998;338(4):232238.
2. Ledley RS, Lusted LB. Reasoning foundations of medical diagnosis. Science. 1959;130(3366):921.
3. Shortliffe EH. Computer based medical consultations: MYCIN. Ann Intern Med. 1976;85(6):831.
4. Ramnarayan P, Tomlinson A, Rao A, et al. ISABEL: a web based differential diagnostic aid for paediatrics:results from an initial performance evaluation. Arch Dis Child. 2003;88(5):408413.
5. Zhang S, Guo M, Duan L, et al. Development and validation of a risk factor based system to predict short term survival in adult hospitalized patients with COVID 19:a multicenter, retrospective, cohort study. Crit Care. 2020;24(1):438.
6. Chen JH, Podchiyska T, Altman RB. OrderRex: clinical order decision support and outcome predictions by data mining electronic medical records. J Am Med Inform Assoc. 2016;23(2):339348.
7. Hao S, Wang Y, Jin B, et al. Development, validation and deployment of a real time 30 day hospital readmission risk assessment tool in the Maine healthcare information exchange. PLoS One. 2015;10(10):e0140271.
8. Park J, Rho MJ, Moon HW, et al. Prostate cancer trajectory map:clinical decision support system for prognosis management of radical prostatectomy. Prostate Int. 2021;9(1):2530.
9. Kohler S, Carmody L, Vasilevsky N, et al. Expansion of the human phenotype ontology (HPO) knowledge base and resources. Nucleic Acids Res. 2019;47(D1):D10181027.
10. Koile D, Cordoba M, Serro MD, et al. GenIO:a phenotype genotype analysis web server for clinical genomics of rare diseases. BMC Bioinform. 2018;19(1):25.
11. Shen F, Liu S, Wang Y, et al. Utilization of electronic medical records and biomedical literature to support the diagnosis of rare diseases using data fusion and collaborative filtering approaches. JMIR Med Inform. 2018;6(4):e11301.
12. Sidiropoulos K, Glotsos D, Kostopoulos S, et al. Real time decision support system for diagnosis of rare cancers, trained in parallel, on a graphics processing unit. Comput Biol Med. 2012;42(4):376386.

13. Rother AK, Schwerk N, Brinkmann F, et al. Diagnostic support for selected paediatric pulmonary diseases using answer pattern recognition in questionnaires based on combined data mining applications: a monocentric observational pilot study. PLoS One. 2015;10(8):e0135180.
14. Dragusin R, Petcu P, Lioma C, et al. FindZebra: a search engine for rare diseases. Int J Med Inform. 2013;82(6):528538.

Internet of Medical Things Systems

6

Contents

6.1 Overview of Internet of Medical Things Systems........ 164
6.1.1 Introduction to Internet of Medical Things and Internet of Medical Things Systems........ 164
6.1.2 Development History of Internet of Medical Things Systems........ 165
6.1.3 Current Research Status of Internet of Medical Things at Home and Abroad... 167
6.1.3.1 Policy Aspects........ 167
6.1.3.2 Technical Aspects........ 168
6.1.3.3 Application Aspects........ 169
6.2 Main Functions and Applications of Internet of Medical Things Systems........ 170
6.2.1 Patient Management........ 171
6.2.2 Remote Monitoring........ 171
6.2.3 Medication Management........ 172
6.2.4 Hospital Supplies Management........ 173
6.2.5 Hospital Logistics Personnel Management........ 174
6.3 Case Studies........ 175
6.3.1 Application of In-Hospital Medical Supplies Management........ 175
6.3.2 Application in Public Health Management........ 177
6.4 Frontiers in Medical Internet of Things Research........ 179
6.4.1 5G Smart Wards........ 179
6.4.2 Unmanned Material Distribution........ 180
6.5 Summary........ 182

With the advancement of technology, the Internet of Things use cases have proliferated across various industries, and the medical field is no exception. Portable Internet of Things devices have brought us more convenient monitoring equipment, enabling longer-term monitoring of indicators for patients, thereby providing a better understanding of their own conditions. Thus, the Internet of Medical Things has emerged. With the support of Internet of Things and big data, coupled with the integration of medical devices, it is possible to construct a perfect Internet of Things medical system, allowing the general public to enjoy better medical services and

J. Li et al., *Healthcare Information Systems*, Innovative Medical Devices,
https://doi.org/10.1007/978-981-97-9551-2_6

address issues such as difficulty in accessing medical care and low efficiency. Additionally, through Internet of Things technology and the support of related medical devices, real-time communication can be achieved via remote networking technology, enabling hospitals to remotely diagnose patients and provide advice and reminders, thereby offering patients more convenient medical conditions.

6.1 Overview of Internet of Medical Things Systems

6.1.1 Introduction to Internet of Medical Things and Internet of Medical Things Systems

The Internet of Things is an information medium based on traditional telecommunications networks and the Internet, enabling all independently addressable physical objects to form an interconnected network. Internet of Things has unified standards and technologies globally, suitable for comprehensive coverage and large-scale applications. Its close integration with emerging technologies such as cloud computing and big data addresses various issues including fragmentation of technology, networks, applications, and industries. The Internet of Medical Things is a healthcare system that applies Internet of Things technology. By connecting various medical devices and sensors, it facilitates the collection, transmission, storage, processing, and application of medical data to improve the efficiency and quality of healthcare.

According to medical scenarios, the Internet of Medical Things system can be divided into four parts: the perception layer, the network layer, the platform layer, and the application layer.

1. Perception Layer: This layer achieves continuous, comprehensive, and rapid information acquisition. It primarily collects necessary data from various medical and health devices, using physical sensors to assist in the collection of medical information. For example, a resistive sensor can convert values of various physical quantities such as temperature, humidity, and displacement into resistance values, thereby completing the information collection.
2. Network Layer: The network layer uses shared or dedicated networks between the identification layer and the platform layer for wired or wireless transmission of information, achieving real time, reliable, and secure information transmission. The access networks of the network layer mainly involve short-range wireless communication technologies such as Wi-Fi, Zigbee, Bluetooth, UWB, Z-Wave, NFC, and IrDA.
3. Platform Layer: The platform layer connects the perception layer through device management and connection management platforms and provides consistent interfaces to service providers through application support platforms. It integrates the management, control, and operation of terminal devices and assets,

achieving accurate, efficient, and intelligent processing of information. Additionally, the platform layer can provide general service capabilities such as data routing, data processing and mining, data simulation and optimization, application development, and equipment maintenance.

4. Application Layer: The application layer aims to achieve more precise, diverse, and personalized information applications. The application layer of the Internet of Medical Things mainly includes three aspects: hospital business management, personal health management, and government decision support. Hospital business management can achieve drug management, medical device management, auxiliary diagnosis, etc., thereby improving hospital management level and medical service quality. Personal health management can manage chronic diseases, health intervention, elderly care monitoring, etc., while promoting remote medical care, health management, and elderly care. The Internet of Medical Things can also provide decision support for the government in public health, medical insurance, and other aspects.

6.1.2 Development History of Internet of Medical Things Systems

On November 17, 2005, the International Telecommunication Union (ITU) formally proposed the concept of the Internet of Things and announced the arrival of the Internet of Things era. In January 2009, IBM introduced the "Smarter Planet" strategy, which received positive approval from the then US President, Barack Obama, bringing global attention to the Internet of Things.

In November 2008, IBM announced the "Smarter Planet" strategy, which proposed integrating Internet of Things through supercomputing and cloud computing. In January 2009, IBM and the Information Technology and Innovation Foundation (ITIF), a US think tank, proposed to the US government that investment in information and communication technology could generate short-term employment and promote long-term development, with support for Internet of Things development mainly focusing on three areas: energy, broadband, and healthcare.

Furthermore, the Internet of Things developed by the European Union introduced new measures against counterfeit drugs by using drug sequence codes in the medical field. Japan and South Korea formulated national intelligence strategies based on Internet of Things in 2004: u-Japan and u-Korea.

From 2010 to 2016, with the popularization of 4G technology, wearable devices gradually entered the medical and health field. During this period, capital and entrepreneurial companies played a significant role, with companies and products such as Jawbone and Fit focusing on sports health emerging. In the healthcare industry dominated by hospitals, Internet of Things Healthcare also emerged, such as Internet of Things respiratory healthcare led by a certain respiratory research institute.

However, this stage can be considered a bubble period because it was mainly driven by capital, and Internet of Things had hardly entered daily life and clinical practice.

In 2017, Huawei began research in the field of Internet of Medical Things by establishing the Wireless Application Scenario Laboratory, internally referred to as X Lab, focusing on future research and incubation. One direction of this research was Internet of Medical Things, targeting hospitals as hypothetical customers, with the goal of applying wireless technology to the medical industry to capture the wireless communication market. Unlike previous approaches targeting ordinary consumers, this research focused on application scenarios within hospitals, including wireless medical applications for clinical use, Internet of Things applications for logistics, and Internet of Things applications for patients. Based on the research results from Huawei's X Lab, the China Academy of Information and Communications Technology, under the Ministry of Industry and Information Technology, played a supportive role. At the 2017 Internet + Medical Health Industry Alliance annual conference, they released the "Wireless Medical White Paper," essentially outlining the research direction and scenarios for Internet of Medical Things in the industry.

In 2018, the General Hospital of the People's Liberation Army (Beijing 301 Hospital) conducted the first remote surgery based on China Unicom's 5G network and Kangda's surgical robot. The surgery involved remotely controlling a surgical robot to perform hepatectomy on a pig in an animal experiment, marking the world's first and only genuine remote surgical operation experiment until 2020. This event sparked widespread industry attention. Similar experiments in remote surgery and many practical tests represent exploration in the field. The success of the surgical experiment also signaled the industry's true entry into the exploration phase. Additionally, the China Academy of Information and Communications Technology held the first "Zhan Fang Cup" competition, generating dozens of innovative application scenarios aimed at the medical industry, initiating the incubation of the industry toward Internet of Medical Things.

The key essence of Internet of Medical Things is to use network connectivity to serve medical equipment in healthcare settings. Over the past few years, the networks used in hospitals have been diverse, with some utilizing wired networks, Bluetooth, Zigbee, Wi-Fi, etc. Some networks are self-built by hospitals, while others are constructed by medical equipment vendors or telecommunication operators. In general, these networks have exposed many issues regarding usability, stability, and maintainability. In 2019, the 5G Network Construction Working Committee, established by industry groups representing hospitals, released the "5G-based Hospital Network Construction Standards." This marks the development of group standards jointly formulated by the medical and communication industries, to some extent, standardizing the requirements for wireless information network construction in hospitals in the 5G era. It is believed that this will help regulate network construction in the future.

6.1.3 Current Research Status of Internet of Medical Things at Home and Abroad

6.1.3.1 Policy Aspects

China

At the national level, based on the overall plan of Healthy China, the development policy of Internet of Medical Things has been incorporated into the policy system of smart healthcare and Internet-based medical policies.

The "Opinions on Implementing the Healthy China Action" proposes to "strengthen technological support, carry out research on major issues affecting health factors and difficult diseases, and provide support from national major science and technology projects and key research and development programs." It also suggests "strengthening information support and promoting the sharing of health-related information among departments and regions." This provides top-level design for Internet of Medical Things.

The "Healthy China Action (2019–2030)" proposes to "give full play to the role of market mechanisms, encourage the research, development, and promotion of health management AI and wearable devices, make full use of Internet technology, and, on the premise of protecting personal privacy, conduct real time and continuous monitoring of health status, achieve online real-time management, early warning, and behavioral intervention, and use health big data to enhance the public's ability for self-health management." This provides a strategic plan for the operation of Internet of Medical Things.

United States

Due to the frequent occurrence of large-scale Internet of Things network attack incidents in recent years, the role of national level policies for Internet of Medical Things has changed. It has gradually shifted from self-organized entities in the private sector to legislative protection by the national government. Since the introduction of the "Innovation Development and Internet of Things Act" in the USA in 2017, which standardized the main procedural architecture and spectrum allocation for Internet of Medical Things, the USA has continued to develop regulations on Internet of Medical Things security. Examples include the "Internet of Things Cybersecurity Promotion Act," which regulates the procurement of Internet of Things devices by government departments and healthcare institutions, and the "Network Shield Act," established by the Department of Commerce, which encourages medical device manufacturers to implement graded labeling certification for the security encryption of their Internet of Things products. These measures aim to strengthen the leadership of the USA in setting international standards. Additionally, the development of Internet of Medical Things policies in the USA continues to focus on data information security. This has increased the complexity of maintaining Internet of Medical Things to a certain extent. However, it also provides more policy market opportunities for Internet of Medical Things operators to improve integration simplicity across Internet of Medical Things architecture layers through integrated Internet of Things service operations. Representative examples include the medical Internet of Things business platform products of Verizon and AT&T.

European Union

In June 2019, the European Union's "Cybersecurity Act" officially came into effect, which proposed network security requirements for the deployment of Internet of Medical Things applications—adopting the framework of the European Network Security Certification System to ensure the network security level of EU medical IoT products and services.

Japan

Japan has entered a highly aging society, with the population aged 65 and above accounting for 28.7% of the total population. There is a strong demand for medical Internet products related to elderly diseases, including implantable Internet of Things products such as pacemakers, artificial heart valves, stents, insulin pumps, and artificial joints. In response to the increasingly widespread application of medical Internet of Things products, the Japanese government has frequently revised regulations on Internet of Things security related to healthcare from late 2018 to early 2019.

6.1.3.2 Technical Aspects

Medical and health Internet of Things has been highly valued as a strategic technology by countries worldwide. Its full application will bring profound changes to the current models of the medical and health industries and provide strong impetus for the industry and society's benign development. Internet of Medical Things is a product of various technologies, including sensor control technology, RFID technology, wireless communication technology, network technology, big data technology, cloud computing technology, and artificial intelligence technology. Based on Internet of Medical Things, medical and health Internet of Things is structured into four layers: perception layer, transmission layer, platform layer, and application layer. The complexity, specificity, and innovation of various new technologies in the Internet of Things era give rise to characteristics distinct from those before, which will inevitably bring new opportunities to the medical industry.

Currently, medical and health Internet of Things has been used in many hospitals and medical care centers in China. However, in regions with lagging medical levels, the utilization rate of Internet of Things in healthcare remains low. To improve the utilization rate, continuous improvement of the top-level architecture, system design, and implementation models are still needed.

The emphasis on health issues can drive the development of the wearable device industry. In 2018, the global market size of wearable medical devices was $10.3 billion. The increase in chronic diseases and mortality rates is a matter of concern for governments and people. Patients are starting to wear 24-h remote monitoring wearable devices. Due to upgrades and improvements in wearable devices, they do not affect patients' daily lives and work. Considering the maturity of devices and technology, it is expected that the demand for wearable devices will continue to grow steadily in the future. In addition, a large number of therapeutic devices, such as smart asthma management devices, wearable pain relief devices, and insulin management devices, are also expected to drive market growth.

Among the various connection methods of medical and health Internet of Things, short-range transmission scenarios are the foundation of medical and health Internet of Things. Moreover, medical and health Internet of Things has high requirements for data reliability. When choosing short-range wireless protocols, security is especially important. Among the available short-range wireless technologies, Bluetooth and Wi-Fi are the most commonly used technologies by medical device developers. Wi-Fi has a larger coverage range and higher transmission rate but is prone to coexistence issues. Bluetooth data has the characteristics of lower transmission rate and shorter transmission distance but is less affected by a large number of RF transmissions in close proximity and has lower power consumption. In medical and health Internet of Things transmission scenarios, each has its own strengths and different applications.

6.1.3.3 Application Aspects

Medical IoT applications are divided into IoT hospital intelligent device management and wearable device health management intelligent monitoring. In Internet of Things hospitals, smart equipment management includes aspects such as nursing management, dynamic management of fixed assets, and logistics management. On the other hand, intelligent monitoring of health management with wearable devices includes monitoring sleep status, body fat, heart rate, blood pressure, blood oxygen level, body temperature, and blood sugar levels.

The widespread application of Internet of Things in various aspects of medical and health fields covers from home communities to hospitals, from disease diagnosis and treatment to health management at various levels of medical services. It achieves intelligent perception, monitoring, decision-making, and management of medical objects, medical and health information, and public health safety. This comprehensive support aims to improve health intervention and management capabilities, enhance the quality of medical services and management, and continuously improve health levels, thus promoting comprehensive health management for all people and throughout their lifecycles.

The application scenarios of smart equipment management in Internet of Things hospitals include both large hospitals and community health institutions. By using medical and health Internet of Things as a medium, through the interconnection of things and people, medical staff's work characteristics are standardized within processes, significantly enhancing work efficiency, strengthening medical technology capabilities, and reducing medical safety risks. Different from the current disease-centric medical model, Internet of Things medical applications have the potential to transform traditional medical care. By combining the health medical model with Internet of Things technology, it is expected to advance disease treatment to disease prevention and health management. Applications of medical and health Internet of Things in large hospitals include automatic collection of patient vital sign data, mobile rounds and nursing, intensive care for critically ill patients, identification and tracking of medical supplies, patient identification and anti-loss measures, management of disinfection items and surgical instruments traceability, management of medical supplies, medical waste disposal, supervision of large medical equipment, and medical robots, among others. Applications of medical and health Internet of Things in community health institutions include monitoring of chronic diseases, care for the elderly, maternal and child health care, electronic health records for residents, health education, etc. Applications of medical and health Internet of Things in home scenarios include remote monitoring of physiological indicators, remote health assessment and intervention, outpatient recovery monitoring, elderly care, personal health management, etc.

6.2 Main Functions and Applications of Internet of Medical Things Systems

Internet of Things technology holds significant potential in the healthcare field, assisting hospitals in intelligent perception of medical subjects, supporting digital data collection and decision-making, digitizing medical information, and achieving closed-loop medical processes. It also standardizes the workflow of medical staff, improves work efficiency, enhances medical technology, reduces medical safety risks, meets the demand for intelligent medical management, and ultimately enhances the overall process monitoring level of medical equipment both inside and outside the hospital. It will ultimately improve the level of full-process monitoring of in-hospital and out-of-hospital equipment, strengthen the ability to build digital hospitals, and innovate to help personalized and precise medical services.

The application scenarios of medical Internet of Things systems mainly include three categories: large hospitals, community health organizations, and households. In large hospitals, medical Internet of Things applications include automatic collection of patient vital signs data, mobile rounds and nursing, monitoring of critically ill patients, identification and tracking of medical supplies, patient identification and anti-loss measures, management of disinfection items and surgical instruments traceability, medical supplies management, medical waste disposal, supervision of large medical equipment, and medical robots. In community health organizations, medical Internet of Things applications include chronic disease management, elderly disease management, maternal and child health care, electronic health records for residents, health consultations, and health education. In household scenarios, medical Internet of Things applications include remote monitoring of physiological indicators, remote health assessment and intervention, outpatient recovery monitoring, elderly care, and personal health management.

The main functions of medical Internet of Things systems can be categorized as follows:

6.2.1 Patient Management

The medical industry is highly regulated, and errors are not allowed in any aspect, making patient identification crucial, especially in emergency situations where medical staff urgently need to match detailed patient information accurately and quickly. Traditional manual registration methods are inefficient and prone to errors.

During hospitalization, patients input their identity information into the hospital's registration system and wear electronic tag wristbands containing personal information. Once the patient wears the wristband, the wireless Internet of Things can detect the information transmitted by the electronic wristband at any time. Medical staff can use the Internet of Things system to obtain the patient's identity, facilitating effective patient management. Additionally, the electronic tags have a long recognition distance. If a patient leaves the nursing area without permission, the electronic tag will upload an alarm message to the monitoring station to ensure proper patient management.

For example, Shanghai Renji Hospital South Campus introduced Internet of Things wristbands that use Bluetooth sensing for identity recognition, replacing the traditional method of scanning QR codes on wristbands. This application can provide patients with a better medical experience, especially when caring for patients undergoing procedures such as injections or deep sleep.

Moreover, managing special patients cannot rely on conventional hospital methods. For example, automatic identification, positioning, and tracking of mentally ill patients are crucial aspects of patient management in psychiatric hospitals. Based on the Internet of Medical Things, the patient area positioning system utilizes RFID technology to keep patients within the range of the reader. The reader can automatically identify the identity tag information of all patients and supervise them in real time. Only authorized patients can enter and exit safely. System administrators can view the entry and exit status of each patient area and the alarm status of each area in real time via computer. Additionally, the patient area positioning system and patient access control management system can be interconnected with the public security Internet of Things platform.

6.2.2 Remote Monitoring

With the improvement of living standards, there is a growing demand for medical and health services. Clinical nurses need to frequently measure and record patients' vital signs such as temperature and pulse. However, traditional medical models have limitations such as long time consumption and low efficiency, making it difficult to meet the real-time monitoring needs of patients 24 hours a day.

The Internet of Medical Things system utilizes physiological sensors to collect important physiological parameter data such as electrocardiogram, pulse, blood pressure, and temperature from the human body and processes it. Wireless Bluetooth technology is used for communication. Smart terminals acquire patient data and real-time location information, which are then sent to the hospital's health monitoring center. Additionally, the Internet of Medical Things system can use wireless communication networks to transmit various physiological information to the corresponding medical monitoring center. Medical staff at the monitoring center conduct timely diagnosis and analysis of patients upon receiving the data to provide real-time assistance. Some hospitals have also developed smart bed monitoring systems, installing Internet of Things sensors on patients' beds to monitor their activities in real time and issue alarms promptly in the event of anomalies to reduce the occurrence of accidents.

As the concept of national health management continues to deepen, the demand for medical services is increasing. However, due to the lack of medical resources, it is challenging to provide personalized and accurate medical consultation services to users. People who have not been diagnosed with a disease cannot fully understand their health status in detail and often wait until they feel unwell before going to the hospital for a check-up, by which time the disease has often progressed to a severe stage. After patients are discharged from treatment, hospitals find it challenging to track and assess their long-term recovery and the effectiveness of hospital treatment methods. Therefore, establishing a remote medical monitoring system based on Internet of Things technology can change the current state of medical services and achieve accurate and effective personal health management.

Mobile health is a new type of medical system derived to meet the current market demand, combining remote medical care with smartphones using Internet of Things. This enables direct communication between doctors and patients, greatly enhancing the portability and flexibility of medical care. Platforms such as Alibaba's Future Hospital and Tencent's WeChat Smart Healthcare enable one-on-one online communication and interaction between doctors and patients. Doctors can assess the risk of chronic diseases remotely based on patients' characteristics without adhering to predetermined care plans or requiring patients to undergo repeated hospitalizations, achieving real-time monitoring and remote assistance for chronic disease patients. Additionally, mobile health can significantly reduce patients' medical expenses and improve the level of national health security.

6.2.3 Medication Management

There are many challenges in the process of drug circulation that urgently need to be addressed. In the pharmaceutical supply chain, changes in environmental factors such as temperature, humidity, and light can alter the properties of drugs, leading to potential loss of effectiveness. Moreover, the circulation of counterfeit drugs poses a significant threat, potentially delaying treatment or endangering lives if not effectively monitored, causing great harm to society. Additionally, frequent incidents of diversion and returns, coupled with the inability to track drugs in a timely and accurate manner, can significantly increase the circulation cost of drugs. Furthermore, if hospitals cannot promptly ascertain patients' medication status during drug usage, they cannot determine whether medication and dispensing times are appropriate.

The Internet of Medical Things system connects patients and healthcare professionals through networked devices and wireless communication technology to collect, store, and track critical medical data. By monitoring medical services and maintaining records of diagnosis and medication, higher-quality medical services can be provided to patients. Identifying and tracking individual drugs in circulation enables timely and accurate data collection and efficient sharing of drug information, facilitating the optimization of drug inspection processes. Internet of Medical Things technology can also be applied to monitor drug intake status to reduce the risk of drug misuse.

In addition to oral medications, intravenous injection is one of the most commonly used treatment methods in clinical medicine. An intelligent infusion monitoring system constructed with Internet of Things technology can monitor changes in infusion time, infusion rate, and fluid volume in real time. If infusion is completed or a malfunction occurs, the system automatically sends an alert signal and prompts medical staff. In the intelligent infusion monitoring system, nurses can monitor the entire infusion process for all patients in the ward in real time, achieving intelligent and automated management, reducing or eliminating medical accidents, reducing the workload of nurses, and improving the quality of medical care in hospitals.

6.2.4 Hospital Supplies Management

The continuous advancement of medical technology provides patients with high-level medical services. However, traditional medical resource management systems have inefficiencies, leading to resource waste and potential medical safety incidents. The implementation of medical Internet of Things systems can enhance hospital resource management effectively, achieving essential functions such as medical equipment positioning management, medical waste traceability management, and intelligent security.

The trend toward scientific and standardized management in hospitals is inevitable, with medical equipment management being a crucial component. Applying radio frequency tracking and automatic identification management systems to medical equipment allows for the storage of equipment information while recording corresponding logs for each maintenance, repair, and inspection session. This can effectively prevent the loss of equipment information due to uncertain factors, ensuring comprehensive understanding of the condition of each machine during inspections and maintenance, thus avoiding oversights in equipment inspections and maintenance tasks. Additionally, the system can identify equipment status, reduce equipment idle time, and improve equipment utilization rates and the efficiency of medical staff.

Managing surgical equipment is crucial to ensuring smooth surgical procedures, and the application of medical Internet of Things can significantly reduce safety hazards associated with instrument usage. RFID-based surgical equipment management and traceability systems greatly mitigate potential safety risks associated with equipment use. By clarifying personnel responsibilities at each stage and recording relevant information, these systems ensure traceability in the event of accidents. Additionally, medical Internet of Things systems can track the location of items, indicating which items healthcare professionals have used and which patients have used them, thereby reducing item loss and waste.

Blood management is an important aspect of medical management. Blood is a transmission channel for various diseases, and variable factors in blood management increase the risk of medical accidents. Applying Internet of Things technology to medical management can effectively enhance blood management. Currently, RFID technology is primarily used to achieve real-time interaction and processing of blood information. This technology comprehensively monitors and manages the blood collection and storage processes, making the entire blood protection process transparent, effectively preventing blood infections, and improving the efficiency of staff.

Medical waste also falls under medical supplies. Medical waste management involves multiple departments, industries, and fields, requiring coordination among different departments to strictly regulate its generation, transportation, and disposal processes. Traditional manual management methods are inefficient, and the medical waste management process is imperfect, making it challenging to promptly identify problems in the processing process. Once human errors occur, they can easily lead to serious medical safety incidents. Medical Internet of Things systems utilize RFID technology to achieve full-process monitoring of medical waste bins. They collect various types of information in real time using mobile terminals and transmit information on each processing process to the monitoring center in real time, ensuring the standardization of the medical waste disposal process and transitioning from traditional manual processing to modern intelligent management.

6.2.5 Hospital Logistics Personnel Management

The logistics department of a hospital is an essential guarantee for all hospital operations to proceed smoothly. Doing well in hospital logistics work can ensure that all medical staff and inpatients enjoy a good medical working and living environment, and can ensure that medical staff have no worries while working in the hospital. More importantly, hospital medical logistics work directly affects the patient experience. Refined project management of medical logistics work not only brings great convenience and help to the medical cause but also more effectively promotes the future development of hospitals. However, with the rapid development of computer technology, relying solely on human resources accumulation is no longer sufficient to fully cover the functions of hospital logistics management. The traditional logistics management model creates obstacles in coordination and communication between the hospital's logistics management and the basic execution level, leading to the inability of logistics management services to be timely and efficiently delivered, failing to meet higher safety and energy-saving requirements, affecting the efficiency of clinical departments and intelligent departments in hospitals, and even affecting medical safety.

The hospital logistics personnel management system developed based on Internet of Things technology first establishes a basic database to input basic information of personnel (including age, gender, job type, years of service, etc.). Logistics personnel are equipped with wristband devices, and the backend management system can obtain information such as the movement trajectory of logistics personnel, retrieve relevant examination and inspection orders from the hospital information system in real time, generate task lists automatically, and intelligently dispatch orders based on the actual conditions such as the busyness of logistics personnel, distance, workload, task routes, etc., achieving optimal order allocation. Combined with big data analysis, the system can continuously optimize the dispatch engine, further reducing the workload of logistics personnel and effectively improving work efficiency. At the same time, key performance indicators (KPIs) for hospital logistics personnel, including indicators such as manual efficiency, completion rate of working hours, average response time, repair rate, average working hours, and satisfaction, can be managed. These serve as their basic assessment indicators, helping hospital management and operations units to grasp the work situation of maintenance personnel in real time.

6.3 Case Studies

6.3.1 Application of In-Hospital Medical Supplies Management

In-hospital medical supplies management includes the management of medications, medical devices, and other supplies. Utilizing Internet of Things technology to enhance the hospital's supply management system, coupled with refined and intelligent management methods, can improve the level of medical services, ensure timely supply of medical materials, increase the utilization rate of supplies, control material costs, enhance overall operational efficiency, reduce operating costs, and align with market dynamics in an orderly manner to achieve cost reduction and efficiency improvement goals.

Currently, the full-process traceability system for medications is fully covered under national supervision. On April 28, 2019, the National Medical Products Administration issued the "Guidelines for the Construction of Drug Information Traceability System" and "Coding Requirements for Drug Traceability Codes." These two standards respectively specify the basic composition of the drug information traceability system and participating parties, as well as the basic requirements and composition requirements for drug traceability codes. The management of medications within the hospital, including procurement, storage, maintenance, unit dose packaging, distribution, storage, and usage, is seamlessly integrated through the information system. Using drug electronic supervision codes (barcodes), RFID technology, and logistics operation equipment, information such as the basic information and transportation and storage information of medications at each link is stored in RFID tags. This achieves full-process information traceability of medications within the hospital. In case of issues with specific medication batches, the distribution of medications and patient information can be quickly located, providing a safety guarantee mechanism for clinical medication. The traceability management mode of medications can effectively reduce inventory management pressure on various departments within the hospital and reduce the workload of clinical staff and clinical pharmacists in logistics.

The full lifecycle of medical devices refers to various stages such as the installation acceptance, daily maintenance, repair, and scrapping of medical devices by the medical equipment management department. Through Internet of Things management methods and the use of RFID, infrared induction, laser scanners, and other information sensing technologies, fixed asset files are established for medical devices. Real-time intelligent identification, positioning, tracking, supervision, and management of medical devices are achieved to provide reliable and efficient data protection for hospital refined management. On December 21, 2020, the State Council's 119th executive meeting revised and approved the "Regulations on the Supervision and Administration of Medical Devices," which came into effect on June 1, 2021. The state has further refined and revised this regulation, putting forward higher requirements and challenges for the use and management of medical devices. All hospitals must meet the following requirements in the four stages of medical equipment management:

1. Installation and Acceptance Stage: Install RFID tags for equipment and write the basic information of the equipment, including equipment manufacturer information, equipment serial number, equipment function introduction, equipment operation precautions, equipment department, equipment personnel, equipment applicability, and equipment maintenance information.
2. Daily Maintenance Stage: According to the set maintenance cycle during installation, the equipment will automatically report maintenance reminders. The personnel responsible for the equipment will record the maintenance content and time in the equipment's RFID tag to ensure that the equipment maintains its optimal working condition. The Internet of Things platform predicts possible failures of equipment based on the data reported by equipment sensors in advance, formulates advance processing plans, prevents accidents, and improves equipment utilization efficiency.
3. Repair Stage: The equipment will send repair warnings to the departments and individuals that may be affected, reminding them to arrange backup equipment to ensure that repairs do not adversely affect normal medical care.
4. Scrap Stage: Use an RFID reader to locate the equipment position and identify the equipment for scrapping, including maintenance information, repair history, and other information. Record the evaluation results of the equipment in the system for subsequent retrieval. Through the full lifecycle monitoring of medical equipment, the working status of equipment is always monitored, unknown risks are effectively prevented, safety hazards are eliminated, equipment reliability is improved, and maintenance costs are reduced.

Internationally, the application of medical device coding is still in the early stages. In 2011, international medical device regulatory agencies completed the coordination of the implementation principles of Unique Device Identification (UDI) and proposed the "Medical Device UDI Standard," recommending the adoption of the Global Standards 1 (GS1) international item coding standard for UDI. In 2013, the International Medical Device Regulators Forum (IMDRF) and the U.S. FDA separately issued guidelines and regulations related to the medical device unique identification system. In 2014, the U.S. FDA implemented unique identification for Class III medical devices. In May 2017, the European Union clarified the regulatory requirements for implementing medical device unique identification. Countries such as Japan and Australia have also begun relevant work. However, the application of regulations and standards has not yet formed a relatively mature application system, and countries like the USA are actively formulating related policies and regulations to promote the implementation of UDI. Medical device management and traceability systems based on RFID technology can eliminate certain safety hazards caused by human factors to a certain extent. They clarify the responsibilities of personnel at each link from hospital admission to discharge and usage of medical devices and record relevant information, facilitating traceability after adverse events. Medical device management based on RFID technology can achieve precise control of "one code for one item," reducing the arbitrariness and subjectivity of manual operations. It enables fast application and distribution between clinical departments, storage, and suppliers, precise inventory management, rapid inbound and outbound processes, quick ordering, logistics tracking, usage registration, scrapping registration, satisfaction evaluation, and intelligent management such as inventory and benefit dosage warning analysis.

6.3.2 Application in Public Health Management

Public health is a public undertaking that affects the health of the people in a country or region. Typical applications of the Internet of Things in public health management include the control and management during the spread of acute infectious diseases, intelligent temperature screening management in public places, and monitoring of the cold chain for vaccines and medicines.

One effective method for preventing and controlling infectious diseases during their spread is to control the transmission routes. By leveraging the advantages of telecommunications big data and combining Internet of Things platforms with artificial intelligence technology, a simulated model of epidemic transmission is created to identify key parameters for controlling the spread of epidemics, assisting governments in epidemic prevention and control work. During the outbreak phase, the best method for controlling transmission routes is to track and isolate individuals who have had close contact with confirmed cases. Traditional methods of tracking contacts rely on interviewing individuals and investigating issues, which is inefficient and risky in large cities. The use of Internet of Things technology (such as RFID, Bluetooth, GPS, and Wi-Fi) can track detailed locations and provide relevant information such as the interaction time and distance between different individuals and confirmed cases. Low-power Bluetooth is one of the most widely used IoT standards, offering relatively high precision in location tracking and various tracking solutions such as Received Signal Strength Indicator (RSSI) and Angle of Arrival (AoA), enabling the classification of tracked contacts and prioritization for data analysis and control of transmission routes.

Another essential aspect of preventing and controlling infectious diseases is controlling the sources of transmission. To prevent the spread of infections, hospitals can provide patients with smart bracelets that record the patients' movement trajectories, Wi-Fi, heart rate, etc. When patients leave the designated area, the electronic fence function on the bracelet will issue an alert, notifying the disease control center and public security system for immediate follow-up. Additionally, the bracelet can provide functions such as medication reminders, periodic checks, and heart rate monitoring.

Since nearly all acute infectious diseases since the twenty-first century cause elevated body temperatures, the use of Internet of Things smart temperature measurement systems can detect suspected cases. Based on Internet of Things technology, smart temperature measurement systems use cameras for facial recognition and infrared detectors for measuring body temperature. Objects with temperatures above absolute zero (−273 °C) emit electromagnetic waves. Thermal imaging cameras collect the infrared electromagnetic waves emitted by objects, convert the infrared signals into electrical signals, calculate the object's temperature based on signal processing systems, and output pseudo-color images that are easy for the human eye to recognize. By setting up Internet of Things smart temperature measurement systems in densely populated areas to screen people for body temperature, suspected cases can be isolated and observed, and confirmed patients can be isolated, subjected to epidemiological analysis, and provided with isolation treatment. The smart temperature measurement system transmits data such as time, geographical location, images of individuals, and body temperature to the backend database. The software management platform of the system can dynamically generate reports based on parameters such as date, time, and body temperature, facilitating data analysis and traceability. If a person's body temperature exceeds the set threshold, the temperature measurement system will automatically trigger an alarm, and security personnel will verify the situation. The smart temperature measurement system enables rapid non-contact screening of body temperature, reducing the risk of infection and ensuring accurate temperature measurement. This system has played a significant role in the prevention and control of the COVID-19 pandemic.

The rapid and widespread vaccination of acute infectious diseases since the twenty-first century requires the use of medical cold chain monitoring for vaccines. Vaccines, as a special type of biological product, are highly sensitive to temperature. Throughout the entire process from production, storage, transportation, distribution to use, deviations from specified temperature requirements may cause vaccines to become ineffective. By utilizing RFID technology and cold chain logistics GPS technology, comprehensive monitoring of drugs and vaccines can be achieved. Sensors installed in cold chain vehicles, cold storage facilities, and refrigerators can detect temperature and humidity in real time and upload the data to servers, enabling real-time monitoring and forming a complete traceable data chain for vaccine cold chain storage and transportation. Manufacturers can trace the flow of drugs through Internet of Things platforms and take urgent measures to stop the spread in case of problems, avoiding harm to the public. The cold chain temperature monitoring system is established through the integration of monitoring equipment and software platforms, covering functions such as cold chain data collection, monitoring, analysis, management, traceability, information alerts, and remote monitoring. All temperature and humidity monitoring devices at various monitoring points can upload data to cloud platform servers via Internet of Things technology and can be uploaded to higher-level regulatory department platforms as needed, enabling 24-hour real-time online unified supervision.

6.4 Frontiers in Medical Internet of Things Research

The value of the Medical Internet of Things comes from three aspects: ① Remote Patient Monitoring (RPM), which remotely collects patient vital signs through Internet of Medical Things systems, saving a significant amount of administrative and medical costs; ② Healthcare and Prevention, where Internet of Medical Things solutions significantly reduce medical costs in healthcare and prevention projects; ③ Operations, where Internet of Medical Things projects contribute to administrative cost savings for some suppliers and greatly enhance consumer experiences for numerous payers. As Internet of Medical Things integrates physical devices and data resources in the healthcare industry, people will achieve better medical care, higher-quality patient monitoring, enhanced customer experiences, and improved overall system operational efficiency. More and more companies are also paying attention to and investing in the Medical Internet of Things, leading to the emergence of cutting-edge Internet of Medical Things solutions such as 5G smart wards and unmanned material delivery technology.

6.4.1 5G Smart Wards

"5G Smart Wards" refer to the intelligent transformation of traditional wards in hospitals around the inpatient care process, leveraging 5G networks, the Internet, artificial intelligence, Internet of Things technology, and smart medical devices. These wards have bedside intelligent interaction systems as core platforms, supplemented by intelligent doctor/nurse station interaction systems and smart ward call systems. Various Internet of Things application devices, such as physical call systems, are used to efficiently collect and utilize medical data, optimize nursing processes for medical institutions, and realize the extension and expansion of HIS into wards to provide intelligent medical services. The characteristics of 5G networks, such as high bandwidth, low latency, ultra-low power consumption, and multi-terminal compatibility, enable a significant improvement in the Internet of Things platform, providing end-to-end data services for smart medical devices in the ward area, meeting various needs for efficient, real time, and stable medical data, and promoting the "Internet of Everything" for intelligent medical devices.

The application scenarios of smart wards cover five different dimensions of business information management systems: diagnosis and treatment, clinical nursing, patient services, drug and item management, and quality management. In hospitals, including nurse stations, corridors, and wards, timely reminders, real-time risk monitoring, and queries are achieved through electronic screens, helping hospitals achieve cost control, efficiency improvement, and reduction of adverse events. The bedside intelligent interaction system, as the central brain of smart wards, collects data generated by intelligent medical devices based on 5G and Internet of Things technologies, connects various management information of the hospital through the hospital network to bedside intelligent terminals, integrates and analyzes them, and displays them uniformly on smart screens in real time.

Using electronic screens, patients and their families can understand the daily diagnosis and treatment plans at any time. For doctors, using mobile terminal devices connected to 5G networks, they can quickly retrieve patients' clinical examination reports such as nursing, examinations, and laboratory tests. The high bandwidth and low latency characteristics of 5G networks ensure that patient medical data and related imaging data can be downloaded within seconds, improving ward rounds efficiency. The reasonable and full utilization of HIS data resources greatly promotes the hospital's informatization construction, presenting timely and accurate information for medical staff and patients, providing more friendly and practical services for doctors and patients. Additionally, a mobile doctor station can be established through the mobile ward round system, allowing doctors to view patients' test results, conduct diagnosis and treatment activities, conduct bedside education, remote visits, and remote consultations, replacing some manual work with information technology, greatly reducing workload, and achieving integrated management of medical care and patient care.

6.4.2 Unmanned Material Distribution

The purpose of unmanned material distribution is to reduce errors that may occur in manual transportation and to achieve full-process informatization and traceability using Internet of Things technology. Additionally, it aims to improve transportation efficiency and reduce transportation costs. The following introduces automated guided vehicle (AGV), medical drones, and automated dispensing cabinet (ADC).

Automated guided vehicles, also known as transport robots, are transport vehicles controlled by computer and Internet of Things sensor technology. They run along predefined paths and can stop at designated locations to complete tasks such as item transportation. All automated guided vehicles are equipped with RFID tags to ensure they reach the correct location. Medical staff can use handheld devices to scan the barcode on the vehicle to verify the correct delivery specifications of medical supplies. Automated guided vehicles are mainly used in six scenarios:

disinfection supply centers, intravenous drug preparation centers, nurse stations, inpatient wards, operating rooms, and warehouses. By integrating robots with hospital HIS, the delivery system of the hospital can achieve informationization, digitization, networking, integration, intelligence, and automation, reducing manual transportation costs and saving transportation time. The use of Internet of Things technologies such as electronic signature and barcode verification effectively reduces the risk of human error. Separate transportation of different materials can effectively reduce the risk of cross-infection or disease transmission. During the COVID-19 pandemic, automated guided vehicles played a significant role in delivering medical supplies such as medical masks and protective clothing to hospitals, entering isolation areas to transport living and medical supplies, solving the problem of the "last mile" in distribution, and avoiding the risk of cross-infection among delivery personnel.

Medical drones are mainly used for emergency medical supply transportation and sample distribution. They have been applied in areas such as emergency blood transfusion and nucleic acid testing sample transportation. As the overall weight of testing samples is relatively light, medical drones are suitable for small-load transportation, which can improve clinical service efficiency. Medical drones can transport medical supplies such as blood, serum, vaccines, and organs between hospitals and blood banks through hospital ground stations. In emergency situations, medical drones have obvious advantages over ground transportation due to their high time sensitivity. They can achieve small-scale, rapid delivery, allowing hospitals and blood banks to transport urgently needed items to rescue areas via medical drones in the shortest possible time. Medical drone technology enables extremely fast point-to-point urban medical services, allowing hospital systems to shorten patient waiting times through centralized laboratories and medical inventory. For example, cancer tissue slices need to be quickly sent to the pathology department for examination after being removed from the operating room, which is crucial for patient safety. Additionally, after extensive use of medical drones, the position of inspection centers can be flexibly arranged. The application of medical drone transportation system logistics can reduce redundant investments in large-scale inspection equipment.

Automated Dispensing Cabinet (ADC) use hospital information system links and Internet of Things sensor technology to achieve closed-loop management of dispensing, replenishment, data maintenance, and dispensing of special drugs. Automated Dispensing Cabinets have their own ADC systems to record the access information and drug information of the cabinets. The prescription is reviewed by the central dispensary center for rationality and suitability. After the prescription is approved, it enters the ADC system. The ADC system can provide prompts, warnings, and controls. Identification of the drug's barcode is required for both withdrawal and storage, effectively controlling drug dispensing and management. Nurses use fingerprint scanning or facial recognition for identity verification to log into the ADC system, select the patient for medication, and verify that the patient information is correct. Each automated dispensing cabinet is equipped with a high-definition camera to ensure transparency and clarity in the withdrawal and storage of medications. The central pharmacy can effectively control the steps of nurse use of Automated Dispensing Cabinets and pharmacist management of ADC drugs. If there are errors in information such as withdrawal time, open storage area, quantity of withdrawn drugs, patient name, or hospital number, the central pharmacy can detect and intervene in a timely manner, effectively avoiding errors. Through the full-process closed management of the ADC system, drug whereabouts can be traced and tracked, reducing safety hazards, improving inventory efficiency, ensuring timely and safe medication for inpatients, and reducing the workload of departmental drug management.

6.5 Summary

This chapter outlined the basic concepts and development history of the Internet of Medical Things, and introduced the current research status both domestically and internationally. It also explained the main functions and applications of Internet of Medical Things systems, including patient management, telemedicine monitoring, medication management, medical supplies management, and hospital logistics personnel management. With the development of Internet of Medical Things technology, RFID technology combined with the Internet, 5G communication, artificial intelligence, and other technologies has formed many complete management systems, providing technical support for hospital refined management and traceable management. The chapter also introduced cutting-edge research on the integration and application of new technologies, including 5G smart wards and unmanned material distribution technology.

Telemedicine Systems and Mobile Health Systems

7

Contents

7.1 Overview of Telemedicine Systems and Mobile Health Systems ... 184
7.1.1 Introduction to Telemedicine Systems and Mobile Health Systems ... 184
7.1.2 Introduction to Mobile Health and Mobile Health Systems ... 185
7.1.3 Development History ... 186
7.1.4 Current Status of Research Domestically and Internationally ... 188
7.2 Components and Related Technologies of Telemedicine Systems ... 190
7.2.1 Composition and Functions of Telemedicine Systems ... 190
7.2.1.1 Telemedicine Diagnostic System ... 191
7.2.1.2 Telemedicine Consultation System ... 191
7.2.1.3 Telemedicine Education System ... 191
7.2.1.4 Telemedicine Monitoring System for Remote Beds ... 192
7.2.2 Technologies Related to Telemedicine ... 192
7.2.2.1 Diagnosis and Clinical Testing Technologies ... 192
7.2.2.2 Information Technology ... 194
7.2.2.3 Network Communication Technology ... 194
7.3 Mobile Health System Compositions and Related Technologies ... 194
7.3.1 Composition and Functions of Mobile Health Systems ... 194
7.3.2 Mobile Health-Related Technologies ... 195
7.3.2.1 Mobile Diagnostic Technology and Applications ... 195
7.3.2.2 Mobile Monitoring Technology and Applications ... 196
7.4 Case Studies ... 197
7.4.1 Case Studies of Telemedicine Systems ... 197
7.4.1.1 Massachusetts General Hospital Telemedicine Center ... 197
7.4.1.2 Huoshenshan (Fire God Mountain) Hospital 5G Remote Consultation System ... 197
7.4.2 Mobile Healthcare System Case Study ... 198
7.4.2.1 Sundray Medical Mobile Nursing ... 198
7.4.2.2 Ping An Good Doctor ... 199
7.5 Frontier Research ... 199
7.5.1 Advancements in Data Exchange Technology ... 199
7.5.2 Virtual Reality Remote Surgery ... 201
7.5.3 5G Pre-hospital Emergency Care ... 203
7.6 Summary ... 204
References ... 205

J. Li et al., *Healthcare Information Systems*, Innovative Medical Devices,
https://doi.org/10.1007/978-981-97-9551-2_7

Telemedicine refers to public health services provided across distances to individuals who wish to maintain their health. It encompasses a variety of medical activities, including disease diagnosis, treatment, prevention, continuing medical education, and medical research and evaluation. Mobile health, on the other hand, involves using mobile communication technologies such as personal digital assistant (PAD), mobile phone, and satellite communication to deliver healthcare services and information. Specifically, mobile health primarily relies on health-related applications on mobile terminal systems and wearable medical monitoring devices. As society advances and people's living standards and levels of informatization improve, the development of telemedicine and mobile health has become increasingly mature. This approach breaks the constraints of time and space, surpassing the traditional singular service model of healthcare. It significantly enhances the efficiency and quality of medical services, making it one of the key directions for the future development of the healthcare industry.

7.1 Overview of Telemedicine Systems and Mobile Health Systems

7.1.1 Introduction to Telemedicine Systems and Mobile Health Systems

Traditional telemedicine refers to a specialized medical practice where basic medical treatment is provided to distant patients who cannot visit the healthcare facility. Currently, it specifically denotes medical service systems facilitated by modern communication technology to provide healthcare services to remote locations.

Telemedicine systems can be functionally divided into three aspects: remote medical monitoring, remote diagnosis and consultation, and remote surgery and treatment. Remote medical monitoring primarily involves real-time surveillance of patients' various physiological indicators (such as heart rate, body temperature, pulse, and blood oxygen saturation), and providing higher quality medical assessments and guidance. These systems are widely used among groups with chronic diseases or those unable to seek timely medical attention. The system can transmit static medical images, diagnostic reports, laboratory results, and physiological parameter readings, allowing doctors to perform remote diagnosis and provide guidance based on this information.

Telemedicine effectively extends the high-quality medical resources, advanced medical concepts, and technologies of large hospitals to broader regions. It is particularly useful for conducting remote diagnosis, treatment, and consultations in underdeveloped areas, remote islands, or on ships, and is applicable to various medical fields such as radiology, pathology, dermatology, and cardiology.

In China, telemedicine has already formed a medical development system driven by urban areas to support rural areas, playing an indelible role in specialized medical treatments. It also holds promise for addressing the issue of uneven distribution of medical resources in the country. With the advancement of information technology, the introduction of cutting-edge technologies (such as virtual reality and augmented reality), and the gradual improvement of relevant laws and regulations, the prospects for the development of telemedicine are indeed bright.

7.1.2 Introduction to Mobile Health and Mobile Health Systems

Mobile health is a new medical model that emerged from the foundation of telemedicine. According to the Healthcare Information and Management Systems Society (HIMSS), mobile health refers to the use of mobile communication technologies such as PDAs, mobile phones, and satellite communications to deliver healthcare services and information. It effectively addresses healthcare service issues in developing countries caused by the shortage of medical resources and human resources, offering a viable solution to the medical human resource shortages in these regions.

The application scope of mobile health can be divided into two main aspects: internal to healthcare institutions and external to healthcare institutions. Internally, it focuses on the electronic and around-the-clock visual management of patients. Externally, its scope is broader and includes the prevention, screening, detection, diagnosis, and treatment of common diseases, such as appointment scheduling, remote data collection, education and notifications, remote monitoring, medical education, tracking and diagnosing disease and epidemic spread, and support for diagnosis and treatment. Mobile technology can comprehensively optimize the entire process of patient care, including registration, consultation, admission, medication, various examinations and tests, surgery, and payment. Mobile applications can efficiently integrate various hospital information systems, making the systems more flexible and agile, thereby further enhancing work efficiency. In the planning and deployment of mobile health services, the USA leads globally, with over half of the world's mobile health services being implemented there. Compared to developed countries, mobile health in China is still in its infancy.

Mobile health has transformed the traditional lifestyle where people could only visit hospitals for medical consultations. It has addressed issues such as the difficulty in registering for appointments and long waiting times. In areas with network coverage, people can access health consultations of interest at any time and obtain professional answers from doctors regarding their personal health issues. With the integration of mobile communication technology, the time cost for seeking medical care is greatly reduced, and the effective utilization of hospital medical resources is improved. This change also transforms public health concepts, encouraging the development of good living habits and shifting the focus from treatment to prevention.

7.1.3 Development History

In the late 1950s, American scholar Wittson first applied two-way television systems to the field of medicine. In the same year, Jutra and others established remote radiology. Since then, there have been continuous efforts in the USA to utilize communication and electronic technology for medical activities, leading to the emergence of the term "telemedicine" [1].

1. First Generation Telemedicine

   The first generation of telemedicine emerged in the early 1960s. However, constrained by the relatively primitive information technology of that time, the amount of information that could be transmitted was limited, thereby impeding the development of telemedicine technology. Consequently, during the more than 20 years from the early 1960s to the mid-1980s, the development of telemedicine technology progressed slowly.
2. Second Generation Telemedicine

   With the rapid development of information and communication technology in the USA and Western Europe in the late 1980s, telemedicine technology in these countries achieved significant advancements. This period saw the emergence of many impactful and influential telemedicine projects, which we now refer to as the second generation of telemedicine. The first commercialized telemedicine system was implemented in the USA, connecting the Massachusetts Medical Center with the Florida Medical Center.

   In 1988, the USA defined the concept of telemedicine systems as an open distributed system, dividing it into several main components: remote diagnosis, consultation of specialists, information service, online examination, and remote studying. This meant that telemedicine should include modern information technologies such as bidirectional audio-visual communication technology, computers, and remote sensing technology, enabling the transmission, storage, and retrieval of medical-related data, texts, images, and the audio-visual information needed for remote consultation systems. Currently, the world's largest and most widely used telemedicine network is the Georgia Statewide Academic and Medical System, which conducts telemedicine activities through cable, wireless, and satellite communications.

   To popularize telemedicine technology, Europe and the European Union organized a large-scale telemedicine system promotion experiment, involving 3 biomedical engineering laboratories, 10 companies, 20 pathology laboratories, and over 100 users. Simultaneously, countries in Asia, Australia, and Africa also conducted a series of telemedicine promotion and practice activities. Notably, in December 1988, with the support and assistance of the US-Soviet Space Physiology Joint Working Group and NASA, a hospital in Armenia, after an earthquake, achieved the first transnational remote joint consultation with four hospitals in the USA.

   The late 1980s also marked the earliest appearance of telemedicine activities in China. As early as 1986, China had already conducted cross-ocean consultations for patients on ocean-going cargo ships via telegraph. By the 1990s, the rapid development of Internet technology in China allowed people to identify their unknown ailments through the Internet. These various applications helped the Chinese truly understand the significance of the telemedicine concept, realizing its uniqueness and advantages, thereby promoting the development of a series of modern telemedicine activities in the country. Between 1988 and 1997, many hospitals such as the General Hospital of the People's Liberation Army, Shanghai Huashan Hospital, and Shanghai Medical University Children's Hospital conducted remote discussions and consultations through satellite technology, telephone lines, and Integrated Services Digital Network (ISDN). During this period, Shanghai Education and Research Network and Shanghai Medical University also launched remote consultation project collaborations and established a telemedicine consultation research lab.

3. Third Generation Telemedicine

   After 2009, China introduced a series of policies related to telemedicine to promote the sharing of medical and health resources. In 2009, the Central Committee of the Communist Party of China and the State Council clearly proposed the concept of "actively developing telemedicine for rural and remote areas" in their "Opinions on Deepening the Reform of the Medical and Health System." In 2010, the National Health and Family Planning Commission put forward the "2010 Remote Consultation System Construction Project Management Plan" and the "2010 Remote Consultation System Construction Project Technical Plan" to advance telemedicine construction at the grassroots level. In 2014, the National Health and Family Planning Commission issued the "Opinions on Promoting Telemedicine Services in Medical Institutions," calling for "actively promoting the development of telemedicine services," eliminating the approval process for telemedicine, and allowing business-to-consumer (B2C) models for enterprises. Remote healthcare began to enter a phase of rapid development.

   In July and September 2015, the State Council successively issued the "Guiding Opinions on Actively Promoting the 'Internet Plus' Action" and the "Guiding Opinions on Promoting the Construction of a Hierarchical Diagnosis and Treatment System" (hereinafter referred to as the "Guiding Opinions"). These documents proposed to fully utilize the efficient and convenient advantages of the Internet to improve resource utilization efficiency, accelerate the development of Internet-based medical services, and promote new models of online healthcare. The "Guiding Opinions" suggested "actively using mobile Internet to provide convenient services such as online appointment booking, waiting time reminders, fee payment, diagnostic report inquiries, and medication delivery. They also encouraged medical institutions to conduct telemedicine services like basic examinations and higher-level diagnostics targeting small and medium-sized cities and rural areas."

   The emergence of "Internet + Healthcare" facilitated a breakthrough in the traditional medical process through "cloud registration," "cloud consultation," "cloud diagnosis," "cloud prescription," and "cloud medication," achieving a completely new approach to medical services.

In 2017, the General Office of the State Council issued the "Guiding Opinions on Promoting the Construction and Development of Medical Consortiums," which called for the vigorous development of telemedicine collaboration networks targeting grassroots, remote, and underdeveloped areas. It encouraged public hospitals to provide telemedicine, remote teaching, and remote training services to primary healthcare institutions.

During this stage, telemedicine services gradually entered communities and households, focusing more on serving individuals and providing targeted and personalized medical services. Particularly after 2015, the rapid development of mobile Internet turned mobile health services based on mobile Internet into a new breakthrough. With the proliferation and advancement of smartphones and breakthroughs in Internet of Things (IoT) technology, cloud computing and cloud services technologies were gradually applied to remote and mobile healthcare fields. This led to the emergence of various intelligent health medical products, such as remote blood pressure monitors, remote electrocardiogram monitors, and even remote fetal heart monitors, providing users with more convenient and efficient daily medical prevention and monitoring services.

4. Remote and Mobile Healthcare Driven by the COVID-19 Pandemic

The outbreak of the COVID-19 pandemic in 2020 brought new opportunities and challenges to remote and mobile healthcare, achieving almost several years' worth of progress in just a few months due to the unique nature of infectious diseases. In the UK, for instance, during the peak of the pandemic, the proportion of telemedicine—using video, telephone, and other electronic communication devices—for general medical consultations increased significantly from about 10% before the pandemic to 75%.

At the J.P. Morgan Healthcare Conference in January 2021, Ascension, the largest private healthcare system in the USA, presented a keynote report revealing that from January to April 2020, the volume of telemedicine services surged 40-fold, and remained highly active in the following months, representing a 20-fold increase compared to pre-pandemic levels.

In China, the pandemic also spurred the development of remote and mobile healthcare. At Wuhan Huoshenshan Hospital, 5G remote medical trolleys were put into use. Additionally, China Mobile launched the "5G Infrared Thermal Imaging Temperature Measurement" application, which allows simultaneous scanning and temperature measurement of multiple individuals.

7.1.4 Current Status of Research Domestically and Internationally

The development of telemedicine is uneven across the globe. Internationally, this field has a history of nearly 40 years, with the USA and Europe being significantly ahead of other countries. Remote healthcare is widely adopted in these regions, with technology maturing and entering a stage of refinement.

According to statistics from U.S. healthcare authorities, over 60% of health service institutions and 50% of hospitals nationwide have implemented telemedicine services to varying degrees. Currently, all states in the USA can provide remote imaging consultation services; 49 states have established remote mental health services; and 36 states have developed telemedicine consultation services centered around family medicine. The core of U.S. telemedicine services is to help patients connect with specialist experts through various communication modes such as telephone, email, audio, and home television, providing them with professional and targeted advice. Remote healthcare is also increasingly used for chronic disease management and post-discharge follow-up care in homes or community hospitals. Using audio-visual equipment and smart applications, doctors can offer remote rehabilitation guidance and disease monitoring, as well as health management, medication compliance evaluation, and cognitive ability assessments for patients.

In China, the mobile health system is still in its developmental stage, and its application in hospitals is relatively limited. Among the more frequently used systems is the mobile nursing system, which helps nurses care for patients in the ward using mobile devices and wireless networks. However, with the rapid development of mobile Internet in China and the growing number of mobile devices and users, there have been significant advances in mobile health. Users can now use mobile apps to book appointments, pay fees, rate services, and check test results, significantly enhancing the healthcare experience and revolutionizing diagnostic and treatment behaviors.

As user habits develop and healthcare policies become more relaxed, the penetration rate of mobile health applications is expected to increase further. The emergence of mobile health is gradually addressing issues such as the uneven distribution of medical resources, irrational medical service processes, and chaotic medical service scenarios. Mobile health is poised to enter a golden period of rapid development.

With increased awareness of mobile health, the use of online consultations and medical e-commerce is driving the expansion of the mobile health market. The rapid market growth and substantial user demand are interrelated; currently, the 35–65 age group represents the largest sub-health demographic. Conditions such as overweight and obesity, dyslipidemia and fatty liver, and hypertension require monitoring and early detection via mobile health devices to facilitate timely treatment. With the aging population, the increase in empty nesters and elderly people living alone makes wearable smart medical devices that can remotely monitor health in real-time highly popular, reducing labor costs. Additionally, the younger onset of chronic diseases and prolonged illness durations are increasing the demand for convenient mobile health services. According to the "China Mobile Internet Development Report (2022)" published by the People's Daily Research Institute, as of December 2021, the number of online medical users in China had reached 298 million. Most provincial hospitals in China have established mobile health systems based on wireless networks, and these systems are developing rapidly.

Currently, there are several issues with mobile healthcare in China:

Data Security Concerns: Mobile healthcare platforms often require users to provide personal information, including not only age and gender but also health and financial status. If these platforms lack proper security protection for user data and privacy in daily use and management, it could lead to serious data breaches, threatening users' personal privacy.

Protection of Doctor Rights: The issue of multi-site practice for doctors involved in mobile healthcare remains unresolved in law. This is one of the significant challenges facing the mobile healthcare industry. Due to the special nature of the medical industry, doctors and hospitals need to bear more responsibilities, especially for patients' lives. Therefore, multi-site practice for doctors may not only increase medical risks but also blur the boundaries of doctors' responsibilities, leading hospitals where doctors originally worked to be reluctant to address such issues. If even mobile healthcare platforms or operators refuse to bear risks and responsibilities for doctors, it will further hinder doctors' willingness to enter the mobile healthcare field. Therefore, to actively promote mobile healthcare, corresponding industry or legal norms need to be established at the national level, such as improving the medical liability insurance system to provide guarantees for doctors' multi-site practice, thus benefiting the general public from the development achievements of mobile healthcare.

Norms for Workplace Order: Currently, China's mobile healthcare industry is still in its early stages. Although the COVID-19 pandemic has accelerated the rapid development of the mobile healthcare market, with the user base reaching hundreds of millions, the public's understanding of mobile healthcare is limited to surface meanings. Most users do not trust mobile healthcare services. Additionally, many mobile healthcare apps for individual users contain various untrue information. People's trust in mobile healthcare is still low. Although there are still deficiencies in laws and regulations related to mobile healthcare, operators involved in mobile healthcare need to strictly comply with the rules and regulations formulated by relevant institutions such as the State Council and the National Health Commission to protect users' rights and interests and ensure the positive development of the market. At the same time, regulatory and market authorities should strictly control audit standards, standardize the behavior of operating platforms and participating doctors, and crack down on illegal activities, ultimately achieving a good ecological environment and positive development prospects for the mobile healthcare market.

7.2 Components and Related Technologies of Telemedicine Systems

7.2.1 Composition and Functions of Telemedicine Systems

All telemedicine systems can be simply defined as consisting of three main components: healthcare service providers, remote seekers of medical services, and the communication network and diagnostic devices used to connect the two. The composition of telemedicine systems is illustrated in Fig. **7.1**.

Healthcare service providers, also known as the source of medical services, are typically located in large urban medical centers with abundant medical resources and diagnostic experience, such as tertiary referral hospitals in the country. Remote seekers of medical services are generally medical institutions lacking sufficient medical capabilities or conditions, home patients, or patients isolated due to contagious diseases, as well as battlefield patients located where doctors cannot reach in time. The primary purpose of telemedicine is to connect these two parties. Therefore, the final part of the medical system consists of the communication network and diagnostic devices used to link them. The communication network may include ordinary telephone networks, wireless communication networks, communication satellite networks, 5G technology, etc., while diagnostic devices may include computer software and hardware, diagnostic instruments, wearable devices, virtual reality (VR) devices, and so forth.

In terms of goals and functionalities, telemedicine systems can be roughly divided into four categories, as illustrated in Fig. **7.2**.

7.2.1.1 Telemedicine Diagnostic System

The telemedicine diagnostic system, aimed at diagnostic purposes, primarily connects a variety of diagnostic devices to the network through portable physiological monitoring devices and other wireless devices. It establishes a wireless network transmission system and integrates with Hospital Information Systems (HIS) and Picture Archiving and Communication Systems (PACS) to quickly obtain various forms of medical records. This enhances the diagnostic and medical level of remote area hospitals, reduces additional costs incurred for accurate diagnosis, and overcomes limitations of time and space.

7.2.1.2 Telemedicine Consultation System

The telemedicine consultation system, aimed at consultation purposes, mainly utilizes network modes in conjunction with in-hospital HIS, PACS, etc., to achieve remote and multi-doctor diagnosis of patients. It eliminates the restrictions of fixed hospital locations and working hours, reducing the time required for doctors to go to hospitals and for patient transfers.

7.2.1.3 Telemedicine Education System

The telemedicine education system, aimed at teaching and training purposes, can achieve remote surgical teaching by synchronously broadcasting expert surgical procedures to teaching rooms in lower-level and grassroots hospitals. It also enables

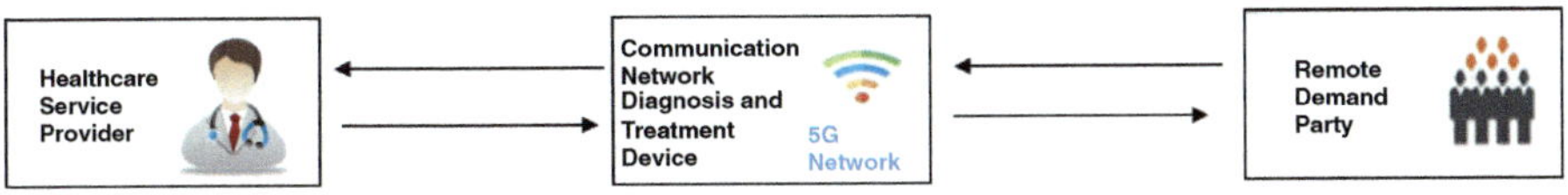

Fig. 7.1 Composition of telemedicine system

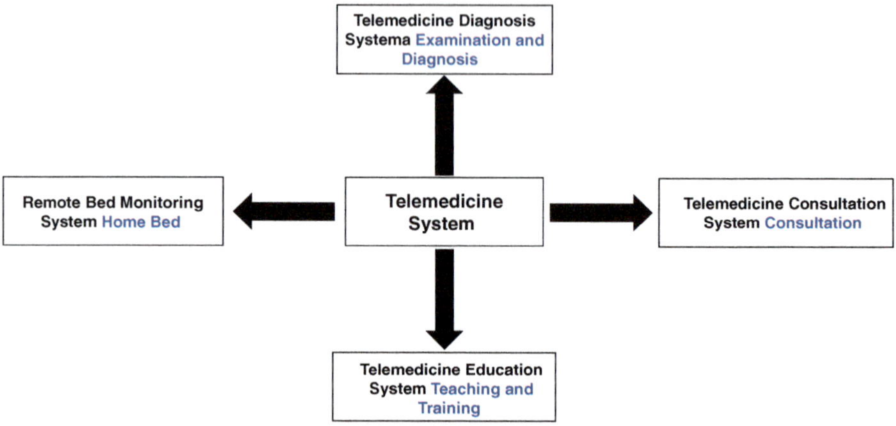

Fig. 7.2 Classification of telemedicine systems

real-time voice communication guidance, online education and training for doctors and nurses, as well as remote interdisciplinary, inter-hospital, and international educational collaboration. This provides doctors with more learning resources and achieves efficient sharing of high-quality medical resources.

7.2.1.4 Telemedicine Monitoring System for Remote Beds

The telemedicine monitoring system for remote beds, aimed at home bed monitoring purposes, utilizes the Internet of Things and 5G technology to allow caregivers to monitor distant patients, elderly, children, etc., in real time through mobile apps, computers, or large screens.

7.2.2 Technologies Related to Telemedicine

Telemedicine is a multi-stage process involving not only traditional medical technologies but also requiring additional information technology and electronic technology, as illustrated in Fig. 7.3.

7.2.2.1 Diagnosis and Clinical Testing Technologies

The starting point of telemedicine remains the personal information of patients, including physiological and electrophysiological parameters such as electrocardiogram, blood pressure, blood oxygen, as well as imaging data such as ultrasound, CT, MRI, and various biochemical indices of blood, urine, and body fluids. The development of medical technology today focuses not only on how to obtain these data but also on the accuracy, efficiency, and convenience of obtaining data. For example, real-time monitoring of patients' physiological parameters such as electrocardiography, blood pressure, and blood oxygen can be achieved through wearable devices. Medical imaging technologies mainly include ultrasound imaging, X-ray imaging, magnetic resonance imaging, and nuclear medicine imaging. The

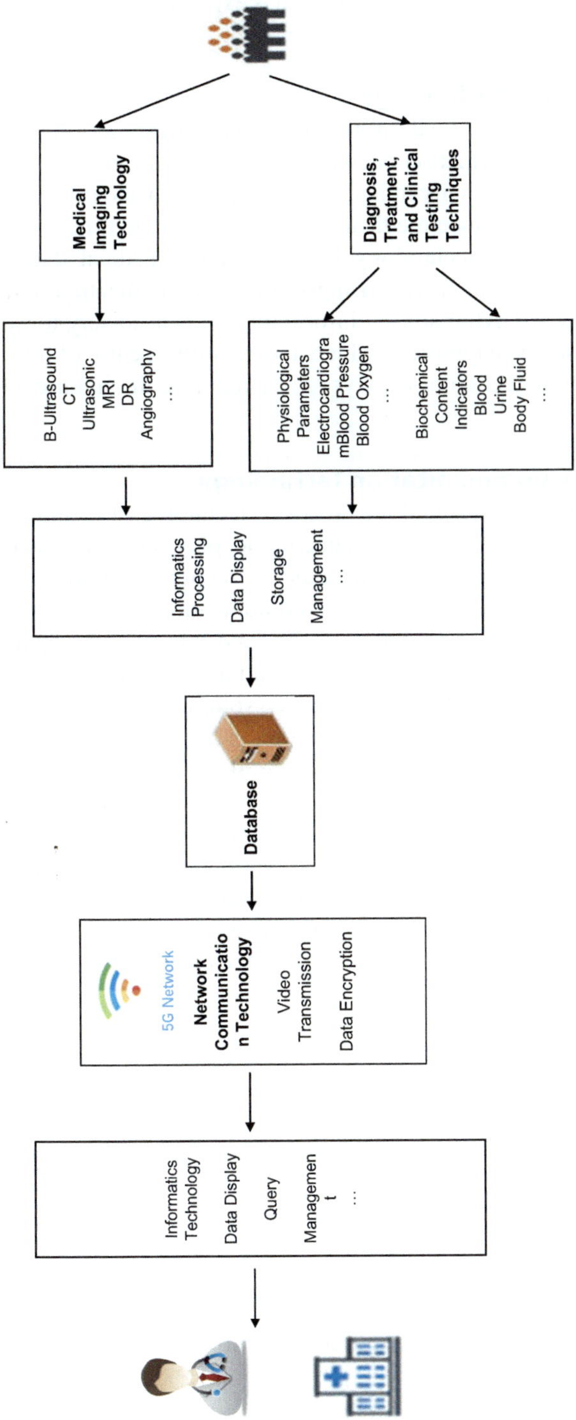

Fig. 7.3 Telemedicine related technologies

development of these imaging technologies has expanded the scope of examinations and improved the diagnostic level of physicians.

7.2.2.2 Information Technology

After collecting various medical information from patients, storing this diverse and voluminous medical information becomes a challenge. Due to the large volume of medical information, especially image data, compression and processing of data are necessary. Additionally, since medical information storage time is often long, reasonable use of database technology is required for medical data management. Furthermore, due to format issues during storage, standardization of data exchange technologies is needed. After storing information, it is necessary to extract and display the compressed data remotely, which also requires the use of information technology. Information technology plays a crucial role in linking all aspects of telemedicine.

7.2.2.3 Network Communication Technology

Network communication technology, as a key technology for implementing, connecting, and ensuring the quality of telemedicine, plays an indispensable role in the overall process of telemedicine. Telemedicine involves multiple important areas such as public safety and emergency communication. The transmitted medical information includes data, text, video, audio, and images. Among them, data and textual information have small data volumes and low communication requirements, while video and audio signal data have larger volumes. Real-time teleconsultation usually requires simultaneous transmission of video and audio signals, as well as some medical imaging information. Therefore, there are high requirements for the timeliness, security, and reliability of information exchange and transmission. With the rapid development of information technology, from private network communication, Wi-Fi, 4G networks to 5G networks, the timeliness of information exchange, data transmission speed, and quality have been significantly improved. Additionally, with the latest data privacy protection methods such as homomorphic encryption, the security of information has also been greatly enhanced.

7.3 Mobile Health System Compositions and Related Technologies

7.3.1 Composition and Functions of Mobile Health Systems

Mobile health systems consist of four parts: information/communication, monitoring, surveillance, and diagnosis, each with the following functions:

Information/Communication: Specifically includes the management of patient-centered appointment reminders, treatment prompts, examination results, and other health-related data.

Monitoring: Monitors patient medication adherence and other conditions through real-time connection with medical supplies or devices.

Surveillance: Public health event monitoring, including disease prevention, disaster relief, determining the location of medical personnel, and minimizing the occurrence of diseases. The disease tracking function of mobile health is often used in disease early warning systems in places like India, supporting public health personnel in monitoring the spread of infectious diseases.

Diagnosis: Divided into diagnostic support and telemedicine. Through mobile health services, patients can receive diagnosis from doctors at home without the need to meet them directly. Of course, patients must have specific software installed on their phones. Patients select symptom text or image information based on prompts from the software, which is then transmitted to the doctor. The doctor provides diagnosis and treatment advice based on the patient's description.

7.3.2 Mobile Health-Related Technologies

Mobile health technology has almost covered various aspects of healthcare. The main application areas currently include: doctor–patient communication tools and doctor tools for healthcare professionals; medication guidelines and drug sales for pharmaceutical companies and pharmacies; telemedicine, mobile ambulance services, health prevention and control, and organizational coordination management for medical institutions; mobile medical devices designed and manufactured for medical equipment; mobile services and cloud services for mobile operators; Internet of Things (IoT) applications for the logistics industry; mobile surveys and health surveys for research institutions. According to the current scope of the medical field, the application of mobile health technology can be divided into three parts: pre-hospital application, in-hospital application, and post-hospital application, mainly corresponding to pre-hospital health monitoring and management, in-hospital mobile health services and safety and efficiency management, and post-hospital health promotion, health education, chronic disease management, and health surveys.

7.3.2.1 Mobile Diagnostic Technology and Applications

Ultrasound Diagnostic System: Ultrasound imaging is a widely used diagnostic method in medicine that has saved countless lives since its inception. However, nearly 70% of patients worldwide still cannot be diagnosed using this technology, especially patients in developing countries with poor medical conditions. The mobile ultrasound diagnostic system integrates a movable ultrasound probe into a smartphone, allowing patients to perform ultrasound scans by handholding the smartphone. The scanned images are then transmitted to the doctor via the network for remote diagnosis. This invention is very suitable for developing countries and underdeveloped areas lacking equipment.

Smartphone Stethoscope: The StethoCloud team in Australia developed an application that installs a special stethoscope on a smartphone to diagnose whether children aged 1–5 years have pneumonia. When pneumonia patients inhale, their lungs make crackling sounds, so a stethoscope is commonly used to diagnose whether children have pneumonia based on lung sounds. To use this device, the specially designed stethoscope needs to be connected to the smartphone's audio interface, and the microphone needs to be pointed at the test location during use. The microphone uploads the collected sound data to the server through the smartphone, and the server diagnoses the sound based on WHO standards and returns the diagnosis to the smartphone.

7.3.2.2 Mobile Monitoring Technology and Applications

Embedded Monitoring in Medicine Bottles: By embedding monitoring chips in medicine bottle platforms, patients' medication status and remaining medicine quantities can be monitored according to medical orders. Automatic medication reminders or medication refill reminders can be sent through alarms, text messages, phone calls, etc. These types of medicine bottles can also record relevant operations, including drug use or refill operations, and periodically upload operation records. Medical personnel or family members can judge whether patients adhere to treatment plans based on the uploaded series of data.

Home Monitoring System: Norway has used embedded mobile technology to embed wireless communication machines into home devices to build a home monitoring system that monitors the living conditions of elderly people living alone using sensors. The system uses IoT technology, including fall detectors, electronic bed sheets, epilepsy alarms, GPS positioning detectors, humidity sensors, etc. When these devices detect that the elderly are about to encounter danger, they immediately send alerts to medical service providers or other family members.

Personal Intelligent Alarm Monitoring System: Vodafone and the Spanish Red Cross have built a personal intelligent alarm monitoring system to help Alzheimer's patients build confidence in independent living. In addition to monitoring patient behavior, the system is equipped with a GPS receiver that records the location every 3 min. If it exceeds the pre-set geographical area, the device will be triggered to raise an alarm.

Blood Glucose Monitoring System: Traditional blood glucose monitoring methods require patients to undergo multiple tests at regular intervals every day, which can cause great inconvenience to patients. The blood glucose monitoring system utilizes implanted sensors to achieve continuous monitoring of human blood glucose within 7 days. Unlike traditional single measurement methods, this system can continuously read blood glucose indicators in real-time and return the data to smartphones and computers for analysis. Patients can adjust their diet and medication doses based on the returned data. In addition, the system also supports low blood sugar alarm functionality.

7.4 Case Studies

7.4.1 Case Studies of Telemedicine Systems

7.4.1.1 Massachusetts General Hospital Telemedicine Center

Founded in 1811, Massachusetts General Hospital, located in Boston, is one of the oldest hospitals in the USA and is affiliated with Harvard Medical School.

The history of Massachusetts General Hospital's development and implementation of telemedicine solutions can be traced back to the 1960s. As early as 1967, Massachusetts General Hospital established the first telemedicine program in the USA. Using a closed-circuit television system connecting Massachusetts General Hospital and Logan Airport in Boston, doctors from the hospital could provide examinations for arriving passengers who fell ill. At that time, the distance between Logan Airport and the hospital was approximately 3 miles. Following this successful attempt, Massachusetts General Hospital collaborated with the U.S. Department of Veterans Affairs to provide remote psychological counseling services for veterans, extending the collaboration to prisons, schools, and other settings. With the development of new projects, the hospital's telemedicine services continued to expand, including adding remote clinical nursing services for acute stroke patients and launching remote healthcare services through partnerships with communities.

In 2000, Massachusetts General Hospital, in collaboration with Brigham and Women's Hospital, initiated the TeleStroke program. Through this program, stroke treatment experts from both hospitals could provide guidance on stroke treatment to doctors at other hospitals using video and image-sharing technology. The program quickly gained popularity in New England and across the USA. Building on the success of the TeleStroke program, Massachusetts General Hospital also implemented telemedicine services for other medical conditions within its own hospital. In 2012, the hospital officially launched the TeleHealth program, offering remote medical services in departments such as cardiology, neurology, psychiatry, and burn care.

In 2017, Massachusetts General Hospital formally established the Telemedicine Center, collaborating with relevant TeleHealth service organizations to further extend and expand remote medical services. According to reports, Massachusetts General Hospital completed over 10,000 remote visits in 2019, totaling more than 36,000 remote consultations.

7.4.1.2 Huoshenshan (Fire God Mountain) Hospital 5G Remote Consultation System

In early 2020, to concentrate treatment for patients with novel coronavirus pneumonia, Wuhan urgently constructed the Huoshenshan Hospital. On the evening of January 31, 2020, Huawei and China Telecom reached a cooperation agreement and jointly completed the network construction and equipment debugging of the first remote consultation platform in Wuhan's Huoshenshan Hospital. On February 3, 2020, the hospital officially admitted patients, and the remote consultation platform was put into use.

The system features high-definition video conferencing terminals supporting 1080P high-definition quality. Even in the extreme network environment with a bandwidth limit of 512 kB, the remote medical system can ensure smooth operation. In the Huoshenshan Hospital, directors of each ward can request consultations at any time based on changes in patients' conditions. With the help of 5G network, video signals can be connected to each ward, bringing medical diagnosis services to each patient's bedside. High-quality medical experts from other places can also conduct consultations remotely via video with frontline medical staff at Huoshenshan Hospital. This platform has alleviated to some extent the problem of tight deployment and overloaded work of frontline medical staff in Wuhan, and it has also reduced the risk for medical experts from other places traveling to and from the epidemic area.

7.4.2 Mobile Healthcare System Case Study

7.4.2.1 Sundray Medical Mobile Nursing

With the rapid development of medical informatization, business areas such as mobile rounds and mobile nursing have seen swift growth. Mobile healthcare, as an essential module in hospital informatization ratings, imposes strict requirements on the stability, security, throughput performance, and roaming effects of wireless networks.

Sundray Technology, a subsidiary of Sangfor Technologies Co., Ltd., was established in 2014 and specializes in enterprise-level wireless, Internet of Things, and switch solutions. In the field of intelligent healthcare, Sundray Technology provides a mobile nursing solution for hospital scenarios. This solution boasts the following three significant advantages:

Seamless Roaming: Ensuring quick and seamless roaming of mobile rounds terminals during movement, utilizing high-speed, high-throughput wireless networks to effectively support image transmission.

Centralized Management: Through the web management interface of the wireless controller, the entire network of access points (APs) can be uniformly managed. Key network operational information such as AP online status and traffic can be viewed, and operations management can be conducted via the app, including real-time monitoring of network operation status, configuration modifications, and security alerts.

Data Encryption: The wireless controller used in the system complies with the requirements of Order No. 82 of the Ministry of Public Security. It can also trace back illegal activities and improper public opinions in real names, ensuring the security of wireless networks.

7.4.2.2 Ping An Good Doctor

Ping An Good Doctor app was launched in April 2015, with doctor resources as its core, providing users with real-time consultation and health management services, including online consultations, medication purchases, and search functions.

Compared to similar mobile healthcare apps, Ping An Good Doctor introduced artificial intelligence relatively early. It has established deep cooperation with many Grade A tertiary hospitals in China, sharing multidimensional data sources of AI doctors in research, diagnosis, and medication. To alleviate the pressure of doctors' heavy and repetitive online consultations, the Ping An Good Doctor app has explored and developed an intelligent auxiliary diagnosis and treatment system, which can be applied in the consultation and guidance process. Additionally, by recording patients' past medical history data, it creates "data-based medical records" and "health files" for patients.

According to platform data, as of the end of 2020, Ping An Good Doctor app has more than 2247 in-house medical teams, with over 21,116 external contracted doctors. The platform has registered users totaling 373 million people, with over 72.6 million monthly active users at the end of the period, making it the top mobile healthcare application in terms of coverage in China. In January 2021, the "Ping An Good Doctor" app was officially renamed "Ping An Healthcare".

7.5 Frontier Research

7.5.1 Advancements in Data Exchange Technology

The FHIR standard is the latest version of the HL7 standard. The HL7 organization was established in 1987, facilitated by Dr. Sam Schultz at a meeting held at the University of Pennsylvania Hospital, and it received accreditation from the American National Standards Institute in 1994. The HL7 standard, or Health Level Seven standard, is a standardized protocol for electronic transmission of clinical and administrative data between different applications used in the healthcare field. It specifies numerous flexible standards, guidelines, and methods to enable communication among various healthcare systems.

The primary application areas of the HL7 standard are Health Information Systems (HIS) and Radiology Information Systems (RIS). Its main function is to standardize communication between HIS/RIS and their devices, involving aspects such as ward and patient information management, laboratory systems, pharmacy systems, radiology systems, and billing systems. The aim of the HL7 standard is to develop and formulate protocols and standards for hospital data information transmission, standardize clinical and management information formats, reduce the cost of interconnecting hospital information systems, and enhance the degree of data sharing among hospital information systems.

The "L7" in the HL7 standard refers to the seventh layer of the Open Systems Interconnection (OSI) reference model, but this does not mean that it strictly adheres to the definition of this layer's data elements. HL7 uses the seventh layer to construct its own abstract data types and encoding rules. It does not specify how to support data from OSI layers one through six. With the addition of many users, vendors, and consultant organizations, the HL7 standard team has grown gradually and established the HL7 Standards Development Group in 2011. This group combines the advantages of HL7 V2, V3, and CDA, supports modern network standards and the latest web technologies, provides unified extension and constraint mechanisms, and focuses on implementability.

SMART is a healthcare application platform that helps healthcare information technology workers quickly create various applications suitable for use by doctors, nurses, patients, and other participants in healthcare processes, covering the entire diagnostic and treatment process or focusing on specific scenarios. Most applications on the SMART platform are based on open source principles and can be directly integrated into HIS or EMR systems that comply with the FHIR standard. We all hope that application systems can be freely chosen, installed, and uninstalled like mobile apps. From the perspective of hospitals, this requirement manifests in the ability to freely choose the same application or functionality among different developers and seamlessly integrate it into the hospital's HIS or EMR system. From the perspective of application developers, this requirement manifests in the ability for applications to be seamlessly integrated into any HIS or EMR system.

To achieve seamless integration between applications, four main challenges need to be addressed:

Data Understanding: Ensure that the same concepts have consistent definitions across applications, such as patients, visits, orders, results, etc.

Data Acquisition: Use consistent technical specifications across different applications to retrieve the same data. Applications do not need to concern themselves with the internal implementation details. For example, retrieving visit information should follow the same approach regardless of the vendor.

Identity Authentication and Authorization: Implement identity authentication and authorization control between applications to ensure data security.

Interface Integration: Utilize standard interface application development techniques to seamlessly embed one application into another.

The SMART app is defined around these four aspects to achieve seamless integration between applications. SMART stands for Substitutable Medical Apps Reusable Technology and revolves around the core concepts of replaceability and reusability. It was launched by a group of ambitious individuals from Boston Children's Hospital and Harvard Medical School as a nonprofit project with the goal of enabling the free loading of apps on top of systems such as electronic medical records.

The SMART app adopts OAuth 2.0 (OAuth is an open protocol that provides a secure, open, and easy-to-use standard for user resource authorization. OAuth is an abbreviation for Open Authorization) as the standard for identity authentication and authorization and uses HTML5 as the UI implementation technology. Additionally, as the FHIR standard matures, the SMART app collaborates closely with the HL7 standard and adopts FHIR as the standard for data models and APIs.

As long as a healthcare institution's HIS or EMR system supports the FHIR standard, the SMART app can be installed and used. The SMART app automatically populates patient-related information and runs predictive models to derive risk prediction results based on the data scope permitted by the user, using FHIR standard interfaces for access.

7.5.2 Virtual Reality Remote Surgery

Some complex surgical cases require real-time assistance from another professional surgeon, yet the on-site efficiency of the surgeon is not high. Researchers have developed several digital technologies for such situations, including video-assisted systems, remote monitoring systems, telemedicine systems, and remote rendering. These technologies aim to support remote collaboration. Over the past few decades, remote surgery platforms have been developed, but due to cost barriers and lack of flexibility, they have not been widely promoted globally.

The point-to-point communication mode of remote consultation and remote surgery requires the transmission of large amounts of medical imaging data. However, the technological conditions under 4G are far from meeting the quality requirements for such data transmission. The emergence of 5G technology ensures the operability of remote surgery in terms of network communication technology. The key to 5G technology lies in high-quality medical imaging data transmission. Medical experts can use this data to remotely guide on-site doctors during surgery. With the concept of remote rendering introduced, 5G technology has become an indispensable part of remote medical applications, such as using VR glasses based on 5G technology to observe virtual scenes in the operating room and using high-precision robotic arms to perform surgery instead of manual operation by doctors. VR technology greatly expands the scope of surgery while ensuring the safety of doctors, such as in cases involving patients with severe infectious diseases or in battlefield environments.

A 5G-based remote VR surgery system generally includes VR glasses, control handles, transmission modules, panoramic cameras, and VR robotic arms, as shown in Fig. 7.4. Through 3D panoramic cameras arranged at the surgical site to collect information on the entire surgical process and environment, and 5G networks transmitting the collected image information to the 3D fusion controller, the fusion controller converts the information into signals visible in VR glasses. Doctors can then intuitively understand the surgical site and patient's condition through VR glasses from a first-person perspective and remotely control VR robotic arms to perform surgery by operating the control handles.

Further realizing remote rendering technology is augmented reality (AR) technology. AR is defined as "a technology that overlays computer-generated images onto a user's real-world view to provide a composite view." AR provides a real-time representation of the real-world environment, where computer-generated images

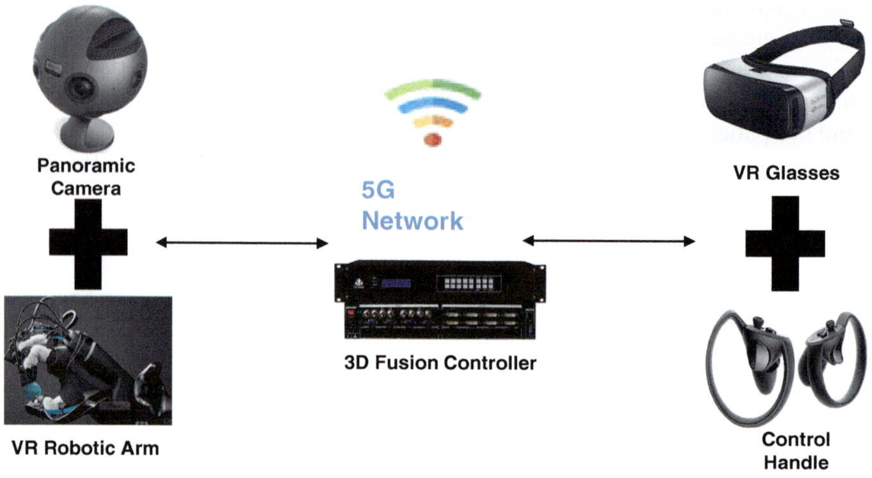

Fig. 7.4 5G based remote VR surgical system

are overlaid onto a continuous visual "canvas," creating an enhanced composite image. Although video conferencing technology has previously been successfully used as an alternative setting for remote guidance, its application in on-site surgery is still limited. In contrast, augmented reality technology allows remote surgeons to use a combination of gestures, annotations, charts, and clinical imaging to outline necessary procedural steps in a step-by-step manner. This technology surpasses simple one-way video or telephone communication: augmented reality elements allow remote surgeons to "show" how to perform surgery rather than simply "tell" remote surgeons how to operate.

Proximie is a secure, cloud-based augmented reality platform overseas that allows local surgeons (operating) and remote surgeons (assisting) to collaborate in real time using a bird's-eye view of the surgical field. The two surgeons communicate via bidirectional audio and utilize many integrated augmented reality features. For example, remote surgeons can use a webcam to insert their hands into the virtual surgical field or use a series of annotation and drawing tools to highlight important structures. In 2016, a surgeon in Beirut, Lebanon, assisted surgeons in Gaza, Palestine, through the platform in reconstructive surgery on an 18-year-old male's hand. Currently, one of the latest technologies is mixed reality, which can meet the essential requirements of remote rendering. The introduction of this technology helps combine the real world and virtual world for remote collaboration. In the case of remote collaboration, mixed reality technology can overcome the limitations of existing technologies and achieve a combination of augmented reality and virtual reality to obtain accurate results. This concept is referred to as the reality-virtuality continuum.

Overall, the application of VR technology and AR technology has made breakthrough progress in the field of remote surgery, allowing remote surgery to no longer be limited to remote consultation and not just remote guidance through images, but also demonstration through remote operation, even directly performing surgery on patients, enabling patients to receive higher quality medical treatment.

7.5.3 5G Pre-hospital Emergency Care

The main processes of pre-hospital emergency care include handling at the accident scene and patient transportation, as shown in Fig. 7.5. Data from pre-hospital emergency care is typically not integrated electronically, and there is a lack of effective communication methods for aggregating, transmitting, and reusing data between ambulances and trauma centers. To address this issue, it is necessary to ensure accurate, comprehensive, real-time, and continuous information sharing between on-site medical personnel, command centers, ambulances, and hospitals. This places extremely high demands on the transmission rate, bandwidth, latency, and stability of network communication. The characteristics of 5G, such as high bandwidth, low latency, and reliable stability, meet the requirements of remote medical applications in pre-hospital emergency care [2].

In 2019, the Second Affiliated Hospital of Zhejiang University School of Medicine conducted innovative exploration in the field of remote medical care in pre-hospital emergency care and pioneered the "multidimensional 5G smart emergency green channel." The "5G Remote Emergency Command Center" within the hospital integrates multiple subsystems, including the in-hospital emergency command center, VR immersive real-time remote command, 5G remote ultrasound, 5G

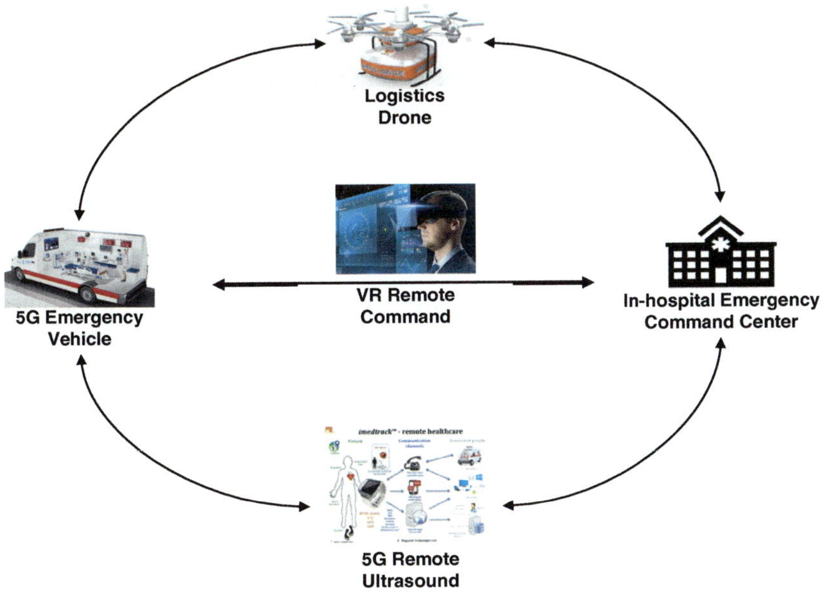

Fig. 7.5 Composition of 5G pre-hospital emergency system

ambulance transportation, and logistics drones, to establish a real-time data exchange and interconnection multidimensional pre-hospital emergency care system through the 5G network.

Through the 5G remote ultrasound system and 5G ambulance, doctors can perform ultrasound examinations on patients during transportation to the hospital and monitor the real-time vital signs of patients (including blood pressure, heart rate, blood oxygen saturation, temperature, etc.), and synchronize medical information in real time to the large screen of the in-hospital emergency command center, achieving real-time monitoring and assessment of patient conditions and reaching the goal of information synchronization. Meanwhile, the introduction of the VR remote command system allows doctors and experts within the hospital to have a complete understanding of the situation inside the ambulance and achieve remote medical guidance, further promoting the standardization of pre-hospital and in-hospital medical quality, saving the overall treatment time for patients, and improving the treatment rate of patients.

After achieving real-time synchronization of patient information, the in-hospital emergency team can quickly determine the required emergency supplies for the patient. Once there is a shortage of supplies, such as blood or small reserves of drugs, emergency supplies need to be quickly deployed from other hospital areas or medical institutions. Given the current traffic conditions, small-scale supplies can be rapidly delivered by drones, and the entire flight process of the drones can be monitored in real-time through the 5G network.

The 5G pre-hospital emergency care system is a comprehensive application of remote medical systems and mobile medical systems. This advancement not only makes comprehensive recording along clinical pathways possible but also ensures essential continuity of care. It also expands remote medical consultations from consultations between hospitals to remote medical consultations between pre-hospital and in-hospital settings, enhancing the coverage of high-quality medical services. This also demonstrates the close relationship between the development of remote medical care, mobile medical care, and the progress of information technology.

7.6 Summary

Telemedicine and mobile health are the products of the integration of multiple disciplines such as medicine, informatics, and engineering, as well as the inevitable outcomes of the development of healthcare. Telemedicine and mobile health are covering various aspects of the entire medical process, extending medical services from hospitals to communities and even to individual homes. With the improvement of information technology, the quality of telemedicine and mobile health has also been technically assured, overcoming the spatial and temporal challenges faced by traditional healthcare. This not only improves the quality of medical services received by patients but also provides greater convenience for doctors.

To better promote the development of telemedicine and mobile health, more national level policies have been introduced, laws and regulations have been continuously improved, and informatization has further developed. More high-quality medical resources have been invested, and China's telemedicine and mobile health have entered a stage of rapid development. However, the current telemedicine services are mainly concentrated in large hospitals and economically developed areas. How to better extend telemedicine services to primary healthcare institutions, optimize the allocation of medical resources, promote the sharing of regional medical resources, enable more people to enjoy telemedicine, and promote the healthier development of telemedicine are all issues that need to be addressed in the future.

References

1. Baker J, Stanley A. Telemedicine technology: a review of services, equipment, and other aspects. Curr Allergy Asthma Rep. 2018;18(11):60.
2. Gaebel J, Bockelmann C, Dekorsy A, et al. Requirements for 5G integrated data transfer in German prehospital emergency care. Curr Dir Biomed. 2020;6(3):912.

Public Health Information Systems

8

Contents

8.1 Overview of Public Health Information Systems 208
8.1.1 Introduction to Public Health Information Systems 208
8.1.2 Development History of Public Health Information Systems 210
8.1.2.1 United States 210
8.1.2.2 Canada 211
8.1.2.3 Japan 211
8.1.2.4 China 211
8.1.3 Current State of Domestic and International Research on Public Health Information Systems 213
8.2 Data Sources and Architectural Composition of Public Health Information Systems 215
8.2.1 Data Sources of Public Health Information Systems 215
8.2.2 Architectural Composition of Public Health Information Systems 218
8.3 Public Health Information Systems and Personal Health Statistics 223
8.3.1 Comprehensive and Lifelong Personal Electronic Health Records 223
8.3.2 Population Statistics Analysis 227
8.3.3 Health Statistics Analysis 229
8.4 Case Study 231
8.4.1 CDC's INPHO System in the USA 231
8.4.2 Australia's Public Health Information System Response to the COVID-19 Transition 232
8.4.3 Infectious Disease Surveillance and Early Warning Platform Based on Big Data in Yinzhou District, Ningbo City 233
8.5 Cutting-Edge Research 236
8.5.1 Early Warning and Efficient Response to Emerging Major Infectious Diseases 236
8.5.1.1 Strengthen Data Sharing and Integration Between Medical Institutions and Health Department Information Systems, Breaking Down Information Barriers 238
8.5.1.2 Improving Infectious Disease Monitoring and Analysis Methods 238
8.5.1.3 Leveraging the Advantages of Joint Prevention and Control to Build and Improve Infectious Disease Monitoring Management Platforms 239
8.5.2 Identification of Occupational Health Risk Factors 240
8.5.3 Public Health Event Early Warning Based on Social Networks 244
8.6 Summary 246
References 247

J. Li et al., *Healthcare Information Systems*, Innovative Medical Devices,
https://doi.org/10.1007/978-981-97-9551-2_8

At present, the public health information systems (PHIS) constructed in our country are mostly applied according to specific fields and scopes, and they are relatively closed systems from each other, thus forming "information islands." This prevents interconnection, interoperability, and information sharing among them. It fails to fully realize digitalization and intelligence at the "group" level and cannot meet the needs of life cycle health management services. Therefore, as an important content of implementing, the national informatization development and an important means of implementing medical reform, accelerating and standardizing the informatization of public health has become a key construction content.

Facing the contradiction between the demand and supply of public health services, medical informatization is a powerful means to improve the capacity of basic public health services and enhance the level of scientific management, the quality and efficiency of health services.

8.1 Overview of Public Health Information Systems

8.1.1 Introduction to Public Health Information Systems

With the development of emerging information technologies on the Internet such as cloud computing, countries have begun to establish public health information systems in the field of public health, aiming to achieve interconnection and data sharing among systems. These systems are committed to monitoring public health factors, improving the health level of the whole population, and enhancing the scientific decision-making and management capabilities for coping with public health emergencies by monitoring disease risk factors, as well as improving the prevention and control capabilities of major diseases and public safety.

The establishment of the public health information system is based on public health information, and when it comes to public health information, it is necessary to clearly define public health first. Public health takes society and groups as the objects, uses macro-control, supervision and law enforcement, and publicity and education as means, takes controlling group diseases and improving the level of public health as the center, and mobilizes social forces to jointly improve the health level of the whole population. Therefore, issues and factors related to population health and diseases can all be included in the research scope of public health, and the corresponding information is public health information. As shown in Fig. 8.1, public health information is mainly divided into the following four parts: disease monitoring and health monitoring related to detection, and medical treatment and command decision-making related to response. Among them, disease monitoring and medical treatment aim at prevention and control, while health monitoring and command decision-making aim at supervision and decision-making.

The public health information system is an essential component of public health infrastructure and an important tool for public health. Public health decision-making largely depends on the timeliness and reliability of information acquisition. The role of the public health information system is to generate, analyze, and utilize this data. With the continuous expansion of public health data sources and the development of

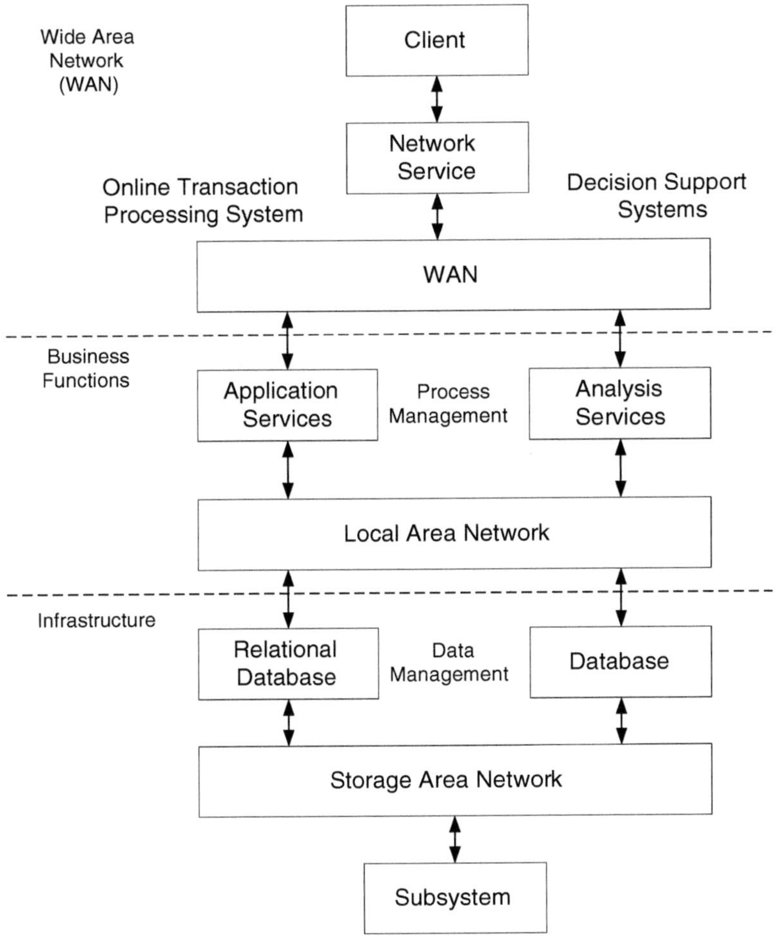

Fig. 8.1 Public health information

Internet technology, the role of the public health information system in public decision-making is becoming more and more important. It provides information for public health services and management decisions, covers various fields of public health, and plays an irreplaceable role in epidemiological monitoring, health outcome evaluation, planning and clinical management, program evaluation and performance measurement, public health planning, and policy analysis.

In practical application, the public health information system has two major aspects: service-based and population-based. First, the information system is used to store and provide service data that reflect the activities of public health organizations and other health-related entities. Second, the information system stores and provides population-based data, which are very important for public health monitoring, program evaluation, policy formulation, and decision-making on priorities. These two common applications are not separate but widely interact with each other.

As a multifunctional platform, the public health information system has a wide range of functions. For ordinary patients, the system can collect, store, and manage their electronic medical records to improve treatment; for clinical doctors, the system can provide multiple patient samples, use the advantages of big data to provide information for research, and support medical solutions; for hospitals, the system can help formulate operation management policies, and also obtain the treatment history of patients in other medical institutions by accessing public health records; for health officials, it can help formulate correct and effective public health policies, especially for public health emergencies that require rapid decision-making. From the national macro perspective, with the help of the public health information system, not only can health data be used to improve the health level of the whole population, but population health trends can also be analyzed and medical costs can be effectively reduced.

In April 2018, the General Office of the State Council issued the "Opinions on Promoting the Development of 'Internet + Medical Health'," which put forward 14 specific opinions from 3 aspects: improving the "Internet + Medical Health" service system, improving the "Internet + Medical Health" support system, and strengthening industry supervision and security. In December 2020, in order to further promote and standardize the construction and application of national public health informatization, the National Health Commission and the National Administration of Traditional Chinese Medicine jointly formulated the "National Public Health Informatization Construction Standards and Specifications (Trial)," which clarified the development direction of China's public health informatization construction for the next 5–10 years.

8.1.2 Development History of Public Health Information Systems

The development and construction of the public health information system in various countries have gone through different stages in accordance with specific national conditions. But in general, after decades of development, developed countries have built a more mature public health information system and are in fierce competition in effective management and technical upgrades. The following takes the USA, Canada, Japan, and China as examples to introduce the development history of the public health information system of each country.

8.1.2.1 United States

The USA began to establish professional public health functional institutions in the twentieth century and started the development of health informatization in the 1960s. However, the real large-scale medical informatization construction started in 1996, when the National Committee on Vital and Health Statistics (NCVHS) began the standardization of medical information. From 1996 to 2004, the United States' medical informatization was still in the exploratory stage. In 2004, President Bush of the United States issued Executive Order No. 13335, setting a clear goal for the USA to achieve electronic medical records within 10 years. In 2005, in order to provide targeted suggestions and implementation plans for medical informatization, the U.S. government established a new advisory committee. In 2009, President Obama of the United States issued Executive Order No. 13507, which clearly included medical informatization in the new U.S. medical reform. After half a century of development, the scope of U.S. public health informatization has gradually expanded, from the stage of independent application of medical institutions to the stage of regional health informatization construction, and then gradually developed to the stage of overall network construction of the national medical and health service system.

8.1.2.2 Canada

The construction of Canada's health informatization has mainly gone through three stages: infrastructure construction stage, information sharing stage, and information application stage. The main strategic goal of the first stage was to formulate the future development goals and gradual plans of the public health information system, and to integrate the construction of medical and health services; the second stage shifted the strategic focus to achieving interconnection between systems, and the construction of electronic files was developed in this stage; the strategic goal of the third stage was to integrate the EMR system on the basis of the second stage, so that it can span different medical entities and achieve its application in different medical institutions.

8.1.2.3 Japan

Due to factors such as economy and technology, Japan's development of public health information systems is leading among Asian countries. In the 1990s, Japan gradually established a national strategy focused on the development of information technology. Driven by this strategy, the "e-Japan Strategy" was formulated and implemented in 2001. The "New IT Reform Strategy" was released in 2006, which further planned the construction of medical and health informatization, emphasizing the promotion of interconnection and information sharing between medical institutions' information systems. In 2009, the "i-Japan Strategy 2015" was formulated, applying digital technology and informatization to medical reform, focusing on the development of telemedicine and electronic health records, paving a new way to solve social issues such as an aging population, insufficient and unevenly distributed medical care resources.

8.1.2.4 China

The development of China's public health information system is also divided into the following three stages.

The first stage was from 1999 to 2009, a decade of data accumulation. In 1999, China took the first step in public medical informatization—the Golden Card Project. This project achieved a breakthrough from 0 to 1 in the informatization of some hospitals in China. However, it was the outbreak of Severe Acute Respiratory Syndrome (SARS) in 2003 that brought the issue of medical informatization to the attention of central and local governments and led to rapid development.

The SARS epidemic exposed many problems in China's public health sector, greatly affecting the prevention and control of the epidemic, with the lack of public health informatization being particularly prominent. In response to this issue, the government began to promote medical informatization nationwide. The Ministry of Health issued the "National Health Informatization Development Plan Outline (2003–2010)" to strengthen the construction of informatization related to disease control. During this period, medical informatization construction was centered on clinical practice, carried out in various medical institutions, building systems such as LIS, PACS, and rational drug use monitoring, while gradually connecting hospitals with local medical insurance and the new rural cooperation systems. Data shows that China's medical informatization market size rapidly developed from about 1.3 billion yuan in 2001 to about 5.8 billion yuan in 2007, with an average annual growth rate of over 20%. Although China's medical informatization developed rapidly during this period, due to weak software and hardware foundations, China's level of informatization was still relatively low compared to foreign countries, and China was still in a stage of data accumulation.

The second stage was from 2009 to 2019, a decade of data integration. After the initial stage of data accumulation, with the rapid development of "Internet +", medical informatization also entered the fast lane. In 2008, medical informatization construction was included in medical reform for the first time, emphasizing the acceleration of the construction of medical and health information systems focusing on resident health files, hospital management, and electronic medical records. In 2011, the Ministry of Health formulated the "2011–2015 Health Informatization Development Plan," and in order to promote and standardize the development of electronic medical records, it successively issued documents such as "Basic Standards and Functional Specifications for Electronic Medical Records," "Basic Architecture and Data Standards for Electronic Medical Records," "Grading Evaluation Methods and Standards for the Level of Functional Application of Electronic Medical Record Systems," and "Technical Solutions for Hospital Information Platform Construction Based on Electronic Medical Records." In 2013, the government issued documents to promote the application of health medical big data, issued electronic medical record application management specifications, and the construction of medical consortiums entered the pilot work. In 2015, the General Office of the State Council issued the "National Medical and Health Service System Planning Outline (2015–2020)," marking the national comprehensive promotion of population health informatization construction, with the core content summarized as "46,312," that is, it is planned to build a 4-level health information platform at the national, provincial, and municipal levels by 2020, 6 business systems including public health, medical services, family planning, medical insurance, drug management, and comprehensive management, 3 basic databases including electronic health records, electronic medical records, and the entire population's personal data, a unified population health network, and 2 systems for information security and information standards. It also requires hospitals to take electronic medical records as the core and interconnect with the population health information platform to achieve information sharing inside and outside the hospital.

A series of policies have greatly promoted the development of the medical information industry. Data shows that from 2008 to 2018, China's medical informatization market size grew from about 7.2 billion yuan to as high as 49.2 billion yuan, with the market size increasing by about 7 times in 10 years.

The third stage is from 2019 to 2029, a decade of data application. With the gradual maturity of information system construction, China's medical informatization construction has entered a new stage. In 2018, the National Health Commission issued the "National Hospital Informatization Construction Standards and Specifications (Trial)," and subsequent policies on specific aspects such as electronic medical records, Internet medical treatment, tiered diagnosis and treatment, and interconnection have clarified the direction for the future development of domestic hospital informatization. In the next few years, with the large-scale deployment of new national infrastructure, medical informatization has great potential in upgrading business-end products and expanding the consumer market. In recent years, policies have continuously promoted the penetration and development of medical informatization from hospital information systems that lead management and payment to clinical diagnosis and treatment informatization, and more clinical data applications and internal and external information sharing will be realized in the future.

8.1.3 Current State of Domestic and International Research on Public Health Information Systems

Research on public health information systems has developed greatly both domestically and internationally, with different focuses in different countries as they develop.

Represented by some developed countries in Europe and America, they have rich experience in building and maintaining public health service systems and information systems. They are often supported by government special funds, using top-level planning and unified standards to achieve business collaboration and interconnection between subsystems.

As a pioneer in medical informatization, the USA is currently in a leading position in the development of public health informatization systems. The USA has established the Office of the National Coordinator for Health Information Technology (ONC), which is responsible for planning medical informatization. In 2014, ONC released the "US Federal Government Health Informatization Strategic Plan (2015–2020)," clarifying the application goals of the US information system construction in the next 5 years: to enhance the capacity of medical services, improve the health level of the public and communities, and promote research and innovation in medical knowledge.

In the construction of public health informatization systems, the USA has always taken data as the core content. The United States Department of Health and Human Services (HHS) manages the national-level health data open platform. As a federal government website, its data content covers various fields of public health, including clinical service quality information, a directory of national health service providers, the latest medical and scientific knowledge database, consumer product data, community health performance information, government expenditure data, etc.

Looking at the current situation of medical informatization implementation, the informatization of US medical services is still in the implementation stage, and the medical informatization strategy formulated and implemented by the government is gradually proceeding; looking at the current situation of medical informatization technology, with the technical advantages of many high-tech companies, the USA is vigorously developing new medical informatization technologies in recent years. For example: Google has cooperated with American medical centers to establish electronic files for millions of community patients, which can achieve remote monitoring by doctors; Microsoft has also launched a new medical informatization service platform to help doctors, patients, and their families understand the latest situation in real-time; Intel has launched a digital medical platform, which helps doctors and patients interact through Internet technology.

The UK has also made information system construction one of the directions for the development of public health. In order to achieve a unified national public health information system, the UK has invested 5.5 billion pounds to build a medical information storage service system, which collects and stores data from more than 23,000 medical information systems in the country, covering medical information for more than 50 million residents, and has served the work of 1.3 million medical personnel.

Similar to the USA, the UK's National Health Service (NHS) has a huge and comprehensive medical data set, including patients' health records and disease data. As of April 2018, the UK's public data official website had 2148 health-related data sets, including general practice medical services, prescription and drug records, the number of registered patients in general practice, hospital data, smoking, drinking, obesity, sports, diet, and other report data. In addition, the UK also has a 200-year national census health record, which can create more value for public health services and medical research and is also of great value for studying the UK's medical health service system.

Japan, in the process of building a public health information system, not only focuses on public health but also pays great attention to the development of the information industry and the control of medical costs. Taking the affiliated hospital of Fukuyama University as an example, the hospital has accumulated more than 17 million medical records, 143 million medication prescriptions, and 3 million disease names. Based on these data and technical support, it can now achieve automatic analysis and matching of prescriptions. In terms of controlling medical expenses, due to the impact of an aging population, it is estimated that Japan's medical expenses will double by 2025 compared to 2012. To this end, since 2015, the government has used the diagnosis and treatment remuneration details in the public health system to control medical expenses, using big data analysis to calculate the composition of wasteful medical expenses, prompting local governments to set specific numbers to control medical costs. The government expects to cut 5 trillion yen in medical expenses by 2025 based on the expected costs, and controlling the public health information system based on big data has become an important means.

Compared with the more mature construction examples of public health information systems in the above-developed countries, China is still in the initial stage in this field. The 2003 SARS epidemic exposed the serious problems of China's lagging public health development and the imperfect mechanism for dealing with public health emergencies. Faced with a series of problems exposed by the public health information system during the epidemic, such as incomplete epidemic information reporting, poor monitoring timeliness, small coverage of health information networks, and poor information integration capabilities, the country has given unprecedented attention to the research, establishment, and improvement of the public health system. During this period, the public health information system has also made great progress.

After years of rapid development, many regions in China have built regional health information platforms. These platforms can be divided into provincial, municipal, and district levels according to the coverage area. The regional health information platform is based on serving the health of residents. On the basis of the regional health information platform, China's public health information system is also gradually developing, but unlike the regional health information platform, which focuses more on blockiness, public health business pays more attention to processes.

Different from foreign countries, the construction of China's public health information system relies on national public data, covering various levels of health administrative units, extending to various urban and rural communities, while also strengthening the construction of legalization and standardization, and standardizing the collection, organization, and analysis of information to ensure information quality. In order to improve the scientific decision-making and emergency command capabilities of public health, China has also established a three-level early warning and emergency command system for national, provincial, and municipal epidemics and public health emergencies.

8.2 Data Sources and Architectural Composition of Public Health Information Systems

8.2.1 Data Sources of Public Health Information Systems

In today's era where "data is king," data is an extremely valuable resource. The core of any public health information system is the data it contains. For a public health information system, whether it is for user diagnosis, disease research, or scientific decision-making, accurate data is needed as support. The implementation of these functions requires not only data collected by a single information system but also association with various types and channels of health data. For example, associating data from disease reports with data on food sales, restaurant inspections, and drug sales can more truly and comprehensively reflect the dietary hygiene of residents. Therefore, the data sources for a public health information system are not limited to the health system but also involve departments such as food and drug, and industrial and commercial departments. Only by obtaining a variety of data and then performing correlation analysis on it can the greatest value of these data be realized.

For these data, it is essential to ensure their accuracy and completeness. Generally, there are two ways to collect data: paper collection and electronic collection. In some health information systems, information is collected on paper through questionnaires and then transmitted to a computer by data entry clerks. In other systems, clinical or technical personnel use electronic methods to collect and transmit data using computers or mobile phones and other devices. There is no absolute advantage or disadvantage to the two data sources. Using electronic data collection methods means faster collection and processing of larger amounts of data, and the probability of data recording errors is lower because paper information is more likely to be lost or damaged irreversibly. However, this also requires the design of a well-functioning electronic system; otherwise, it would be counterproductive, causing difficulties in data collection or even data loss.

Based on the determination of the collection method, a specific analysis of the data to be collected is carried out. However, it is important to note that when analyzing the data to be collected, it is necessary to combine business needs at the same time, and divide the necessary data into different modules according to their characteristics. Taking the monitoring of infectious disease outbreaks as an example, the necessary data modules to be collected include the patient's demographic characteristics, basic contact methods, basic information of the hospital/medical institution, basic information of the patient's symptoms, basic information of the patient's diagnosis and treatment, laboratory test information, basic information of epidemiological investigation, and review information. For each module, it is necessary to analyze and determine the required data items separately. These data items must meet the business needs of the corresponding module. These complex data may have more complex sources, as shown in Fig. 8.2. From the perspective of the unit they belong to, they can come from various levels of medical centers, physical examination centers, health and health committees, and various regional medical centers; from the perspective of each subsystem, they can come from common disease grading systems, targeted therapy systems, vaccination systems, etc.

In different levels of the information system, the demand and supply of data change in a complex way. As shown in Fig. 8.3, as the level gradually develops toward a higher and more macro level, the functions of the public health information system also gradually transition from specific implementation to strategic decision-making. Correspondingly, the data required at each level is different, and the data sources are also different. At the individual and community level, effective clinical management and home visits can obtain information that meets community needs. At the provincial and municipal level, public health information should enable

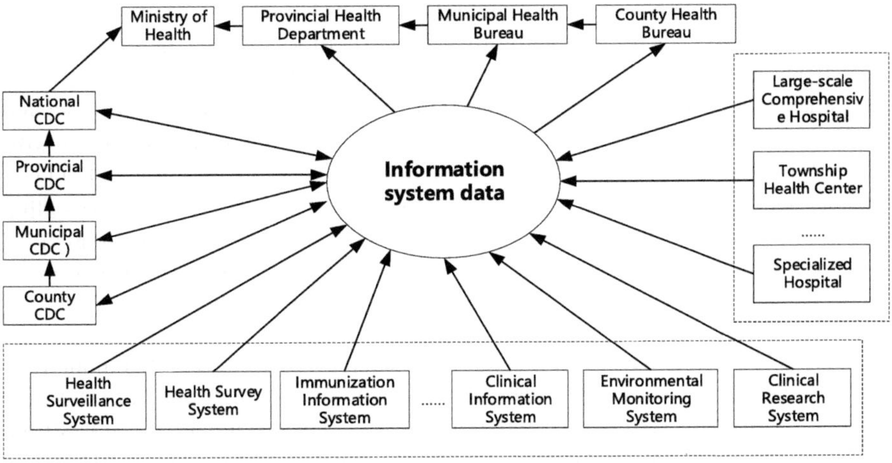

Fig. 8.2 Data sources of public health information systems

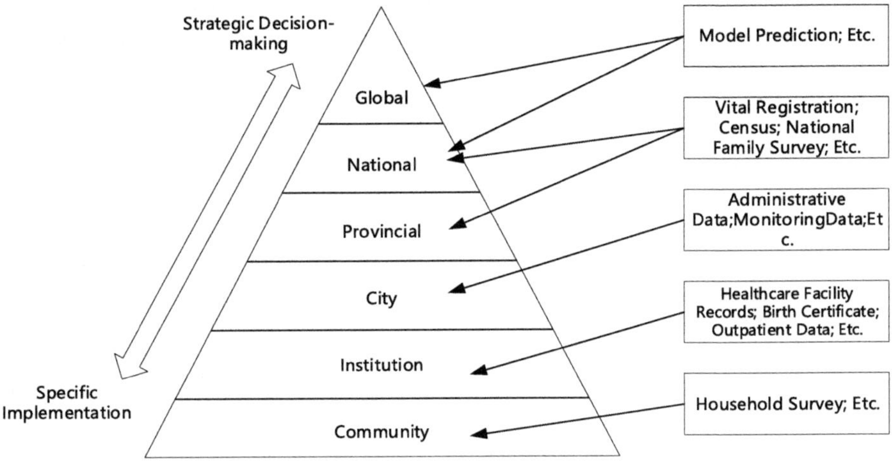

Fig. 8.3 Data sources vary by different levels

health administrators to instantly grasp the operation of health facilities and the entire health system. At a higher level, health information should serve strategic decision-making and resource allocation. There are different data needs and sources at each level, but these data are closely linked together. For example, the census is planned by the country, but the data is generated by individuals. Population data is analyzed and used at both the national and subnational levels.

Traditional public health information systems are generally government-led. Due to different organizational departments and scope of application, they have formed their own independent closed data systems. These systems still use a centralized data model that is reported layer by layer, resulting in data systems between departments that are basically "parallel relationships," unable to connect and communicate directly. Therefore, there are some difficulties when a large-scale real-time dynamic data collaboration is needed in the face of public health emergencies and other scenarios. With the development of new technologies, data collection sources have also undergone tremendous changes. Distributed information systems can expand the collection range of public health data to every citizen in society through the integration of the Internet of Things and other technologies. The daily information that this system can collect includes the population's mobility status and geographical location, etc. Based on this data, public health emergencies can be prevented early, or the response and intervention efficiency can be improved after the event occurs.

It should be noted that unlike the unified and standardized data structure in financial application scenarios, large-scale data collection in public health scenarios will inevitably involve a variety of heterogeneous data. These data have complex relationships and numerous attributes. This means that the data collection dimension must also develop toward a refined direction, gradually transitioning from large particles to small particles. Taking the collection of basic health information of citizens as an example, the traditional public health collection dimensions are nothing more than relatively static large particle fields such as gender, age, and occupation. Although these dimensions are closely related to individual health status, collecting only this data means losing the diversity and difference information of each individual within the group. This approach is difficult to statically simplify and summarize the health status and geographical location of individuals that make up the group, and it is precisely these dynamic changes that constitute the basis of public health prevention, monitoring, and decision-making. Therefore, in the construction of public health information systems, it is necessary to realize that the dynamic behavior of the group needs to be included in the monitoring. When making public health decisions, it is necessary to consider the complex and dynamic social behaviors of the group. The real-time data fluctuations generated by these behaviors, especially those that can reflect changes in location and environment, should be an important source of system data.

8.2.2 Architectural Composition of Public Health Information Systems

The fundamental network architecture principle of China's public health information system is "vertical to the end, horizontal to the side." The "vertical" aspect establishes a five-level network and three-level platform, while the "horizontal" aspect creates a regional public health information network. As shown in Fig. 8.4, the five-level network relies on the national public data network to establish a bidirectional information transmission network connecting township, county (district), city (prefecture), provincial, and national levels of health administrative departments and healthcare institutions, forming a virtual private network for the national PHIS; the three-level platform involves establishing three levels of public health

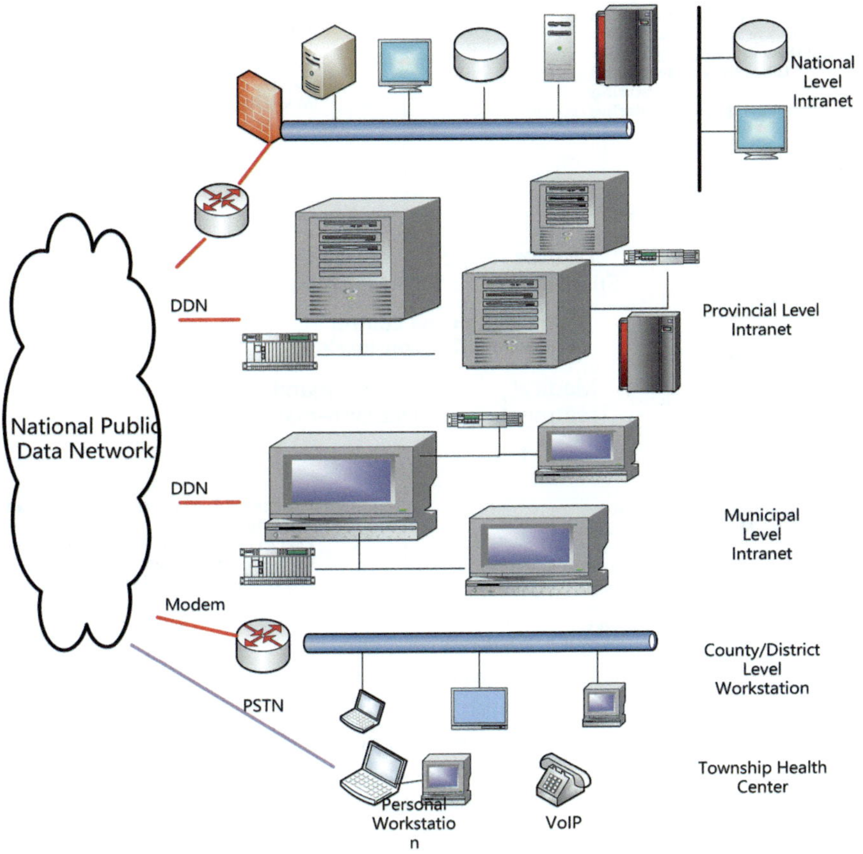

Fig. 8.4 China's five-level network of public health information systems

information network platforms at the prefecture (city), provincial, and national levels [1].

"Horizontal to the side" means, in accordance with regional health planning requirements and the principle of local management, on the basis of constructing the prefecture (city) level public health information network platform, various health administrative departments, disease prevention and control departments, community health information systems, and various medical institutions at all levels within the region, in accordance with unified requirements, rely on the national public data network to access the prefecture (city) public health information network platform, forming a regional health information network.

Looking at the network architecture, as shown in Fig. 8.5, the information system is generally divided into three layers: WAN, LAN, and SAN. The bottom layer provides infrastructure for the tiered architecture, maintained by technical support teams and data analysts, and must ensure high reliability of data, with features such as disaster recovery, disaster relief redundancy, and communication guarantees. At

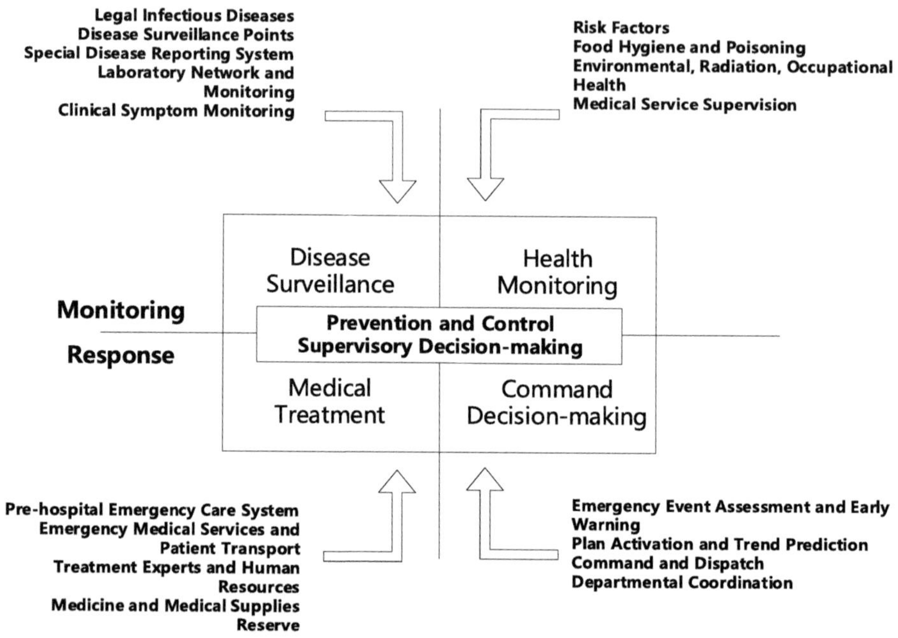

Fig. 8.5 Network architecture of public health information systems

the same time, it is necessary to define public interfaces, information exchange protocols, access control, etc., to ensure authority, achieve information integration between different subsystems, and support data reuse. The middle layer provides business support for the tiered architecture; businesses are often concentrated in scenarios such as hospitals and health supervision departments that require rapid response. The use of LAN can achieve interconnection within the department, ensuring the security and speed of data transmission. The top-level application scenarios cover almost all fields of public health, focusing on the collaborative effect between various fields, and meet the information needs of all parties through the wide area network to achieve public health decision-making.

Public health information systems can be divided into the following three types according to the deployment method.

The first structure: The system deploys applications and data in a hierarchical manner, and information sharing between levels is achieved through data exchange.

In this structure, operational data generated at lower-level applications is transmitted to upper levels based on demand. Lower levels have control over the data, including the scope, timing of uploads, and the ability to modify uploaded content. Data security is high, and each level of institution has high accessibility to data, as shown in Table 8.1. With applications deployed at lower levels, these institutions can integrate various applications through the regional health information platform, enabling data sharing, event-driven processes, and single sign-

Table 8.1 Characteristics of three application and data deployment structures

Structure	Data security	Data accessibility	Application convenience	Business rule consistency	Construction cost
1st	High	High	High	Low	High
2nd	Moderately high	Moderately low	Moderately low	High	Moderately low
3rd	Low	Low	High	High	Low

on functionalities. Integrating applications reduces redundant logins and data entry, while enhancing prompts and warning capabilities. This structure improves system flexibility; however, since applications and data control reside at lower levels, integration methods and structural rules may lack uniformity, necessitating constraints from higher level institutions. As each business process may be segmented across several levels, achieving business process alignment between levels requires substantial time. Hence, this structure incurs the highest development costs and longest construction cycles.

The second structure: The system centrally deploys applications and data at a certain level, and information sharing between levels is achieved through data exchange.

In this structure, data is centralized at a particular level, increasing security but potentially reducing accessibility of data across levels. Upper levels can control the scope and timing of data from lower levels. Because applications are concentrated at one level, integration with applications at the same level may not be possible, reducing structural flexibility. However, business logic can be uniformly controlled, leading to higher consistency in business rules. Compared to the first structure, construction costs are significantly lower. This structure represents a compromise between the first and third structures, balancing various indicators across different aspects.

The third structure: The system centrally deploys applications and data at a higher level, and if the application provides an export function, lower-level institutions can obtain relevant data.

This structure is known as the "cloud" structure, and it is also the structure most familiar to public health workers adopted during the "national major epidemic." Data being completely controlled by upper levels enhances data security but reduces accessibility of data across lower-level institutions. Business logic consistency, application convenience, and characteristics similar to the second structure are maintained in this structure. However, since this structure is built in the cloud, construction costs are minimized.

These three structures each have their own characteristics, as given in Table 8.1. There is no one-size-fits-all structure; each has its features suitable for different occasions. When facing different system applications, a comprehensive consideration is needed to determine the most suitable structure. Some business processes interact less with other systems' data and require higher internal data security. In such cases, adopting the third structure is most appropriate, such as for a mental health management system. Conversely, other businesses may have moderate security requirements but involve numerous internal entities and closely relate to diagnostic and treatment systems, demanding high application convenience. In these scenarios, the first structure is more appropriate, such as for managing diabetes or hypertension.

Currently, the development direction of public health information systems is the "Internet +" model, building a service platform with big data as the infrastructure and medical big data as the core content, for use by residents, doctors, medical companies, health management institutions, and other parties. To ensure the reliability and stability of the system, the current system architecture design often introduces the "middle platform" concept. The role of the "middle platform" is to extract reusable basic services within the system to form a separate guarantee platform, providing better service protection for the system while reducing reusability. Separating each core business line from the "middle platform" can lay a good foundation for the independent development of each business line. The overall system design using this architecture generally has three levels: back-end, middle platform, and front-end. The "back-end" is for information management personnel, covering the information of various business lines of public health, used to handle business logic; the "middle platform" is also for information management personnel, providing protection for the basic services needed for the operation of the "back-end," resource pooling the data and systems required by the back-end, and supervising these resources to ensure the normal provision of services; the "front-end" is for end-users, providing services to doctors, patients, and other audiences through web clients, mini-programs (apps), etc., and needs to pay attention to issues such as interactivity and esthetics.

The construction of the "middle platform" is the foundation of Internet + public health services, which specifically includes the "data middle platform," "technology middle platform," and "business middle platform." The "data middle platform," as the name suggests, is mainly responsible for data collection, exchange, governance, and utilization. The main role of the "technology middle platform" is to complete the construction of technical resources in the platform, supporting the release, operation, and supervision of public health services on the "business middle platform."

With the development of new generation technologies such as blockchain, the introduction of these technologies has greatly improved the stability and reliability of public health information systems. As shown in Fig. 8.6, using blockchain technology to build a distributed architecture is more reliable than other network architectures. Applying it to public health information systems can not only expand the data collection range of information systems but also increase social participation. Moreover, it can reduce the vulnerability of a single key node in traditional architectures through a distributed multi-node approach. In other words, even if some nodes in the system fail, the overall network can still operate normally, and the system can still work effectively, effectively overcoming the common "single point of failure" challenge in traditional information systems. In addition, the internal data of systems using blockchain technology are backed up in real-time by multiple nodes, so the system has strong resistance to attacks, and data is difficult to tamper with, allowing the system to recover quickly.

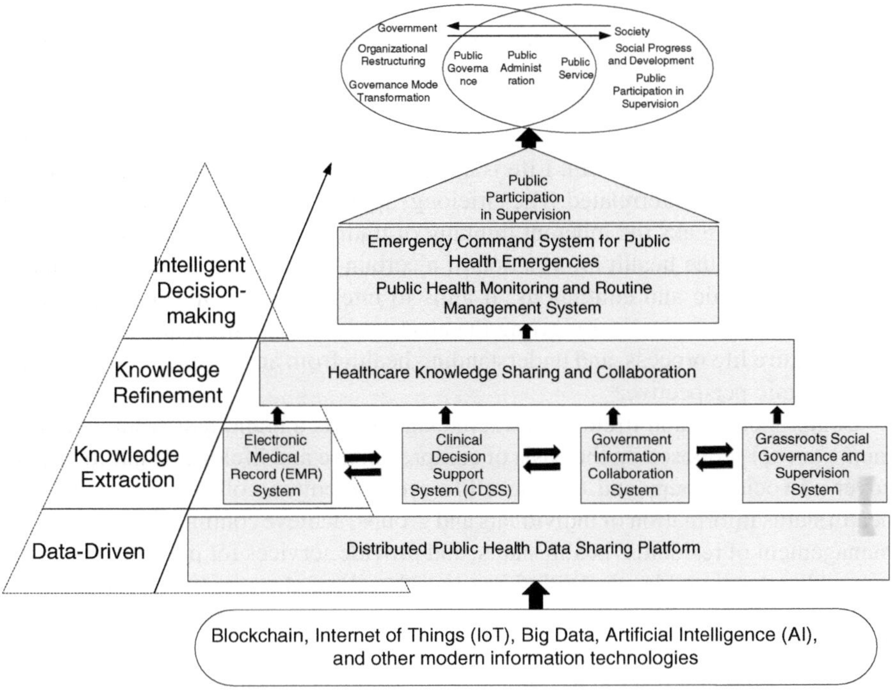

Fig. 8.6 New national public health information system construction model

8.3 Public Health Information Systems and Personal Health Statistics

8.3.1 Comprehensive and Lifelong Personal Electronic Health Records

Comprehensive and lifelong health refers to the process of an individual's good adaptation to physiological, psychological, and social states throughout the entire life course from birth to death. It is a dynamically changing phase. For a group, it is a summary of the health status of the entire societal group.

"Comprehensive" includes not only all health-related factors and health conditions of an individual but also the health status of all individuals in society. It is a comprehensive reflection of the health status of the entire social group. Compared to traditional health concepts, comprehensive and lifelong health is an expansion and sublimation from point to surface, from individual to whole, and from part to whole. It is more comprehensive and perfect. It extends the scope of health from individual to group, which is more in line with the characteristics of public health information field research that takes the group as the object. It is conducive to the analysis and development of various fields such as clinical medicine, social medicine, and preventive medicine, and helps the exchange and sharing of information between health supervision departments, health service departments, and other health service units at all levels, providing reference information for the rational allocation of health care resources.

"Lifelong" refers to the entire life process of an individual, covering the entire life course from birth to death. Life is a continuous and gradual process, and adjacent life stages are interrelated. The "lifelong" in the concept of comprehensive and lifelong health breaks the inherent thinking of traditional health concepts that only pay attention to the health information of a certain life stage. It makes the concept of health dynamic and continuous. It aims to integrate the health information of each life stage organically, reflecting the changes in health characteristics throughout the entire life process, and understanding health from an overall, developmental, and dynamic perspective.

Comprehensive and lifelong health management is a brand-new health management concept proposed on the basis of comprehensive and lifelong health. It aims to cover all social groups and the entire life cycle, monitor, collect, and analyze the health status information of individuals and groups, achieve continuous and dynamic management of residents' health status, and provide services for public health at the regional and national levels. With the proposal of the concept of comprehensive and lifelong health management, using computer technology and network information technology to build comprehensive and lifelong personal electronic health records is an inevitable trend in the development of China's medical and health undertakings. The overall framework of the regional health information platform based on comprehensive and lifelong personal electronic health records is shown in Fig. 8.7.

"Lifelong" includes ten life nodes of an individual's life cycle: fetal period, newborn period, infant period, toddler period, preschool period, school-age period, adolescence, young adulthood, middle age, and old age. "Comprehensive" includes 11 subsystems: Resident Health Record Subsystem, Immunization Planning Subsystem, Rehabilitation Medical Subsystem, Minor Health Care Subsystem, Women's Health Care Subsystem, Basic Medical Subsystem, Family Planning Technical Guidance Subsystem, Chronic Non-communicable Disease Special Management Subsystem, Communicable Disease Special Management Subsystem, Health Education Subsystem, and Life Event Registration Subsystem, with specific functions as follows.

1. Resident Health Record Subsystem This system combines personal, family, community, and regional health records to achieve dynamic management of residents' continuous and comprehensive health records. The personal health record (PHR) includes demographic information, lifestyle habits, medical history, current illness, physical examination information, and medical consultation information of residents. The personal health record, combined with family information, forms a family record, which, combined with community characteristics, forms a community record, and finally converges to the regional health information service platform.

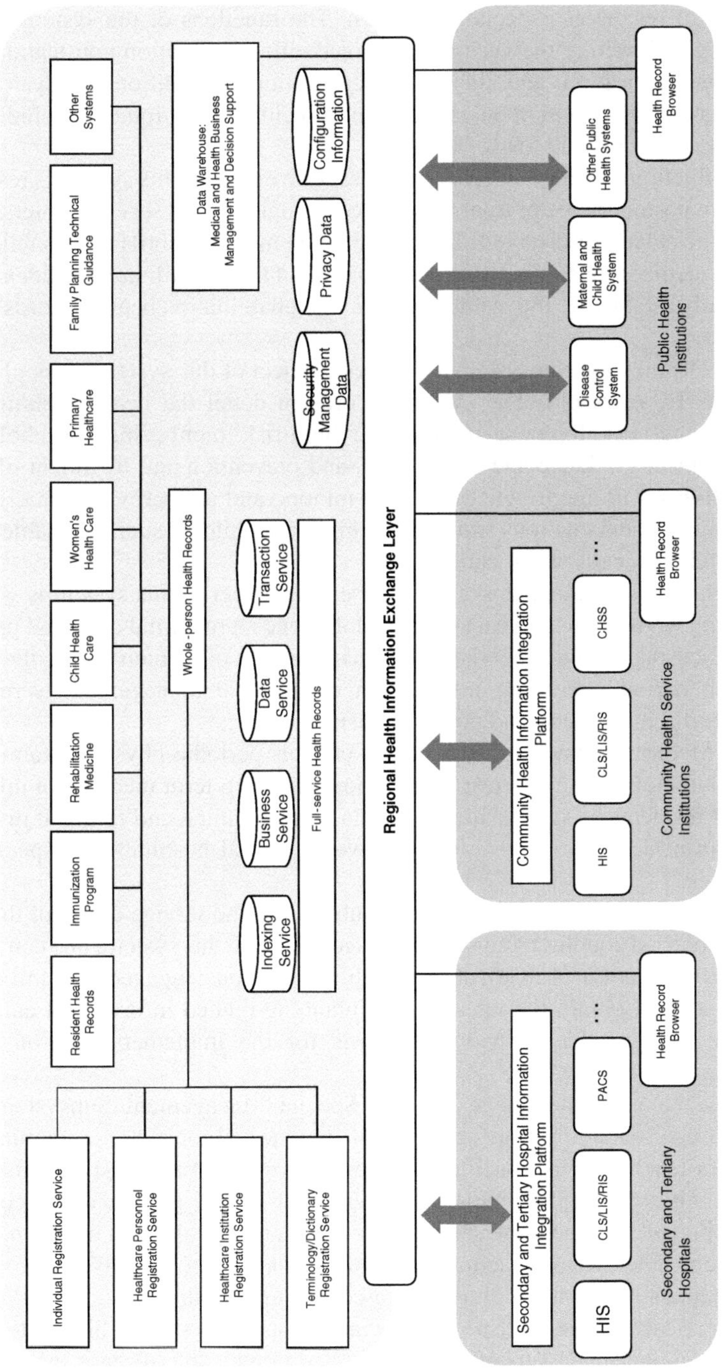

Fig. 8.7 Regional health information platform overall framework

2. Immunization Planning Subsystem This system manages the vaccination information of residents, especially children. The functions of the system include creating and writing the vaccination target's file, vaccination notification, vaccination registration, and side effect registration. In addition, the system can also manage information on vaccines and vaccination equipment, including the storage, issuance, and loss of vaccines.
3. Rehabilitation Medical Subsystem The service object of this system is residents who are postoperative or transferred to community health service centers, especially the elderly or disabled. The system dynamically records the rehabilitation needs, methods, and effectiveness evaluation of the rehabilitating residents, and gradually establishes the residents' personal rehabilitation health records in this process.
4. Minor Health Care Subsystem The service object of this system is people from birth to 18 years old. The system records in detail the health examination, growth and development monitoring, high-risk monitoring, psychological development guidance and assessment, and prevention and treatment of common diseases in the growth process of minors, and also provides timely early warning for the dangerous situations of high-risk children such as disabled children and physically weak children.
5. Women's Health Care Subsystem The service object of this system is women, covering women's health care during adolescence, premarital care, and prenatal care, focusing on the supervision and management of women during the childbearing period, recording information on prenatal management, screening, (childbirth) midwifery, and postnatal visits.
6. Basic Medical Subsystem This system collects periodic physical examination information, biochemical test information, and long-term medication information of residents, assists residents in managing common and frequent diseases, and can achieve two-way referral between general hospitals and specialized hospitals.
7. Family Planning Technical Guidance Subsystem The service object of this system is married couples of childbearing age. Through this system, one can timely grasp the situation of medical and health institutions engaged in family planning services, obtain the latest family planning-related information and technology, and provide a theoretical basis for the implementation of family planning technology.
8. Chronic Non-communicable Disease Special Management Subsystem This system can manage the information of common chronic non-communicable diseases (such as hypertension, diabetes, tumors, etc.) among residents, track and monitor the health status of residents for a long period, and record the development, treatment measures, and effectiveness evaluation of chronic non-communicable diseases, achieving a transformation from individual to group management methods for chronic non-communicable diseases.
9. Communicable Disease Special Management Subsystem This system can achieve digital management of residents' communicable disease information. Community health service centers are responsible for collecting and reporting

all residents' communicable disease information within the regional scope, including the occurrence, development, and treatment of communicable diseases, meeting the needs of various institutions such as hospitals, disease prevention and control centers, and community health service centers.
10. Health Education Subsystem This system is used to collect and record the health education information of residents in the community, and provide information related to various health and disease issues, imparting correct medical and health knowledge to families and individuals, helping residents develop good health habits, and promoting the healthy development of the entire society.
11. Life Event Registration Subsystem The Life Event Registration Subsystem primarily documents the births and deaths of residents. This information facilitates the timely identification of cases that may be fatal due to infectious diseases, providing early warning data to disease control centers to enable the prompt formulation of appropriate response measures. Additionally, the system can analyze the distribution of causes of death and monitor dynamic changes, offering valuable insights for disease prevention efforts.

8.3.2 Population Statistics Analysis

Population statistics analysis involves the examination of population numbers. By organizing and analyzing demographic data, one can identify patterns in population dynamics and describe the relationships between population factors and various socioeconomic elements. This process reveals the causes of specific population events or changes in population status, shedding light on underlying societal patterns. The aggregation of individual electronic health records within a region yields a wealth of demographic information. Utilizing this data for statistical analysis can provide a comprehensive understanding of the community's overall health and hygiene conditions. It can even offer risk warnings for certain diseases, which is invaluable in current public health monitoring.

One common method of demographic analysis is cohort analysis, which focuses on populations with shared characteristics. Based on electronic health records (EMRs), researchers have developed various algorithms and parameter settings for cohort studies, as given in Table 8.2. To date, the most successful EMR research has utilized well-defined databases from healthcare systems in the UK and the USA, where patient populations receive the majority or entirety of their medical services.

Researchers using EMRs can construct standard cohorts and group patients with specific diseases. For example, Kaiser Permanente in the USA has established multiple EMR-based cohorts, including the Diabetes Study of Northern California (DISTANCE). This study involves 20,000 diabetic patients and addresses numerous medical issues, such as diabetes in Asians and Pacific Islanders and the relationship between socioeconomic status and the risk of hypoglycemia [2].

An increasing number of researchers from health systems are conducting multi-system, multi-center cohort studies. A US cohort study on chronic hepatitis combined data from over 1.6 million adults across 4 healthcare systems to identify a

Table 8.2 Selected samples from electronic health record studies (population data from cohort studies)

Data source	Sample size range
Single Psychiatric Inpatient Ward	728–2010
Specialty Center/Clinic	544–10,017
Prison Network	370,511
Single Hospital	467–55,492
Multiple Hospitals	1074–25,241
Multiple Primary Care Institutions	7925–345,143
Healthcare System	2537–919,873
Consortium	8709–233,844
Centralized Anonymous Database	923–524,402

group of patients with hepatitis B and C. According to the chronic hepatitis cohort data, a study by Mahajan et al. found that among patients who died with documented liver disease and were hepatitis C positive, only 30% had hepatitis C recorded on their death certificates, indicating a significant underestimation of hepatitis C-related mortality in the USA.

Researchers have also collected study population data from centralized, anonymized databases, including the Clinical Data Analysis and Reporting System in Hong Kong, China, and the Clinical Practice Research Datalink (CPRD) [3], the Health Improvement Network (THIN), and QResearch studies in the UK [4]. The CPRD gathers data from over 500 general practitioners in the UK, with information on more than 5 million active pediatric and adult patients. These databases provide researchers with standardized, longitudinal data, facilitating cohort construction and statistical analysis.

With the proliferation of EMRs and increasing public concern over obesity, researchers have begun leveraging vast EMR datasets to construct cohorts and conduct demographic and population health research. Researchers are using large EMR datasets to re-evaluate conclusions drawn from previous smaller-scale studies. For instance, many small studies have reported a positive or inconsistent association between body mass index (BMI) in middle age and the risk of Alzheimer's disease in later life. Iwagami et al. used longitudinal CPRD data from two million individuals and found that higher BMI in middle age was associated with a lower risk of Alzheimer's disease, suggesting that obesity may protect against Alzheimer's or that weight loss may be a result of early Alzheimer's disease, both of which are important areas for future research [5]. In another study, Hibbard et al. used EMR data from the Consortium on Safe Labor (with 233,844 deliveries) to control for factors missing in previous birth outcome studies, such as the medical conditions of the mothers. They found that late preterm infants had an increased association with respiratory morbidity compared to full-term infants, but the association was smaller than reported in previous smaller-scale studies. Similarly, studies with small samples from fertility clinics have previously linked celiac disease to infertility [6]. Dhalwani et al. calculated the incidence of infertility in over two million UK women and found no evidence of such a link.

Research on rare diseases can also benefit from the large volume of EMR data. Thomas et al. used four UK EMR databases to study varicella as a risk factor for stroke. Stroke is a rare event in children, and using patients as their own controls, they observed a fourfold increased risk of stroke in children within 0–6 months after varicella. This study identifies future research pathways exploring the link between infections and vascular damage and their roles in stroke.

Cohort analysis based on electronic medical records has yielded a wealth of significant research findings and will continue to grow with the expansion of EMR use, decreasing costs, and increased linkage to other health records and improved accessibility. Moreover, as new technologies allow for the capture of patient data without the assistance of healthcare professionals, opportunities for such research will also increase.

8.3.3 Health Statistics Analysis

Monitoring the development of key diseases and health status indicators within populations, and conducting health statistics analysis, aids in promptly grasping the overall health level of the public. This also alerts public health institutions to take action to prevent and control diseases. The widespread adoption of personal electronic medical records (EMR) for public health monitoring enhances the timeliness and completeness of this monitoring. More broadly, personal EMRs offer a unique opportunity to expand the role and scope of current surveillance efforts. Rich in data, EMRs can assist public health departments in monitoring the prevalence, healthcare utilization, treatment patterns, and outcomes of a range of diseases, including obesity, diabetes, hypertension, and kidney disease, in a timely and effective manner. Leveraging these emerging opportunities can significantly improve the ability of public health departments to monitor population health, guide public health initiatives, and measure the impact of interventions, as detailed in Fig. 8.8. Additionally, EMRs have the potential to foster closer collaboration and better integration between clinical care and public health. Tightening the connection between these two domains is expected to improve and enrich both, leading to better health outcomes for individuals and populations.

As previously mentioned, EMRs record and store residents' health data, including demographic information, medical history, current illness, laboratory test results, immunizations, pathology reports, and treatment reports by healthcare providers. Beyond conveniently providing this information to healthcare providers, EMRs also offer additional functionalities, such as accessing clinical and public health guidelines and receiving reminders about routine screenings or disease reporting responsibilities. The rapid development of EMRs in clinical medicine presents opportunities for advancing public health agencies in conducting public health statistics analysis. Standard computer algorithms can be designed within EMR systems to identify disease cases that require surveillance and automatically transmit reports to public health agencies. This approach complements traditional disease reporting triggered solely by abnormal laboratory results and can also strengthen monitoring of common chronic diseases, such as cardiovascular diseases and asthma, which are defined through clinical criteria found in EMRs rather than laboratory tests. For diseases first reported to health departments via EHRs, the

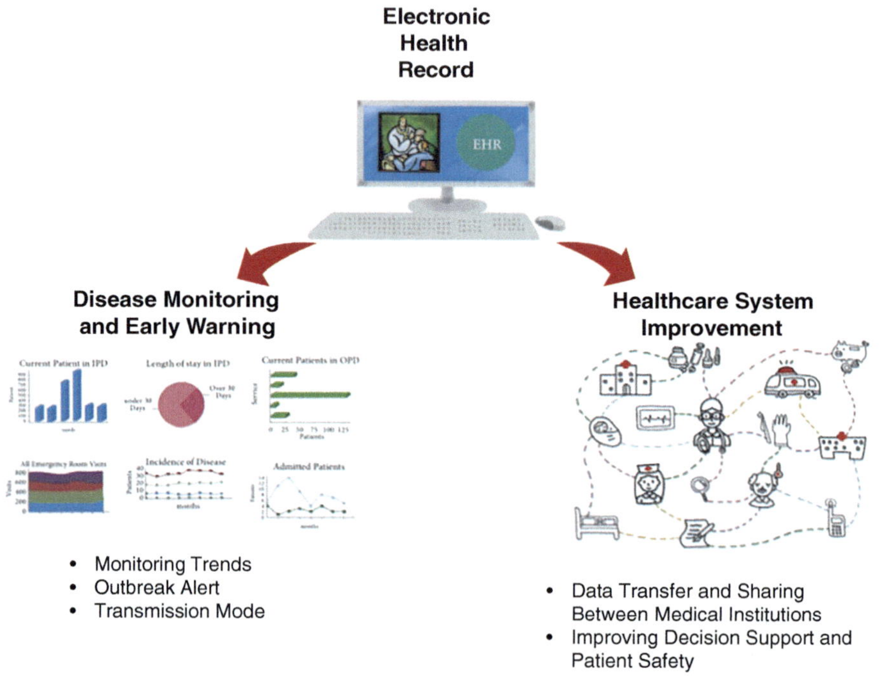

Fig. 8.8 The role of electronic health records in public health

system can automatically send clinical parameters and risk factors associated with the disease, providing reference background information for the report and expediting the collection of clinical data and risk factors for public health monitoring personnel. Ultimately, the electronic link between health departments and EMR providers can be bidirectional, with health departments also supplying information to EMR providers, i.e., healthcare workers, such as the latest updates on active disease outbreaks, diagnostic and treatment recommendations, and guidance on managing significant public health conditions.

ESPnet (Electronic Medical Record Support for Public Health) is a system developed by the Harvard Center for Excellence in Public Health Informatics and the Massachusetts Department of Public Health, funded by the U.S. Centers for Disease Control and Prevention, for public health surveillance using electronic medical records. Employed in four major clinics in Massachusetts and Ohio, the system serves nearly two million people in collaboration with their respective state health departments. ESPnet features a standalone server independent of the main EMR system, allowing compatibility with various EMR systems and preventing additional computational burdens on the main EMR system. The main EMR system can transmit structured data for each patient to ESPnet overnight or even in real-time. This data encompasses demographics, diagnostic codes, laboratory tests and results, prescriptions, vaccinations, and social history. ESPnet employs algorithms to identify cases relevant to public health, with results organized into individual case reports for reportable diseases or aggregated reports for chronic diseases and influenza-like illnesses (ILI) and transmitted to the state health department [7].

ESPnet utilizes physician diagnostic coding, laboratory test results, vital signs, and prescriptions to identify public health-related conditions. Presently, ESPnet includes modules for reportable diseases (such as active tuberculosis, chlamydia pneumonia, gonorrhea, syphilis, Lyme disease, pelvic inflammatory disease, whooping cough, and acute hepatitis A, B, C), chronic diseases (asthma, type 1 diabetes, type 2 diabetes, gestational diabetes, prediabetes, obesity, hyperlipidemia, etc.), ILI, and vaccine adverse reactions. Algorithms for each disease must be calibrated to maximize sensitivity and positive predictive value while minimizing false positive reports to reduce the burden on public health departments. ESPnet relieves providers of the responsibility to report to the health department and provides detailed clinical information with initial reports, potentially simplifying surveillance investigations.

8.4 Case Study

8.4.1 CDC's INPHO System in the USA

The Centers for Disease Control and Prevention (CDC) initiated the construction of the Information Network for Public Health Officials (INPHO) in 1992. The CDC has been committed to creating a network that connects local and state public health information with federal agency information. This type of information network is increasingly indispensable for disease surveillance activities, especially in the event of potential localized disease outbreaks on a regional and national scale. In this way, health information systems can help establish and maintain effective inter-organizational relationships among public health organizations.

CDC WONDER is software designed by the U.S. CDC to quickly and easily deliver key information into the hands of public health managers. Initially a personal computer (PC)-based system, it can now be used on any computer connected to the Internet, solving the problem of workstations dedicated to specific databases. Through WONDER software, the public can search for weekly summary articles on morbidity and mortality and prevention guidelines published by the U.S. CDC. They can also access dozens of digital datasets on the U.S. CDC mainframe and other computers, such as public-use datasets on mortality, cancer incidence, hospital discharge rates, behavioral risk factors, diabetes, and many other topics, and can easily summarize and analyze the requested data [8].

The INPHO system is a framework developed based on an advanced telecommunications network to facilitate the liaison of public health information, part of the strategy to strengthen public health infrastructure. Three important concepts in the INPHO system are linking, information access, and data exchange. First, the U.S. CDC collaborates with state and local health agencies to establish local area networks (LANs) and wide area networks (WANs). Second, the U.S. CDC extends the "virtual network" by using CDC WONDER, providing access to data in the U.S. CDC's public health databases. Lastly, the U.S. CDC encourages states to network and obtain information.

There are multiple public health information systems in various states across the U.S., often maintained systems include computerized immunization registries, lead toxicity tracking, early intervention databases for children with disabilities, congenital disease registries, as well as vital statistics data, Medicaid usage, and disease reporting.

Georgia was the first site to implement the CDC's INPHO system. Through a unique state agency alliance formed with academic health partners and IT partners, Georgia rapidly became a model site. Members of this alliance included the Medical College of Georgia, the Georgia Center for Advanced Telecommunications Technology, and Emory University's Rollins School of Public Health. The project was initially funded by the Robert Wood Johnson Foundation. The foundational units of the project included 81 clinics and 59 county health departments. Georgia's INPHO system included LAN and WAN computer networks, office automation and email, public health calendars, administrative personnel information systems, and electronic notifications for public health emergencies. Before the project began, the state public health office operated 13 small, disconnected LANs. With the implementation of the INPHO project, hardware and software were integrated into an integrated network system.

Cornerstone is a management information system developed by Illinois to integrate maternal and child health services. This system is a state information system that integrates several related programs, where risk assessments and demographic information only need to be captured once to be used for multiple projects. This information system can be used to assist in information exchange, risk assessment, follow-up assurance, and referral services.

8.4.2 Australia's Public Health Information System Response to the COVID-19 Transition

By the end of 2020, certain regions in Australia, particularly Queensland, had successfully controlled the infection rate of COVID-19 to a level manageable by the health system. This achievement has been recognized globally as a successful model in combating the pandemic. The COVID-19 pandemic posed significant challenges to traditional public health information systems, which often relied on paper-based workflows, spreadsheets, and isolated databases. The intense public focus on the virus, coupled with demands from both political and public spheres for accurate and real-time reporting of case numbers, as well as the rapid spread of information and the 24-h news cycle, placed considerable strain on these traditional systems.

The government deemed it essential to transition the workflows and data management for COVID-19 response from traditional, isolated information systems, clinical registries, and paper-based processes to creating real-time integrated digital data streams. The usual processes and structures of large-scale digital transformation projects, such as staff and end-user involvement during project planning, extensive consultation, and detailed workflow training, were not feasible under the crisis conditions of the pandemic. Implementing such large-scale digitization of public health workflows to provide real-time data was challenging, but it was crucial to minimize the incidence and mortality rates of COVID-19 within the jurisdiction.

The health department implemented real-time integrated digital and data workflow solutions on top of the existing information systems to support effective multi-agency management of the COVID-19 outbreak in Queensland, Australia. The main features included: (1) A significant shift in workflows (moving clinical staff from paper-based and isolated information systems to rapidly evolving digital workflows); (2) Identifying the actual sources of infection for patients infected with COVID-19; (3) A cultural and governance shift across government, centralizing data collection from individual agencies and departments to the infected patients themselves. The integrated program on the public health information system is known as the Digital Coronavirus Application (DCOVA), which is a key component of the digital health information system and has contributed to Queensland's successful containment of COVID-19 [9].

The system employed a "pair programming" approach to expedite the development process, with clinical informaticists (with backgrounds in medicine and nursing) collaborating with developers in real-time to build the application, significantly speeding up the work. Development took place within the Microsoft Powerapps environment, which allows for configuration on both mobile and desktop devices. An internal development team of eight people followed a low-code strategy, keeping costs minimal as existing personnel and resources were redirected to COVID-19 development efforts. The system adopted a continuous improvement methodology, with ongoing iterative enhancements. Given the rapid changes in government policy and frequent adjustments to quarantine standards (which needed to be immediately reflected in DCOVA), development flexibility was vital. This flexibility was achieved by having a dedicated development team on standby in the crisis environment of the infectious disease outbreak.

DCOVA is a web-based application that securely captures information from individuals required to be isolated, creating a secure, multi-agency database. Individuals identified by the database as being at an increased risk of infection, such as those from areas with severe outbreaks or in close contact with known cases, are legally mandated to undergo a 14-day quarantine. DCOVA enables public health officials and police to assist those in isolation, ensuring their safety and access to necessary services. It also integrates with other digital systems within a cloud-based data warehouse for broader reporting purposes. Queensland Health, Queensland Police, and the Department of Housing and Public Works have all implemented DCOVA.

8.4.3 Infectious Disease Surveillance and Early Warning Platform Based on Big Data in Yinzhou District, Ningbo City

Since 2004, a national infectious disease direct reporting system has been established in China, achieving nationwide monitoring and reporting of infectious disease cases. However, the monitoring scope did not cover all diseases and medical institutions, thus the system's early warning capability for emerging major infectious diseases was insufficient. Yinzhou District in Ningbo City has established an infectious disease surveillance and early warning platform based on big data, building upon the existing comprehensive health information platform and health big data platform.

The Comprehensive Health Information Platform in Yinzhou District includes 532 health management service organizations and various levels of medical institutions' HIS, PACS, LIS, chronic disease follow-up management, infectious disease reporting, etc., achieving interconnectivity and data exchange among these systems. The system, taking the electronic health records of residents as the carrier, integrates all medical and public health information systems in the region, breaking down the barriers of "data silos" and promoting the development of regional medical and health.

In 2009, Yinzhou District established a Health Big Data Platform, achieving interconnectivity and data exchange of health data from all medical institutions within the jurisdiction, constructing a unified terminology system, and realizing the standardization of data structures. This has improved the quality of medical data and advanced the development of public health. The platform adopts big data management technology systems that are layered, graded, and domain-based, configurable data quality repair and fusion technology data catalogs, data control technology for bloodline tracing, and other data governance technologies, as well as technologies centered on patients for automatic identification of the entire chain of disease characteristics. It has achieved collaborative medical and health applications within the region and the integration of health information data across platforms. Currently, the platform has covered the personal health information of 95% of the permanent residents in Yinzhou District and has successfully implemented multiple tasks, including chronic disease management and infectious disease surveillance.

The data for the infectious disease surveillance and early warning platform comes from the aforementioned Health Big Data Platform, covering all medical and health information generated by residents in clinical diagnosis, treatment, and public health service activities. This includes residents' demographic data, electronic health records, inpatient and outpatient electronic medical records, drug use data, laboratory test data, imaging data, and other clinical data; public health data such as tumor registration data, immunization data, infectious disease report data, and death registration data that are docked or automatically imported by CDC institutions; demographic information data and student group characteristic data automatically imported by other departments such as the education and statistics departments. These data form the foundation for multidimensional, joint prevention and control of disease surveillance and early warning.

The early warning platform implements classified monitoring for permanent and key populations. The early warning route is shown in Fig. 8.9. The warning route is divided into three stages: First, analyze historical infectious disease surveillance data reports, consult public health experts, and determine the types of infectious diseases and surveillance indicators to be monitored; second, process the data required for system monitoring using technologies such as multi-source heterogeneous data fusion, and prioritize the establishment of thematic databases for infectious diseases such as influenza, dengue fever, tuberculosis, and COVID-19; finally, for these themes, establish respective clinical case definition standards for syndrome

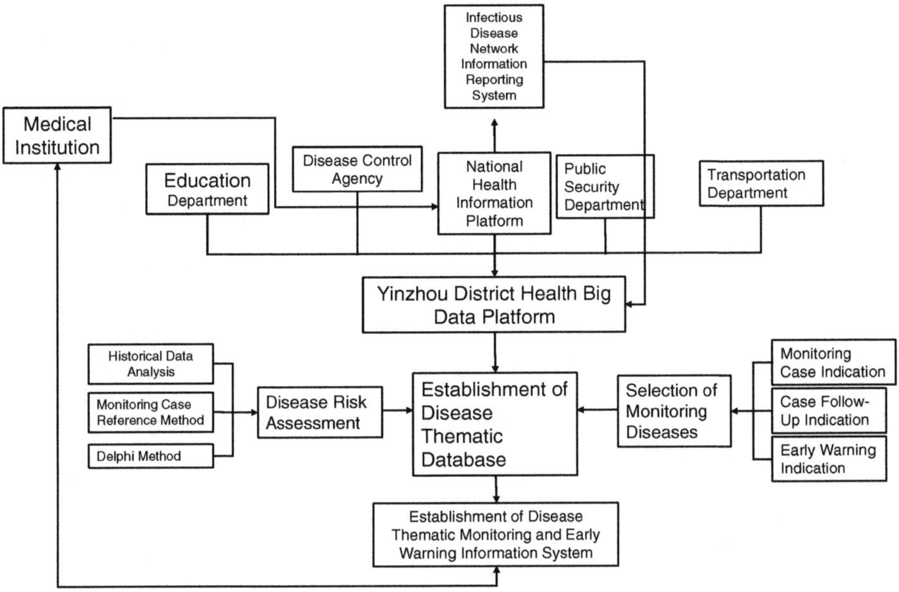

Fig. 8.9 Technology roadmap for big data-based infectious disease monitoring and early warning

clusters, construct individual case monitoring and group early warning models, and develop corresponding early warning information systems, with various medical institutions within the region carrying out specific offline disposal work, ultimately establishing a response mechanism that combines online monitoring and early warning with offline investigation and follow-up.

For individual case monitoring, the system first pushes individual cases' syndrome clusters that match clinical cases to the corresponding medical institution staff within the region. Staff verify the case situation through home visits or telephone follow-up and complete the corresponding information collection, promptly entering the information into the monitoring and early warning platform system for regional group monitoring and early warning. For regional group monitoring and early warning, the system pushes group monitoring and early warning signals to the regional public health department staff. Staff assess the authenticity of the warning signals based on past experience and guide the corresponding health departments and disease control centers within the region to take appropriate early warning measures. At the same time, if the monitoring event is severe and urgent, the health department and disease control center will report in a timely manner and activate the public health emergency plan.

For individual case monitoring and early warning, during the dengue fever outbreak in 2019, the system identified a total of 1278 cases that matched the clinical syndrome cluster. Through on-site verification by staff, combined with laboratory screening and epidemiological history analysis, three positive cases were ultimately confirmed. After the outbreak of COVID-19, according to the prevention and control plan issued by the country, the system added corresponding clinical syndrome cluster matching case detection standards. From January to March 2020, a total of 1595 cases matching the clinical syndrome of COVID-19 were identified. Through on-site verification by staff, combined with laboratory screening and epidemiological history analysis, five confirmed cases were ultimately confirmed. For group monitoring and early warning, between October and December 2019, the system identified a total of 77,664 influenza-like cases, detected 5 suspected influenza event early warning signals during the monitoring process, conducted 3 on-site investigations by staff, and ultimately verified 1 cluster outbreak in the region.

8.5 Cutting-Edge Research

8.5.1 Early Warning and Efficient Response to Emerging Major Infectious Diseases

It is estimated that out of the approximately 60 million people who die globally each year, at least 25% are related to infectious diseases. Neglected infectious diseases claim more than 500,000 lives annually and lead to chronic infections in at least 1 billion people, causing immeasurable suffering. Throughout history, the disasters caused by emerging infectious diseases have been persistent. In today's globalized world, the spread of emerging major infectious diseases has become one of the main threats to public health. One of the primary methods for humans to combat infectious diseases is to establish surveillance and prevention systems to detect risks early and minimize them as much as possible. Over the past 20 years, strengthening global public health surveillance and early warning systems has become a consensus among scientists both domestically and internationally.

Traditional public health emergency response procedures, as shown in Fig. 8.10, face increasing difficulties in meeting actual needs due to the growing severity of infectious disease prevention and control. Traditional monitoring methods have increasingly failed to meet practical requirements in terms of information acquisition, overall efficiency, and predicting infectious disease outbreaks. One major reason for these issues is that, in the current market economy environment in China, infectious disease information is mainly obtained through the health direct reporting system. Many patients have the mindset of "not going to the hospital unless the condition is severe," resulting in delayed data that is less effective for early warning purposes. This system generally only reflects already erupted epidemics and fails to provide timely alerts for early-stage or impending outbreaks. Traditional infectious disease monitoring methods rely mainly on static and qualitative analysis, which lack sensitivity and are overly simplistic.

Internationally, developed countries place great emphasis on pathogen analysis and early warning in bacterial infectious disease monitoring. They achieve early warning through the integration of pathogen detection technology, networked laboratories, field investigations, and data analysis. For example, the USA has established the PulseNet system for bacterial disease surveillance and the FoodNet

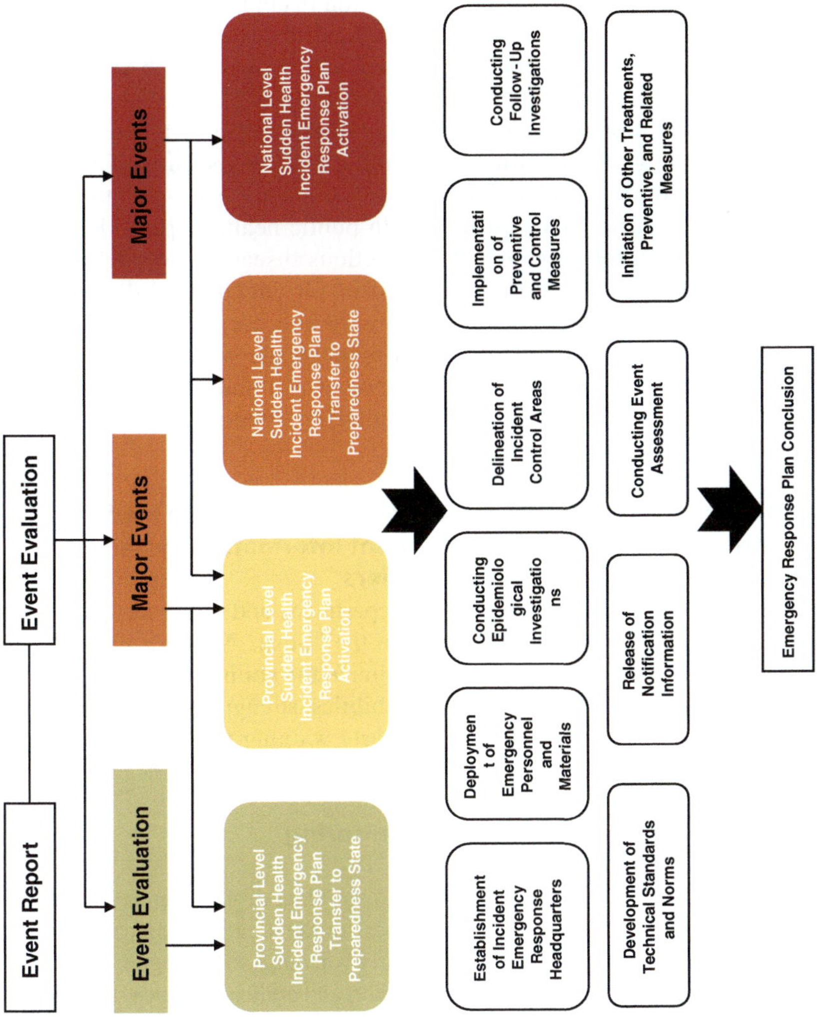

Fig. 8.10 Traditional public health emergency response procedures

system for active foodborne disease surveillance. The Global Emerging Infections Surveillance and Response System (GEIS) focuses on integrating global surveillance systems, capacity-building projects, epidemic investigations, and routine training, covering 92 countries. It has played a significant role in global biosurveillance, particularly in controlling H1N1 influenza and malaria.

On February 3, 2020, the National Health Commission issued a notice emphasizing the importance of leveraging informatization in epidemic control. It called for enhancing data collection and analysis applications (network direct reporting, information linkage with other departments, regional health information platform coordination), promoting telemedicine services, standardizing Internet diagnosis and consultation services, deepening "Internet+" government services, and strengthening network infrastructure upgrades and cybersecurity. On June 2, 2020, President Xi Jinping emphasized the need to enhance early monitoring and warning capabilities during a symposium with public health experts. He called for improving the monitoring system for infectious diseases and public health emergencies, refining the monitoring mechanism for unexplained diseases and abnormal health events, increasing the sensitivity and accuracy of monitoring and assessment, establishing intelligent multi-point trigger warning mechanisms, and enhancing real-time analysis and comprehensive judgment capabilities. There are measures to Enhance Early Monitoring, Warning, and Response Capabilities:

8.5.1.1 Strengthen Data Sharing and Integration Between Medical Institutions and Health Department Information Systems, Breaking Down Information Barriers

Data sharing and integration includes cross-department and cross-sector integration, dismantling "data silos," and focusing on the "Smart Network Project." By centering on big data, we can continuously optimize the ability of various medical institutions to fulfill their public health responsibilities, strengthen medical and preventive collaboration, and achieve intelligent early warning for syndromes, unexplained diseases, and abnormal health events.

8.5.1.2 Improving Infectious Disease Monitoring and Analysis Methods

Disease modeling uses mathematical methods to simulate disease spread in the real world. By reconstructing transmission dynamics, models can assess transmission potential, predict outbreak sizes, and provide early warnings to management departments, aiding in the development of new prevention and control policies. Identifying the epidemiological characteristics of infectious diseases is a primary task. Models based on real data and statistical analyses play a crucial role in understanding infectious diseases and the socioeconomic issues related to outbreaks. Statistical descriptions of raw data can provide basic epidemic information, while deeper insights rely on statistical models. Model construction and parameter setting are major challenges, requiring identification of specific disease transmission chains and sufficient data collection on transmission nodes.

8.5.1.3 Leveraging the Advantages of Joint Prevention and Control to Build and Improve Infectious Disease Monitoring Management Platforms

With the improvement of public health monitoring systems, the sources of infectious disease monitoring data are also expanding. The foundation of infectious disease monitoring and early warning is big data. Depending on the source of big data, current monitoring and warning systems primarily rely on network big data, social and environmental big data, medical big data, and pathogen monitoring big data. Without effectively integrating big data from different fields, the early monitoring and warning capabilities of health information systems will be limited. Infectious disease monitoring management platforms need to establish and improve information monitoring coordination mechanisms, utilizing the advantages of joint prevention and control to ensure information is efficiently transmitted to decision-makers. Although medical institutions in China have clear organizational divisions of labor, issues such as unclear departmental roles and insufficient proactiveness of local governments still exist. Given China's large population, it is crucial to fully leverage the roles of local governments and grassroots medical institutions under the central government's coordination for regional public health emergency responses. Additionally, an abnormal public health event reporting platform can be established, allowing doctors, nurses, medical students, and even ordinary people to report abnormal health events in their vicinity through this platform. The platform should be equipped with professional public health experts to review and transfer suspicious events to the national public health infectious disease monitoring platform.

Effective surveillance systems are key to rapid intervention and control of infectious disease outbreaks. In addition, comprehensive population surveillance information is needed to complement current clinical data. Current surveillance systems have several limitations in dealing with rapid population growth and environmental changes. Geospatial technologies and wastewater-based epidemiology (WBE) are newer epidemiological research tools that could potentially serve as supplementary methods to existing infectious disease surveillance systems and early warning systems for disease outbreaks.

The increasing demand for mapping, analysis, and visualization in the public health sector over the past 20 years has spurred the continuous development of information age technologies for infectious disease surveillance and epidemiology. This ongoing public health burden, coupled with advances in information technology and spatial data, has enabled the emergence of visual systems that provide disease data in space and time. Geospatial technology offers public health professionals and decision-makers with visualization and analysis tools to implement disease control programs in affected and/or suspected areas, making analyses and predictions that were technically unfeasible before possible. Advances in information technology and spatial features have promoted the development of geospatial technology, which is crucial for mapping, monitoring, predicting outbreaks, identifying clusters, and analyzing the spread patterns of infectious diseases that may become epidemic or pandemic within communities and across territories [10]. Geospatial technologies include Geographic Information Systems (GIS), Global Positioning

Systems (GPS), and satellite-based technologies such as remote sensing (RS). GIS plays an increasingly vital role in the field of public health, especially in infectious disease surveillance and modeling strategies. GIS can provide dynamic maps to understand the geographical distribution of diseases, facilitating the analysis of case frequency, disease mapping, spatial clustering of diseases, associations between diseases and environmental factors, and network analysis. With such visualization and analytical capabilities, GIS technology has seen widespread development in the field of public health, providing information support for the surveillance, early warning, and response to infectious diseases.

WBE is an emerging method that can provide comprehensive health information about communities. Wastewater is an important medium for water fingerprinting studies, containing a rich source of biological and chemical information. Epidemiological research based on wastewater can provide an unbiased reflection of community health and lifestyle habits. With a multitude of endogenous chemical and biological urinary markers related to diseases, WBE clearly has great potential for monitoring the spread of infectious diseases and epidemics at the community level. WBE can serve as a supplementary monitoring technique, providing rapid and reliable information about the population, helping to understand what diseases are present in the community, and aiding in the surveillance of disease outbreaks. A schematic diagram of epidemiological monitoring based on WBE is shown in Fig. 8.11.

A research group in Japan utilized fluorescent quantitative polymerase chain reaction (PCR) and nested PCR techniques to test a large number of sewage samples collected from wastewater treatment plants for the novel coronavirus, providing a strong reference for epidemiological investigations and research based on sewage. The research group believes that WBE research is conducive to the early warning of the COVID-19 pandemic because WBE research can cover asymptomatic infected individuals and those infected before symptom onset, predicting the overall state of the epidemic without medical bias.

8.5.2 Identification of Occupational Health Risk Factors

Public health information systems also play an indispensable role in monitoring occupational health risks. For instance, during the fight against the COVID-19 pandemic, public health information systems can not only provide effective protection for combating the epidemic but also analyze the occupational health risks of medical and health personnel, further promoting positive research on occupational health policies for medical and health workers in our country.

The European Union and other related regions have monitoring systems for the occurrence of occupational diseases, which are used to identify occupational diseases and assist patients with these diseases in obtaining compensation. In 2012, the European Agency for Safety and Health at Work (EU-OSHA) compiled a report that identified the priorities for occupational safety and health (OSH) research from 2013 to 2020 to promote the coordination of EU OSH.

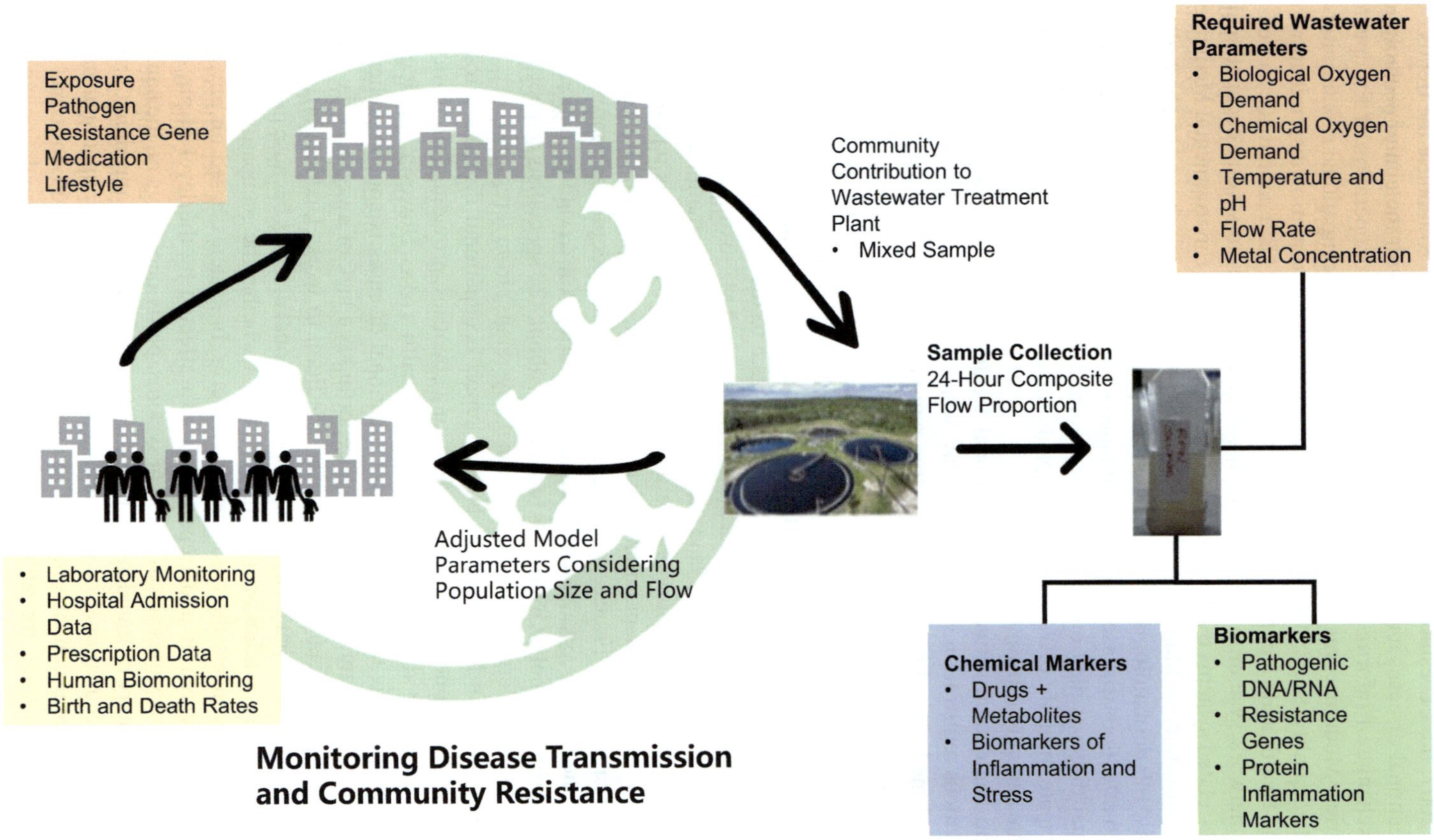

Fig. 8.11 Schematic diagram of epidemiological monitoring based on WBE

In 2007, the EU established a network called Modernet to monitor the trends of occupational diseases and track new or emerging risks, with the aim of promoting the exchange of information and knowledge through the cooperation of European countries. Modernet was set up to address four issues in occupational risk monitoring: data quality, trend analysis, new risk analysis, and information dissemination.

The Health and Occupation Research Network (THOR) is a nationwide surveillance network system in the UK, which was integrated from several occupational health-related systems by the Centre for Occupational and Environmental Medicine at the University of Manchester in 2002. The system includes about 415 chest physicians, 149 dermatologists, 283 occupational physicians, 231 general practitioners, and 26 infectious disease control consultants who voluntarily report any new occupational diseases they encounter in their normal clinical practice. Physicians can participate monthly (10% of all participants) or choose a month at random to participate annually (90%).

The National Institute of Occupational Health (NIOH) registry is a national anonymous registration system in Norway, where any physician from the six occupational medicine clinics (based on large regional hospitals) reports cases of suspected occupational diseases to the registry.

The health department of the French Institute for Public Health Surveillance (InVS) proposes monitoring programs for work-related musculoskeletal diseases, mesothelioma, asthma, and other diseases. Voluntarily participating physicians can report cases they see in their daily clinical practice to the system. Musculoskeletal disease monitoring (troubles musculo-squelettiques, TMS) is reported by occupational physicians, surgeons, and neurophysiologists. Mesothelioma monitoring (programme national de surveillance du mésothéliome, PNSM) is reported by all specialists (pathologists, pulmonologists, oncologists, occupational disease specialists) in 21 regions of France, covering about 18 million people, or approximately 30% of the French population. Asthma monitoring (observatoire national des asthmes professionnels, ONAP2) is reported by about 420 specialists (pathologists, pulmonologists, allergists, and occupational physicians) from 6 regions.

Most systems in Modernet are built to report occupational diseases across all geographic and economic areas of participating countries, providing information on existing or newly discovered occupational health risks. However, participants widely acknowledge that reporting on occupational diseases is not comprehensive. One of the main factors leading to underreporting is a lack of awareness, i.e., individuals and/or physicians not linking the condition to work. Underreporting may also occur in systems that compensate for occupational diseases because individuals are unaware of the availability of compensation or whether the occupational disease they suffer from meets the compensation criteria. In systems based on physician reporting, the degree of underreporting is also affected by the level of physician participation. This varies across different systems, partly depending on the nature of reporting (voluntary or mandatory), but other factors, such as the physician's workload, level of occupational health training, and closeness to occupational health, also affect the comprehensiveness of reporting. Many systems do not cover freelancers, who account for about 15% of the EU working population and the proportion is rising. Moreover, these systems have limited coverage of the workforce in specific sectors; it is well known that in the UK, occupational physicians tend to be allocated more toward the public sector and larger industries. However, some systems have taken steps to quantify the population covered by the system, enabling the calculation of more accurate occupational incidence rates.

The Finnish job-exposure matrix (FINJEM) was established in the 1990s and covers major occupational exposures that have occurred in Finland since 1945. Table 8.3 summarizes epidemiological studies using FINJEM as an exposure assessment tool, most of which are about cancer. FINJEM has been applied in epidemiological studies in Sweden, the Netherlands, Australia, Spain, and Germany. These studies are mostly large case-control studies based on the general population with occupational histories spanning a long period and covering the entire occupational spectrum. Health outcomes include various types of cancer, sleep apnea, and Alzheimer's disease. Different chemical agents are often used for treatment studies, but there is little research on physical, microbial, physiological ergonomic, and psychosocial factors [11].

In a meta-analysis of pancreatic cancer, FINJEM was used to classify chemical exposures in epidemiological studies, and meta-relative risks were calculated using a simple random model and a stratified Bayesian model. To achieve the purpose of monitoring occupational risks, FINJEM provides a document outlining the degree and level of accessible physical or chemical reagents. When Finland conducts national-level chemical hazard monitoring, indicators such as the number of exposed workers and the level of contact with reagents are used. FINJEM can serve as an exposure assessment tool for occupational epidemiology, especially in large population cohort studies, providing information for national-level hazard monitoring. The system can identify occupations with the highest average chemical exposure, thus helping to determine the order of occupational hazard prevention. National estimates of exposure doses and their trends over time help assess the immediate and future health risks associated with relevant occupations. However, the effectiveness of using this system for chemical or physical hazard monitoring in the

Table 8.3 Application of FINJEM in occupational disease epidemiological research

Disease	Exposure substance	Study design	Country
Lung cancer	Silica	Population census, cohort study	Finland
Nasal cancer	Wood dust, formaldehyde	Population census, cohort study	Finland
Esophageal cancer	Chemical agents	Case-control study	Spain
Pancreatic cancer	Chemical, physical factors, etc.	Case-control study	Spain
Bladder cancer	Polycyclic aromatic hydrocarbons	Mixed analysis	Six European countries
Alzheimer's disease	Psychosocial factors	Case-control study	Germany
Intervertebral disc disease	Psychosocial factors	Population census, cohort study	Finland

workplace is limited; the system's exposure estimates for different occupations are based on average levels, mainly helping to plan national or regional preventive measures, and cannot identify worker groups with different exposure levels in the same workplace.

8.5.3 Public Health Event Early Warning Based on Social Networks

Traditional public health event early warning involves doctors or laboratory personnel reporting known infectious diseases to government agencies either mandatorily or voluntarily. This method offers good accuracy and completeness, providing a wealth of demographic and influencing factor information for risk factor analysis. However, traditional early warning systems have certain issues, such as the time needed for case confirmation and information transmission, leading to a lag in warnings; information mainly comes from hospitals or third-party laboratories, which can miss many cases during monitoring; and for emerging infectious diseases without historical experience, timely early warnings cannot be issued. Major public health events in recent years, such as the SARS-CoV in Asia, the global H1N1/09 influenza virus, the *E. coli* O104:H4 outbreak in Germany, and the global COVID-19, have prompted governments and international health organizations to improve infectious disease surveillance methods. To address the limitations of traditional public health event early warnings, public health monitoring methods based on social media and the Internet have gradually developed.

Standard public health event monitoring methods include indicator-based monitoring and event-based monitoring. Indicator-based monitoring systems collect and analyze structured data based on established surveillance and monitoring protocols for each disease (used to calculate incidence rates, seasonality, and disease burden) to understand population-related information, detect changes in population trends or distribution, which is the traditional public health event early warning method mentioned above. In contrast, event-based monitoring refers to the organized and rapid acquisition of information on events that may pose a threat to public health. This information often relies not on official reports but directly from eyewitnesses at the scene of the event or indirectly from various communication channels (such as social media or established routine alert systems) and information channels (such as news media, public health networks, etc.). Event-based monitoring can determine events more quickly than indicator-based reporting procedures and can discover events occurring in populations that cannot be reported through formal channels. Public health monitoring methods based on social media and the Internet are an essential part of event-based monitoring and the most focused source of many existing event-based monitoring systems. Existing event-based monitoring systems include search functions that allow epidemiological experts and public health scientists involved in monitoring to quickly obtain information compiled from many media and news sources.

Health information technology using social media and the Internet as data sources is an important driver of global surveillance innovation, which can accelerate the collection and dissemination of information for a faster and better response to public health events. A study has shown that using Internet data (especially emails and online news) for event-based surveillance can identify warning trends comparable to those using indicator-based surveillance methods.

The Global Public Health Intelligence Network (GPHIN) system developed by the Canadian Department of Public Health uses the Internet and the latest global health event news reports to create a unique early warning outbreak detection form. GPHIN has created a new monitoring technology that breaks the national boundaries of epidemic reporting while creating new possibilities for global epidemic response. By incorporating news into the emerging global infectious disease surveillance mechanism, GPHIN effectively addresses the challenge of global media to official national epidemic reports, enhancing the effectiveness and credibility of international public health. The system detected the SARS outbreak in Guangdong Province, China, as early as November 2002, more than 2 months earlier than when the World Health Organization publicly released detailed information on new respiratory disease cases. In 2009, Google used its Google Flu Trend (GFT) service to track flu-like cases in the population by analyzing a large number of Google search query data, which could accurately estimate the current weekly influenza activity level in each region of the USA, with only a 1-day lag.

The innovative use of mobile health and social media is beginning to have a significant impact on public health practice. With the continued growth of Internet usage, people use mobile technology and social media to search for health information and post their personal health information. Wilson and others explored the use of mobile technology to establish personal immunization registries to assist travelers in providing proof of vaccination required for specific countries. In addition to mobile technology, many people also use social media to find and share health information. Online community platforms for specific diseases are evolving toward social media applications, providing researchers with opportunities to capture new and monitor different types of data. Social media also shows promise for emergency preparedness professionals in disaster risk reduction and management.

However, despite the significant development of public health event monitoring technology based on social networks, which saves more manpower, material resources, and financial resources compared to traditional methods and greatly improves timeliness, the current social network-based monitoring system has not yet been widely accepted and included in mainstream use by national and international health departments. The limitations of this technology are mainly reflected in the following aspects.

1. The information provided by social networks is abundant but of low quality, leading to a high rate of false positives in early warnings. Unlike traditional monitoring systems where information sources are all officially released, most of the information provided by social networks comes from the public and social

media, which is not credible. During the H1N1 influenza outbreak in 2012–2013, Google used the GFT service for influenza trend prediction, but due to excessive media attention, its predicted values were much higher than the estimates of traditional monitoring.
2. It is difficult to obtain user location information on social networks, and the system cannot conduct monitoring at the spatial level. Although social apps like Weibo provide users with location information functions, most users do not enable this feature, making it impossible to obtain user location information.
3. The information collected from social networks has not been effectively filtered before being passed on to epidemiological experts. For most epidemiological experts, the process of collecting data from the Internet is complex because it includes text mining (searching for health-related content from websites or social media), preparation (extracting and filtering health-related information), and presenting only the most relevant content (disseminating information). Data acquisition and processing are either automated or done manually, and results often depend on the technology with which users interact with data, often leading to significant differences in results.

Although there are still some issues with the public health event early warning technology based on social networks, its superiority in timeliness cannot be ignored. If this technology can overcome a series of problems such as a high rate of false positives in the future, the social network-based monitoring system will help with early disease warnings and play a very important role in the field of public health information.

8.6 Summary

Public health information systems are an essential link and bond in establishing and improving disease prevention and control systems, public health emergency mechanisms, and health law enforcement and supervision systems. The system consists of national, local, and grassroots public health institutions, including emergency centers, health epidemic prevention institutions, health care institutions, and disease prevention and control institutions, playing roles in disease monitoring, health monitoring, medical treatment, and command decision-making.

The development and construction of public health information systems have gone through different stages in different countries according to specific national conditions and periods. China's public health information system has also formed a relatively complete system after decades of development. The current public health system needs to strengthen data sharing and integration between central and local governments and between medical institutions and health departments, break down information barriers, and continue to build and improve an integrated platform that combines infectious disease monitoring, health monitoring, and medical treatment.

References

1. Johansen MA, Henriksen E. The evolution of personal health records and their role for self management: a literature review. Stud Health Technol Inform. 2014;205:458–62.
2. Moffet HH, Nancy A, Dean S, et al. Cohort profile: the diabetes study of northern California (DISTANCE): objectives and design of a survey follow up study of social health disparities in a managed care population. Int J Epidemiol. 2016;1:38–47.
3. Emily H, Gallagher AM, Krishnan B, et al. Data resource profile: clinical practice research datalink (CPRD). Int J Epidemiol. 2015;3:827–36.
4. Hippisley Cox J, Stables D, Pringle M. QRESEARCH: a new general practice database for research. J Innov Health Inform. 2004;12(1):49–50.
5. Iwagami M, Qizilbash N, Gregson J, et al. Blood cholesterol and risk of dementia in more than 1.8 million people over two decades: a retrospective cohort study. Lancet Glob Health. 2021;2(8):e498–506.
6. Hibbard JU, Wilkins I, Sun L, et al. Respiratory morbidity in late preterm births. Obstet Anesth Dig. 2011;31(3):419.
7. Lazarus R, Klompas M, Campion FX, et al. Electronic support for public health: validated case finding and reporting for notifiable diseases using electronic medical data. J Am Med Inform Assoc. 2008;16(1):18–24.
8. Friede A, Reid JA, Ory HW. CDC WONDER: a comprehensive on line public health information system of the centers for disease control and prevention. Am J Public Health. 1993;83(9):1289–94.
9. Sullivan C, Wong I, Adams E, et al. Moving faster than the COVID 19 pandemic: the rapid, digital transformation of a public health system. Appl Clin Inform. 2021;12(2):229–36.
10. Saran S, Singh P, Kumar V, et al. Review of geospatial technology for infectious disease surveillance: use case on COVID 19. J Indian Soc Remote Sens. 2020;1:1121–38.
11. Kauppinen T, Uuksulainen S, Saalo A, et al. Use of the finnish information system on occupational exposure (FINJEM) in epidemiologic, surveillance, and other applications. Ann Occup Hyg. 2014;3:380–96.

Big Data Technology and Healthcare Informatics

9

Contents

9.1 Overview of Big Data Technologies 250
9.1.1 Introduction to Big Data 250
9.1.2 Introduction to Big Data Technology 252
9.1.2.1 Cloud Computing 252
9.1.2.2 Distributed Database Systems 252
9.1.2.3 Big Data Processing Tools 253
9.1.3 Medical Information Systems Require Big Data Technology 254
9.1.3.1 Electronic Health Record (EHR) Data 254
9.1.3.2 Clinical Notes Data 255
9.1.3.3 Medical Imaging Data 255
9.1.3.4 Clinical Trial Data 255
9.1.4 Development of Big Data Technology in Medical Information Systems 255
9.2 Fundamental Technologies of Medical Big Data 257
9.2.1 Data Storage Management 257
9.2.2 Efficient Data Processing 258
9.2.3 Data Analysis Techniques 259
9.2.4 Data Visualization 260
9.3 Construction of Medical Big Data Platform 263
9.3.1 Platform Construction Philosophy 263
9.3.2 Big Data Platform Ecosystem 264
9.3.2.1 Data System 264
9.3.2.2 Technical System 266
9.3.2.3 Policy System 266
9.3.3 Big Data Platform Implementation Standards 268
9.3.3.1 Data Standardization Norms 268
9.3.3.2 Data Technical Standards 269
9.3.3.3 Platform Security Specifications 269
9.4 Case Analysis 270
9.4.1 Medical Information System Based on Cloud Platform 270
9.4.2 Multi-Center Intelligent Medical Information Platform 271
9.4.2.1 Observational Health Data Sciences and Informatics (OHDSI) 271
9.4.2.2 Zhijiang Laboratory Multi-Center Intelligent Medical Information Platform 273

J. Li et al., *Healthcare Information Systems*, Innovative Medical Devices,
https://doi.org/10.1007/978-981-97-9551-2_9

9.5 Summary........ 274
References........ 274

9.1 Overview of Big Data Technologies

9.1.1 Introduction to Big Data

Big data refers to massive information assets that are so large in volume, grow so rapidly, and are too complex in type that they require "new processing models" to enhance decision-making capabilities and provide deeper insights. Specifically, big data refers to the type of information that traditional methods cannot collect, store, manage, or process effectively due to the sheer scale of the data sets which exceed the processing capacity of conventional methods, often requiring more powerful tools for handling.

IBM identifies five characteristics of big data, summarized by the five "Vs":

Volume. The unit of data size in big data has leaped from terabytes (TB) to petabytes (PB), affecting not only data storage and processing but also necessitating technological upgrades in data preparation, data recovery, and data management.

Velocity. Big data is characterized by rapid data growth and processing speeds, requiring high timeliness. For example, search engines need to make news from a few minutes ago available for user queries, and personalized recommendation algorithms must perform recommendations in real-time. This is a significant distinction of big data from traditional data mining.

Variety. Big data solutions need to support different formats and types of data. Data can roughly be categorized into structured data, unstructured data, and semi-structured data. Structured data follows a standard model and is often stored in tables within relational databases. Unstructured data, which makes up over 80% of real-world data, does not follow a uniform data model and includes text and binary files, usually stored as BLOBs in database tables if placed in relational databases. Semi-structured data lies in between, having some structure and consistency constraints but essentially lacking relational characteristics, commonly stored in text files like XML and JSON.

Veracity. Veracity refers to the quality and fidelity of data. Data entering the big data environment needs to be processed to eliminate noise and false data. Only genuine data can be transformed into useful information and knowledge.

Value. The value of big data stems from its veracity; the higher the veracity, the greater the value. Additionally, since data is time-sensitive, its value also depends on the speed of data processing—the shorter the delay in accessing processed data, the higher its value.

The lifecycle of a big data analysis project can be divided into nine stages, as shown in Fig. 9.1.

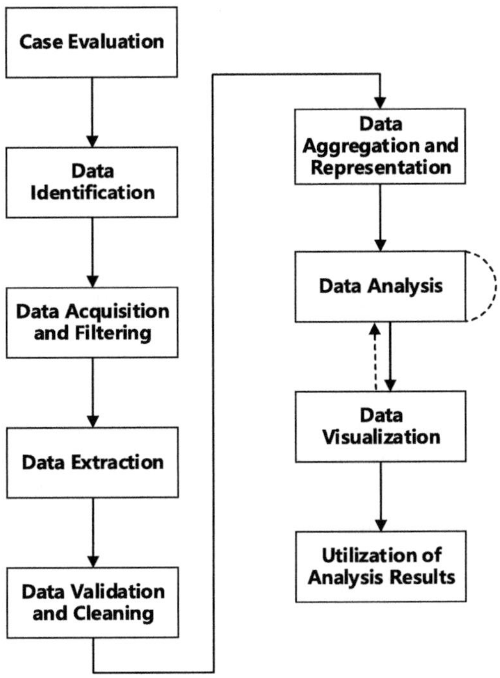

Fig. 9.1 The nine stages of the big data analysis lifecycle

1. Case Evaluation. Determine the reasons, motivations, and objectives for conducting the analysis based on SMART criteria. SMART stands for Specific, Measurable, Attainable, Relevant, and Timely.
2. Data Identification. This stage involves identifying the datasets and resources required for the analysis project. These datasets and resources may vary greatly in source, structure, and content, thus requiring further processing.
3. Data Acquisition and Filtering. In this stage, acquired data is filtered and categorized to remove contaminated and valueless data for the project.
4. Data Extraction. Having acquired the necessary data in the previous stage, the purpose of this stage is to convert this input data into a format that can be processed in subsequent operations.
5. Data Validation and Cleaning. Generally, invalid data can distort and falsify the results of the analysis. The aim of this stage is to integrate validation rules across different datasets and remove known invalid data.
6. Data Aggregation and Representation. In big data analysis projects, data needs to be propagated across multiple datasets, so this stage involves connecting these datasets through the same domain to obtain a unified view.
7. Data Analysis. Typically, the analysis phase of a big data project can be divided into confirmatory analysis and exploratory analysis. Confirmatory analysis involves proposing a hypothesis and then using data analysis methods to validate or refute it, providing clear answers to specific questions. Unlike confirmatory analysis, exploratory analysis is closely tied to data mining and involves generat-

ing an understanding of the causes behind phenomena through data analysis, usually without providing definitive answers but offering a general direction.
8. Data Visualization. In this stage, data visualization techniques and tools are used to clearly and richly display the results of data analysis.
9. Utilization of Analysis Results. The results of big data analysis can determine the best ways and links to ensure maximum value from the processed analysis data, which can be used to improve the logic of the entire project.

9.1.2 Introduction to Big Data Technology

Big data technology refers to the techniques used to quickly extract valuable information from various types of data. Generally speaking, big data technology mainly involves tools required for big data collection, storage and management, analysis and mining, interpretation, and application. The following sections will introduce big data technology from three aspects: cloud computing, distributed database systems, and big data processing tools.

9.1.2.1 Cloud Computing

The concept of "cloud computing" was first introduced by Google CEO Eric Schmidt on August 9, 2006, at a search engine conference. It is a product of the integration of traditional computing technologies such as distributed computing and parallel computing with network technology. It allows for the breakdown of massive data processing programs into countless smaller programs via the "cloud" network, which are then processed and analyzed by a system composed of multiple servers to produce results that are returned to the users. Initially, cloud computing was simply distributed computing, mainly addressing task distribution and the merging of computation results. Today's cloud computing refers to a mix of technologies including distributed computing, utility computing, load balancing, parallel computing, network storage, hot backup redundancy, and virtualization. Technically, big data storage and processing inevitably require a distributed computing architecture, and cloud computing provides powerful storage and computing capabilities for this purpose.

Currently, mainstream cloud service providers both domestically and internationally include Alibaba Cloud, Tencent Cloud, Huawei Cloud, Baidu Intelligent Cloud, Microsoft's Azure, and Amazon's AWS (Amazon Web Services). They provide users with Infrastructure as a Service (IaaS), Platform as a Service (PaaS), and Software as a Service (SaaS).

9.1.2.2 Distributed Database Systems

Traditional relational databases are mainly used to store structured data. However, in big data projects, data is often unstructured or semi-structured, and traditional databases cannot adequately meet the needs of big data for high concurrency read/write performance, high storage performance, and high scalability. Consequently, NoSQL (Not Only SQL) databases have emerged. These databases offer scalability, high concurrency read/write performance, flexible data models, and high availability. Depending on the structuring method and application scenarios, they can be categorized into the following three types:

Document-oriented NoSQL databases, with MongoDB as a primary example. MongoDB is an open-source database system written in C++ that is based on distributed file storage. It can add more nodes under high load to ensure server performance, thus maintaining good query performance while storing massive amounts of data. MongoDB stores data as documents, with data structures consisting of key-value pairs. Documents are similar to JSON objects, and field values can include other documents, arrays, and document arrays, supporting the storage of complex data types. MongoDB's syntax is similar to that of object-oriented query languages, and it can perform most of the functions of single-table queries in relational databases. MongoDB mainly addresses the efficiency issues of accessing massive data, showing significant performance improvements over relational databases when the data size exceeds 50 GB.

Key-value databases oriented toward high-performance concurrent read/write, with Redis as a primary example. Developed by Salvatore Sanfilippo, Redis is a cross-platform NoSQL database written in ANSI C and adheres to the Berkeley Software Distribution (BSD) protocol. Redis supports memory-based, distributed, optionally persistent databases and provides APIs in multiple languages. Often referred to as a data structure server, Redis allows field values to be strings, hash tables, lists, sets, and sorted sets. Redis can load the database into memory for operations, which is very fast, enabling read speeds of up to 110,000 operations per second and write speeds of up to 81,000 operations per second. However, because it runs in memory, there is a need to balance memory for high-speed read/write operations on different datasets. Thus, Redis is mainly used for high-performance operations and read/write of small capacity data sets.

Distributed databases oriented toward high scalability, with Cassandra, developed by Facebook, as a primary example. Cassandra is a hybrid non-relational database that combines Google's BigTable column-family data model with Amazon Dynamo's fully distributed architecture. Read and write operations in Cassandra are replicated to other nodes, making it highly scalable and well-suited for scenarios where node scale changes quickly.

9.1.2.3 Big Data Processing Tools

The immense value contained in big data has driven some companies to develop platforms and tools for data processing. The mainstream platforms or tools currently include the Hadoop framework developed by the Apache Foundation, the Apache Storm framework open-sourced by Twitter, and the Spark framework developed by the University of California, Berkeley. This section mainly introduces the Apache Storm framework, with the other two frameworks to be detailed in subsequent chapters.

Apache Storm is a distributed real-time big data processing system. It is designed to handle large volumes of data in a fault-tolerant and horizontally scalable manner.

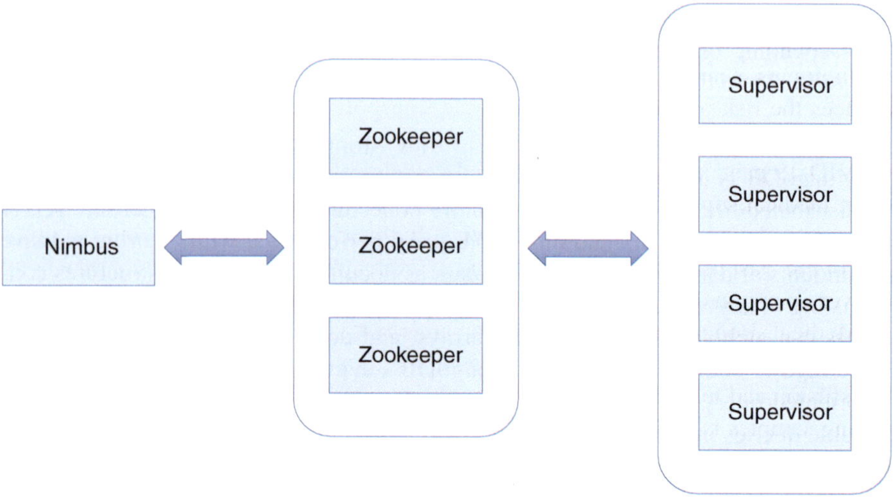

Fig. 9.2 Apache Storm Cluster Structure

Apache Storm is a stream data framework that processes tens of thousands of messages per second across the cluster, featuring the highest access rates and very low latency. As the load increases, it can maintain performance by linearly increasing resources, offering high scalability. Thanks to Apache Storm's excellent real-time processing performance, it is widely used in information flow processing, continuous computation, and distributed remote procedure calls.

The cluster structure of Apache Storm is shown in Fig. 9.2, with two types of nodes: Nimbus (master node) and Supervisor (worker node). Nimbus is the core component of Apache Storm, whose main job is to run the Apache Storm topology. Nimbus analyzes the topology and collects tasks to be executed, then assigns tasks to available Supervisors and monitors for faults. Supervisors have one or more worker processes, and Supervisors delegate tasks to worker processes, which produce as many Executors (executors) as needed and run tasks. The ZooKeeper framework uses a cluster (node group) to coordinate the work status of Nimbus and Supervisor nodes, helping them interact.

9.1.3 Medical Information Systems Require Big Data Technology

Data in the medical field mainly includes data generated during disease research and treatment processes, and these data come in various types. Data in medical information systems mainly come from sources such as electronic medical records, clinical notes, medical imaging data, and clinical trial data.

9.1.3.1 Electronic Health Record (EHR) Data

Electronic Health Records are a fundamental healthcare technology, with data encompassing various levels of medical institutions. The content mainly includes: basic patient information, demographic data, admission and discharge records, diagnoses, treatments, prescriptions, laboratory tests, physiological monitoring data, clinical notes, etc. In most cases, EHRs are text-based and consist largely of semi-structured and unstructured data.

9.1.3.2 Clinical Notes Data

Clinical notes, also known as case reports, are part of the electronic health record and typically include medical orders, summaries of admissions and discharges, and other descriptive analytical reports. Clinical notes often contain special symbols and abbreviations, and different doctors may use different expressions to describe the same concept. Additionally, a substantial portion of clinical notes contains duplicated or copied content.

9.1.3.3 Medical Imaging Data

Medical imaging is a multi-technique and processing approach to non-invasively capture images of the human body and its internal tissues, and to perform inverse problem deduction. The technologies involved include diagnostic imaging, radiology, endoscopy, medical thermal imaging, medical photography, microscopy, electroencephalography, and magnetoencephalography, such as X-ray examinations, CT scans, ultrasounds, gastroscopy, angiography, magnetoencephalography, etc. Medical imaging data mostly exists in the form of images, which are large in volume and complex in image feature representation. Currently, medical imaging data accounts for over 90% of the data within medical information systems, with many hospitals' medical imaging-related data reaching petabyte levels.

9.1.3.4 Clinical Trial Data

Medical information systems also store a vast amount of medical, pharmaceutical, and nursing-related randomized controlled trial data, which is primarily used to test the effectiveness of certain therapies or drugs.

Data in medical information systems have unique characteristics such as privacy, heterogeneity, incompleteness, redundancy, and non-obvious data representation. Medical information system data is like an untapped oilfield, requiring the rational use of big data technology for its management, research, and mining, in order to extract useful information and improve healthcare conditions.

9.1.4 Development of Big Data Technology in Medical Information Systems

If we take the implementation of the world's first electronic medical record system as the starting point, medical information systems have developed for over 50 years. In these five decades, a vast amount of related data has been accumulated in medical information systems, and big data technology has been evolving rapidly. This section will briefly introduce the development of big data technology in medical information systems, using artificial intelligence as an entry point.

The 1960s and 1970s marked the initial exploration stage of medical artificial intelligence. In 1968, the artificial intelligence expert system Dendral was applied in the field of biochemical medicine to help researchers deduce the structure of organic molecules by analyzing mass spectrometry data. In the early 1970s, researchers began exploring the application of artificial intelligence technology in the medical field. In 1972, the University of Leeds developed AAPHelp, one of the earliest medical expert systems for assisting in the diagnosis of abdominal pain and related surgical needs. During the same period, Stanford University developed the expert system MYCIN for diagnosing blood infections, which could help doctors diagnose patients and prescribe antibiotics. Although MYCIN was not used in practice, studies showed that the treatment plans it proposed were highly acceptable. Many early medical diagnostic and advisory expert systems referenced MYCIN's technology, making it one of the most influential expert systems. In 1979, Stanford University developed PUFF, the first artificial intelligence system applied in clinical settings, used for interpreting pulmonary function test reports. Due to the high complexity of medicine, early applications of medical artificial intelligence systems were mostly unsuccessful, but this also initiated the exploration and development of artificial intelligence in the medical field.

From the 1980s to the end of the twentieth century, the development of medical artificial intelligence entered a stage of cumulative growth. Due to the complexity of the research subjects and the practicality of the outcomes, medical artificial intelligence became an important branch of the artificial intelligence field and received widespread attention. In 1985, the first conference on medical artificial intelligence was held in Italy, followed by the establishment of the journal *Artificial Intelligence in Medicine*. Medical artificial intelligence achieved cumulative and breakthrough developments in fields such as knowledge engineering, machine learning, uncertain systems, ontology and terminology, natural language processing, distributed cooperative systems, and image and signal processing. In the 1980s, George Washington University developed APACHE, the first commercial medical decision system used to predict patient mortality. Subsequently, a large number of researchers devoted efforts to medical expert systems, and various medical expert systems emerged like bamboo shoots after a rain. This phase marked a period of accumulation and breakthrough in medical artificial intelligence knowledge, technology, and practical experience.

In the twenty-first century, medical artificial intelligence entered a phase of rapid and vigorous development. Various technologies such as big data mining, deep learning, and artificial neural networks were applied to the research of medical artificial intelligence, analyzing key mechanisms contained in biomedical data, establishing effective clinical auxiliary diagnostic systems, promoting clinical drug research and development, developing auxiliary therapeutic robots, and advancing toward precision medicine. In the twenty-first century, bioinformatics emerged as a new subfield of medical artificial intelligence and developed rapidly. In China, the medical artificial intelligence industry also received extensive attention; in the recorded year of 2017 alone, the total financing in related industries exceeded 1.7 billion RMB. In the fight against the COVID-19 pandemic in 2020, technologies such as comprehensive analysis and auxiliary diagnosis systems for COVID-19 CT images, artificial intelligence and COVID-19 virus drug intelligent development screening, intelligent biometric recognition and intelligent medical testing systems, remote consultations, and robot nursing played unique roles. In the future, medical artificial intelligence and medical big data will continue to develop vigorously.

9.2 Fundamental Technologies of Medical Big Data

9.2.1 Data Storage Management

With the continuous growth of medical big data, higher demands have been placed on the data storage management of hospital information systems. This section introduces the application of data storage management in hospital information systems using Hadoop as an example.

Hadoop is an open-source software framework that supports data-intensive distributed applications and operates on large clusters built with commercial hardware. All Hadoop modules assume that hardware failures are common and should be automatically handled by the framework. Thus, the Hadoop architecture is characterized by high reliability, scalability, efficiency, fault tolerance, and low cost. It is widely used in various big data storage management scenarios, including medical big data applications.

The core design of Hadoop includes the Hadoop Distributed File System (HDFS) and the MapReduce workflow. HDFS stores the location of all storage nodes within the Hadoop cluster and is the foundation of Hadoop. It employs a master/slave architecture, consisting of the NameNode, DataNode, and Client (Fig. 9.3). There is only one NameNode in HDFS, which internally provides metadata services. Its functions include managing the cluster configuration and namespace information of HDFS, managing file information, and storing DataNode information for files. DataNodes store data in blocks and are also known as slave nodes; they store actual data in HDFS. The Client is responsible for sending requests between the NameNode and DataNodes. Above HDFS is the MapReduce engine, which performs splitting operations on raw data and partitions the data, distributing it to different Map tasks for processing. The data is then converted into a collection of key-value pairs for output. Finally, the Reduce function merges the results and outputs them in various formats such as text, binary, and databases. HDFS, in conjunction with MapReduce, allows Hadoop to be perfectly applied to data batch processing. In addition to these two main components, Hadoop also includes a series of sub-projects such as Pig for data analysis and assessment, the Hive database for structured query capabilities, ZooKeeper for coordination services, the distributed database HBase for data mining, the distributed data collection system Chukwa, and the data serialization system Avro.

Taking the hospital information system as an example, the system saves the existing data files in Hadoop data nodes at the lowest data layer and uses them to follow the data for sharding management and load. The system stores structured

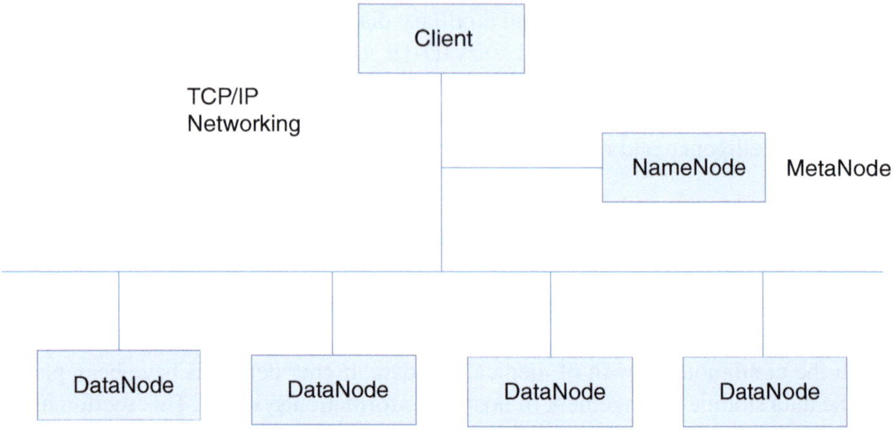

Fig. 9.3 Illustration of a simplified structure of the HDFS cluster

data in the Hive database, setting thresholds for data storage capacity and performing secondary sharding for data exceeding these thresholds. For unstructured data, the system stores it in the HBase database. It has been found that using Hadoop for distributed data storage and management results in higher operational efficiency compared to traditional single-node databases.

9.2.2 Efficient Data Processing

Medical big data processing can be divided into batch processing and stream processing modes. Batch processing is primarily used for handling large volumes of static data sets, returning results once computations are completed. It is particularly suitable for computational tasks that require access to a complete set of records. Hadoop is a framework specifically designed for batch processing. However, batch processing can be time-consuming when dealing with very large data sets. Stream processing, on the other hand, computes data as it continuously enters the system. Unlike batch processing, it does not operate on the entire data set at once but processes each data item as it passes through the system. As such, stream processing can handle almost unlimited amounts of data but only processes one item at a time (true stream processing) or a small batch of items (micro-batch processing), maintaining minimal state between different records. Stream processing shows superior performance in advanced medical big data processing techniques such as deep learning.

Graphics processing units (GPUs) are currently favored in the era of big data and intelligent computing, dominating the hardware landscape in intelligent computing fields. From a hardware perspective, a GPU's execution units are composed of stream processors, which provide substantial computational power by stacking a large number of homogeneous stream processors. From a software perspective, the core execution mode of a GPU is a typical data stream execution mode, where the execution sequence of different cores is determined by the readiness of resources and input/output data. Thanks to the internal design of GPUs, a large number of threads can exist simultaneously, providing optimal performance in machine learning and deep learning on large data sets.

Apache Spark is an open-source cluster computing framework originally developed by the AMPLab at the University of California, Berkeley. Its core model, Resilient Distributed Datasets (RDDs), is a data flow model characterized by automatic fault tolerance, location-aware scheduling, and scalability. Unlike Hadoop's MapReduce, which stores intermediary data on disk after completing tasks, Spark employs in-memory computing technology, allowing data analysis and computation directly in memory before data is written to disk. Spark can run programs in memory up to 100 times faster than Hadoop MapReduce and even 10 times faster when running programs on disk. Spark allows users to load data into cluster memory and query it multiple times, making it highly suitable for machine learning algorithms to analyze massive data sets. The Spark Streaming module enables real-time computation by organizing stream processing into batches executed at regular intervals over small time windows, achieving millisecond-level batch computation of data sets.

In conclusion, the processing of medical big data is inseparable from the application of GPUs and related stream processing architectural models. Medical information systems combining GPU and Spark technologies are continuously being developed and refined.

9.2.3 Data Analysis Techniques

Traditional big data analysis techniques include quantitative analysis, qualitative analysis, text mining, machine learning, and semantic analysis. Given the characteristics of medical big data, the most commonly used techniques in medical big data nowadays are machine learning, natural language processing (NLP), and text mining.

Machine learning is a branch of artificial intelligence primarily focused on designing and analyzing algorithms that enable computers to learn automatically. Machine learning algorithms are a type of algorithm that automatically analyze data to discover patterns and use these patterns to make predictions about unknown data. Currently, the most common analyses in medical big data are clustering analysis and pattern recognition, typically using artificial neural networks, decision trees, perceptrons, support vector machines, clustering algorithms, and Bayesian classifiers. Machine learning has been widely applied in natural language processing, biometric recognition, medical diagnosis, DNA sequencing, and other areas.

Natural language processing (NLP) is a branch of computer science and an interdisciplinary field concerned with the effective processing of natural language for direct use by computers. NLP includes various aspects and steps, covering cognition, understanding, and generation. The cognition and understanding of natural languages involve transforming the input language into symbols and relationships containing information, which are then processed according to specific goals.

Natural language generation systems convert computer data into natural language. After developments in statistical machine translation, supervised learning, unsupervised learning, and semi-supervised learning algorithms, NLP has now entered the realm of deep learning and has achieved significant results in language modeling and syntactic analysis. In the biomedical field, NLP is mainly used for biomedical information extraction, privacy information identification, text summarization, building biomedical question-answering systems, and biomedical knowledge discovery, achieving notable results.

Text mining, also known as text data mining or text analytics, is a process of analyzing unstructured text data to extract information and knowledge of potential use that users care about or are interested in. Text mining extends traditional data mining, which focuses on structured data; however, traditional data mining methods are generally not directly applicable to text mining. The unstructured nature of text data necessitates the use of NLP techniques to extract features from text data during the knowledge discovery process. Typically, in processing input text, an analysis of the data is conducted, along with the addition of linguistic features and noise reduction, to generate structured data. Typical text mining methods include text classification, text clustering, concept/entity mining, precise output classification, sentiment analysis, document summarization, and entity relationship modeling.

9.2.4 Data Visualization

Visualization refers to any technique used to create images, diagrams, or animations to communicate information. Since the dawn of humanity, visualization through visual images has been an effective way to convey both abstract and concrete ideas. Using visualization to present information is not a new phenomenon; maps are a classic example of data visualization, but it wasn't heavily emphasized until the publication of "Visualization in Scientific Computing" in 1987. Concepts such as data visualization, information visualization, and knowledge visualization have gradually gained attention since then. Data visualization refers to the use of computer graphics or general graphics to process data obtained from large-scale computer computations, transforming it into graphics or images focused on specific data characteristics and expressed in an intuitive manner. Data visualization is driven by data, and its research focus is on how to express numbers more intuitively.

Information visualization relies on large-scale data, originally created by the user interface research group at Xerox PARC, aiming to provide dynamic, demand-compliant visual results. Knowledge visualization evolved from data and information visualization, focusing on the direct display of data and analytical results, with a research emphasis on more intuitively presenting internal knowledge.

Currently, the most prevalent form in medical data visualization is still data visualization. Medical data can be divided into spatio-temporal data and non-spatio-temporal data, as shown in Fig. 9.4.

Spatio-temporal data refers to data that has geographical locations and time labels. Data with spatial coordinates is referred to as spatial data, where a scalar

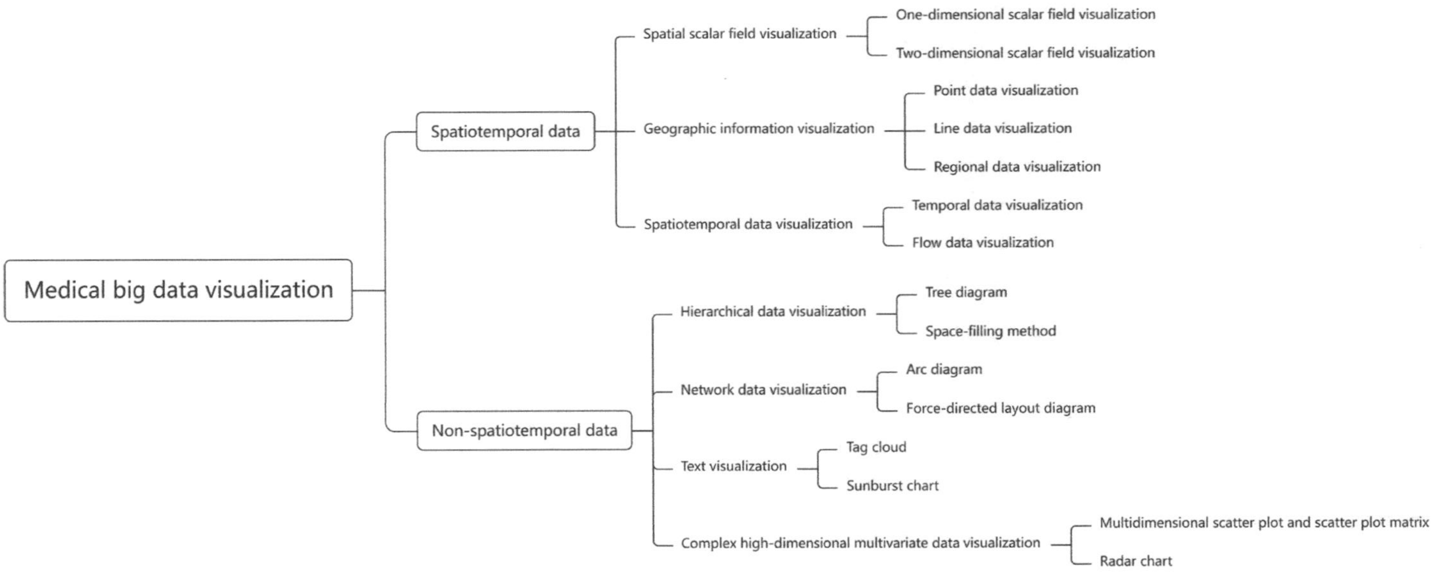

Fig. 9.4 Medical big data visualization classification

field records a single scalar at spatial sampling locations. One-dimensional scalar field visualization uses line graphs to represent data distribution patterns along a path, typically used for displaying various biochemical test results. Two-dimensional scalar field visualization shows scalar data distribution characteristics on a two-dimensional plane, with common X-ray images being a prime example. Some spatial data, such as geographic location information from wearable sensor detection devices, can also be plotted on maps by combining this geographic information. Visualization can be categorized into point data visualization, line data visualization, and area data visualization based on different data object representations. Point data visualization can represent data characteristics through the density of discrete points, and the color and size of data objects. Line data visualization can connect two or more locations with lines or paths to show the distribution of diseases within a region, a common method being flow maps. Area visualization can depict data distribution and relationships with geographic regions through area mapping, useful for detecting regional genetic diseases. Some data are temporal and change over time. First, using time as an axis to plot line graphs can be suitable for analyzing daily outpatient business flow and other scenarios. For continuously increasing stream data: one method is to use an infinite length time axis, employing a sliding window to observe and convert stream data into static data for local analysis; another method is to overlay new data on historical data to monitor changes over time, which can be used to predict upcoming prevalent diseases.

For non-spatio-temporal data, it can be further divided into hierarchical data, network data, text content data, and complex high-dimensional multivariate data. Hierarchical data is typically displayed using tree diagrams, which can be less effective when there are many leaf nodes at the bottom. Another method for displaying hierarchical data is the space-filling approach, using rectangles to represent nodes within the hierarchical structure, and expressing the hierarchical relationship between parent and child nodes through the nesting of rectangles, making full use of screen space. For grid data that does not have a bottom-up or top-down structure, arc length linkage diagrams and force-directed layout diagrams are generally used. Both use nodes to represent data, but the former arranges nodes along a linear axis or in a circular form, connecting nodes with arcs, suitable for medication analysis and routine disease monitoring. The latter loosely distributes nodes across a diagram, connecting related nodes with straight lines, typically used for gene association analysis. Text content is a typical representative of unstructured data types in the big data era and an important form of big data. The significance of text visualization lies in visually expressing the semantic features contained in the text. Depending on different forms, methods such as tag clouds, where tag size is influenced by weight, and sunburst diagrams, which show the proximity of keyword relationships, can describe the importance of related concepts. For complex high-dimensional multivariate data visualization, two-dimensional or three-dimensional scatter plots, as well as scatter plot matrices or radar charts, can be used to display its significance in multidimensional space, thereby allowing for a visual observation of data changes under different influencing factors.

9.3 Construction of Medical Big Data Platform

9.3.1 Platform Construction Philosophy

With the continuous improvement in medical informatics and automation levels, medical big data in China has been growing explosively. Correspondingly, the demand for the application of medical big data in the healthcare industry is also increasing. As a valuable fundamental strategic resource, the ability to integrate these medical big data securely and efficiently, and to use appropriate medical data analysis technologies and tools for mining and analysis, is of great significance for the advancement of China's health and medical field.

Although the governance and application of medical big data have been underway in China for many years, they are still in the early stages of industry development. A large amount of information resources in hospitals, constrained by non-standard data collection, integration, and management, remain "asleep" in databases, and the efficiency of data utilization is low. It is also worth noting that medical information is highly sensitive. The current lack of a secure and efficient data-sharing mechanism between major medical institutions has led to the creation of many "information islands." Institutions that possess data are reluctant to share, and those in need cannot access the data, severely limiting the governance and application of medical big data in China. Therefore, the construction of a medical big data platform capable of managing, analyzing, and applying medical big data is urgent.

A medical big data platform refers to a comprehensive information platform with various functions such as medical data collection, data storage, data analysis, and data presentation. It is a powerful tool for managing, analyzing, and applying medical big data. The former National Health and Family Planning Commission (now the National Health Commission) has provided the following explanations for the standards of a medical big data platform in the "Hospital informatics Construction and Application Technology Guidelines (Trial)":

Data exchange and aggregation. Various data collection access technologies enable the parsing, aggregation, and sharing of multi-source heterogeneous data such as internal data from medical institutions, data from related medical departments, health data, and Internet data.

Data storage. Based on columnar databases, file databases, distributed databases, clusters, and other file storage technologies, it supports the distributed storage of structured, semi-structured, and unstructured files.

Distributed computing. Based on a distributed computing framework and utilizing cluster resources, it performs distributed parallel execution of computing tasks, improving the computational efficiency of multi-source heterogeneous massive data.

Data visualization. Based on a unified spatio-temporal framework and using interactive visualization interface methods, it achieves a comprehensive display of large health data.

For medical staff, the establishment of a medical big data platform can use big data technology to structurally process medical records, meeting the data collection needs for clinical research. It also allows for efficient searching and establishing precise research cohorts. The platform can also provide medical services supported by medical big data, offering auxiliary diagnostic and treatment services for various diseases, analyzing related conditions deeply with past cases and various data sources, and recommending the best treatment plans, laying the foundation for personalized medicine.

For patients, the establishment of a medical big data platform enables patients to actively participate in the medical process, which is beneficial for doctors to provide personalized medical care by integrating patients' medical history and health data, making more accurate disease diagnoses. This medical model respects the individual characteristics and needs of patients more. The medical big data platform can also more efficiently coordinate and integrate different professional medical services, ensuring the continuity and accessibility of medical services, thereby enhancing the quality of medical care.

For management personnel, the medical big data platform can provide a unified visual analysis tool, achieving refined management of the hospital. Through the medical big data platform, data such as the volume of outpatient surgeries, bed occupancy rates, admission/discharge numbers, equipment utilization rates, and disease maps can be efficiently integrated and analyzed to provide objective and reliable data support for hospital operation-related decisions. At the same time, through the comparative analysis of data from different periods, management personnel can accurately assess the current operational conditions of the hospital and quickly identify weak links in the operational process, thereby making targeted improvements.

With the development of big data integration governance and analysis mining technology through the medical big data platform, the productivity of medical institutions can be enhanced, and the re-utilization of historical medical resources can be realized. More importantly, research on big data thinking and methods can be conducted, thus breaking through problems that traditional thinking and methods cannot solve, achieving efficient retrieval, structuring, and analytical computation of medical data. At the same time, promoting the construction of an efficient, secure, and stable medical big data platform and realizing the secure interactive sharing of medical big data will increase the usage value of data, while also providing reliable and effective services and assistance for medical workers, clinical researchers, management personnel, and patients themselves.

9.3.2 Big Data Platform Ecosystem

9.3.2.1 Data System

Medical big data refers to the data generated during the diagnosis and treatment processes by doctors for patients. It encompasses basic patient data, diagnostic data, electronic medical records, medical imaging report data, medical management, economic data, and data from medical devices and instruments. Besides having the general characteristics of big data, medical big data also possesses inherent features specific to the medical field such as temporality, privacy, and incompleteness. Large volume, high quality, and standardized medical big data form the data foundation for the construction of medical big data platforms.

The diverse, heterogeneous, and non-unified nature of medical big data results in a standard system that differs from traditional national or industry data standards. Different types of medical big data often require localized and more flexible data standards; hence, it is important to actively promote the construction of a standard normative system for the utilization of the value of medical big data.

To actively promote the construction of a standard normative system for the utilization of medical big data, it is first necessary to refine and clarify the stakeholders involved in medical big data, including the service providers and consumers within the medical big data platform, as well as other stakeholders and responsible parties involved in the data circulation. By sorting out these data-related stakeholders, the business and technical requirements of each data circulation stage can be identified, collectively forming the overall needs of the big data platform. This assessment helps in evaluating the reasonableness of the standards for the utilization of medical big data. Furthermore, the standard normative system for the utilization of medical big data should be constructed from both the data flow dimension and the IT service dimension: from the data flow perspective, the value of data is realized through data collection, integration, analysis, and the use of results; from the IT service perspective, the value of data is achieved through platform IT services, which ensure the consistency, security, and accuracy of the medical big data platform, thereby effectively leveraging the data value.

Based on factors such as the interests of data-related parties, data circulation stages, and platform service agreements, actively promoting the construction of a standard normative system for the utilization of medical big data through a use case-driven approach is key to establishing a solid data foundation for the medical big data platform. It is also a crucial element within the ecosystem of the medical big data platform.

By adopting a use case-driven approach, we can align the construction of standards with practical scenarios and requirements. This entails identifying specific use cases where medical big data can be applied and understanding the needs and constraints within those scenarios. By doing so, the standard normative system can be tailored to support actual operational workflows, data exchange, and value extraction from the data.

The establishment of such a system not only facilitates the structured growth and integration of various data types and sources within the medical big data platform but also ensures that the platform can serve the needs of different users effectively. This includes healthcare providers who require accurate and timely data to make informed decisions, researchers who need comprehensive data for studies, and policy-makers who rely on data for health system planning and monitoring.

In conclusion, building a standard normative system that can adapt to the unique characteristics of medical big data and address the ecosystem's diverse needs is essential for maximizing the value of the data. This system should foster interoperability, maintain privacy and security, and provide a framework for the ethical and effective use of medical big data.

9.3.2.2 Technical System

The Information Professional Committee of the Chinese Hospital Association released the "Construction Guide for Medical Big Data Platforms in Medical Institutions" in 2019, which points out the current primary needs for constructing medical big data platforms as follows:

Stable Big Data Platform: Through big data-related technologies and frameworks, the platform can provide stable and efficient data collection, data integration, data mining, data computation, data analysis, and data governance functionalities.

Diverse Big Data Collection: The platform should support various data collection methods, including full-table collection and incremental extraction, and should also support log management and anomaly monitoring.

Effective Big Data Governance: The platform should support unified modeling for both structured and unstructured data, centralized and distributed data; it should support data governance activities such as data anonymization and cleansing; and it should normalize data from multiple heterogeneous sources according to unified data standards.

Rich Big Data Applications: The platform should be able to utilize the big data resources of the data center to support auxiliary decision-making applications in medical services, scientific research management, and hospital governance.

Flexible Big Data Presentation: Provide visualization configuration for big data models and visualized display of big data analysis results.

Secure Big Data Services: The platform should ensure the security of big data storage, access, and transmission services. It should be capable of conducting security assessments and monitoring data flows to prevent the leakage of private data.

Faced with the challenges of massive data volumes, diversified data types, dynamic data systems, and significant data value, traditional technical methods no longer meet the six major needs mentioned above. Traditional storage and computation modes struggle to cope with the current scale of data and its complexity, and traditional data analysis methods find it difficult to deeply mine the potential value of data. Therefore, constructing a more advanced technical system capable of addressing the current challenges of medical big data is an indispensable part of the medical big data platform ecosystem.

9.3.2.3 Policy System

Currently, the nation is increasingly emphasizing the governance and application of medical big data, as well as the construction and promotion of medical big data platforms. Relevant policies are actively being introduced to guide these efforts.

In September 2015, the State Council issued the "Notice of the State Council on Printing and Distributing the Action Outline for Promoting the Development of Big Data (State Council Document [2015] No. 50)" (hereinafter referred to as the "Notice"). The "Notice" pointed out the need to comprehensively promote the application of big data in the medical and health field. Health and medical big data, as a crucial foundational strategic resource for the country, will bring profound changes to the health and medical model. It will help stimulate and deepen the motivation and vitality for reforming the pharmaceutical and healthcare system, improve the efficiency and quality of health and medical services, expand resource supply, and continuously meet the multi-level and diverse health needs of the people.

In 2016, the General Office of the State Council issued the "Guiding Opinions on Promoting and Regulating the Development and Application of Health and Medical Big Data (State Council General Office Document [2016] No. 47)" (hereinafter referred to as the "Guiding Opinions"). The "Guiding Opinions" further pointed out the need to explore new service models and cultivate new business forms through "Internet + Health and Medical," striving to build a healthcare system that satisfies the people and provides strong support for the construction of a Healthy China. Health and medical big data, centered around residents' electronic health records, electronic medical records, and electronic prescriptions, and integrating personal health data resources generated by wearable devices and smart health electronic products, aims to build a population health information resource database. The "Guiding Opinions" require starting from the goal of ensuring the health of the entire population, eliminating "information silos," building a health and medical big data platform, and promoting the sharing and application of health and medical big data. Medical big data, as an important component of health and medical big data, primarily aims to analyze patient disease information based on clinical medical data and medical professional knowledge, providing precise medical services to patients. To promote the application of medical big data, it is necessary to build a medical big data platform to lay a solid technical foundation for clinical medical care, medical research, and personal health management.

In April 2018, the Planning and Information Department of the National Health Commission issued the "National Hospital informatics Construction Standards and Specifications (Trial)" (referred to as the "Standards and Specifications"). The "Standards and Specifications" put forward construction requirements for the development of hospital informatics applications nationwide over the next 5–10 years, requiring hospitals to achieve information sharing and business interaction, data standardization, and business normalization. They also put forward clear requirements and basic functional descriptions for the application of big data technology in medical operations. The "Standards and Specifications" clarify that medical institutions need to use medical big data platforms to manage, analyze, and utilize medical big data to achieve the goals of enhancing the efficiency of medical research and application, and promoting the development of smart healthcare. By building a medical big data platform and using big data analysis and mining technology, medical institutions can, to a certain extent, utilize historical medical resources to enhance competitiveness and use big data thinking and methods to conduct research.

This can help overcome tasks that were previously impossible with traditional thinking and methods, achieving efficient retrieval, post-structuring, and computational analysis of medical data.

In September 2018, the National Health Commission issued the "National Health and Medical Big Data Standards, Security and Service Management Measures (Trial)" (referred to as the "Trial Measures"). The "Trial Measures" clarified the definition, connotation, and extension of health and medical big data, as well as the purpose, basis, scope of application, principles to follow, and overall ideas for formulating the measures. They clarified the boundaries and responsibilities of health and health administrative departments at all levels, the responsibilities, rights, and interests of various types of medical and health institutions and corresponding application units, and standardized these three aspects. Regarding standard management, the "Trial Measures" clarified the principles for carrying out health and medical big data standard management work and the work responsibilities of health administrative departments at all levels. They advocate for multi-party participation in standard management work, improving the health and medical big data standard management platform, and stipulating the standard management process, incentive and restraint mechanisms, application effect evaluation, development, and application. Regarding safety management, the "Trial Measures" clarified the scope of health and medical big data safety management, established and improved relevant safety management systems, operating procedures, and technical specifications, proposed storage requirements for data grading, classification, and zoning, and put forward clear requirements for key links such as network security level protection, critical information infrastructure security, and data security assurance measures. Regarding service management, the "Trial Measures" clarified the responsibilities of relevant parties and the principles for implementing health and medical big data management services, implementing a management system of "unified hierarchical authorization, classified application management, and consistent rights and responsibilities," and strengthening the sharing and exchange of health and medical big data. At the same time, in terms of management and supervision, the "Trial Measures" also emphasized the daily supervision and management responsibilities of health and health administrative departments and proposed safety monitoring, evaluation, and accountability systems for big data applications.

9.3.3 Big Data Platform Implementation Standards

9.3.3.1 Data Standardization Norms

As a crucial foundational strategic resource for the nation, health and medical big data have been emphasized in the "Trial Measures" issued by the National Health Commission in 2018. These measures clearly state the need to expedite the development of health and medical big data standards and encourage participation from major healthcare institutions, research and educational units, relevant industry associations, and social organizations in the formulation of these standards. Currently, although there are some mature health and medical big data standards, the data collected and aggregated from multiple institutions lack a unified national or industry standard. Different medical big data platforms adopt different standards, and even within the same region, different hospitals may use different data standards. Such inconsistencies in clinical medical data, including diverse data types, weak integration and analysis technologies, and significant heterogeneity between institutions, severely hinder the conduct of large-scale, high-quality clinical data research. The absence of unified health and medical big data industry standards within the medical information sector can, to some extent, restrict the data quality and governance effectiveness of medical big data platforms.

9.3.3.2 Data Technical Standards

The "Guidelines for Hospital informatics Construction and Application (Trial)" provides the following explanations regarding the data technologies that medical big data platforms should possess:

Data Mining and Modeling.

Provision of services for massive data reading, data processing, and data computation based on big data architecture, supporting data mining and analysis services through visual data exploration tools, data mining models, and simple model training.

Data Application Services.

Support for rapid data integration, online data retrieval, and multi-user collaboration tools, offering services for the retrieval, consolidation, and other applications of big data.

Data Governance.

Through standardized processes and rule libraries, a unified and configurable data processing workflow—including data transformation, cleansing, comparison, association, and integration—is constructed based on a process engine. This enables the processing and production of heterogeneous, massive, and discrete data resources into analyzable, usable, and shareable data.

The medical industry differs from other sectors, and medical big data platforms need to select relevant data technologies based on the specific requirements of medical big data rather than blindly copying from other industries. In critical stages such as data collection and data mining, the technologies must meet the actual needs of hospitals.

9.3.3.3 Platform Security Specifications

Health and medical data are sensitive, necessitating extra caution in developing health and medical big data while ensuring data security and patient privacy. The National Health Commission has outlined a security assurance framework for data platforms that should involve tiered security protection across three areas: computing environment, communication network, and regional boundaries. Additionally, a centralized security management center must be established to centrally manage the security policies and mechanisms deployed in these three areas.

In terms of computing environment security, the data platform should achieve the requirements of a level-two enhanced computing environment, including identity authentication, security auditing, access control, as well as data confidentiality and integrity. Furthermore, based on actual conditions, backup and storage recovery measures for data should be established to ensure quick recovery of data, systems, and operations in case of a security incident. Regarding communication network security, the data platform should realize the requirements of a level-two enhanced secure communication network, which includes communication confidentiality, integrity protection, network device security protection, and network device redundancy. For security in regional boundaries, the data platform should meet the requirements of a level-two enhanced regional boundary, which includes firewall isolation, security auditing, intrusion prevention, and malicious code detection and filtering.

9.4 Case Analysis

9.4.1 Medical Information System Based on Cloud Platform

Cloud computing is the result of the development and integration of traditional computer technologies and network technologies such as distributed computing, parallel computing, grid computing, virtualization, load balancing, and network storage. By utilizing large-scale, low-cost computing units connected via IP networks, it provides users with various computing and storage services, characterized by large scale, easy scalability, resource sharing, dynamic allocation, and cross-regional capabilities.

The 454th Hospital of the People's Liberation Army, as one of the pilot units for the digital hospital construction project based on cloud computing in the Nanjing Military Region, completed its cloud-based digital hospital information infrastructure platform in July 2012. Within 3 months of the platform's completion, 20 new business information systems, including the new version of electronic medical records and electrophysiology, were put online. This marked the transition from the traditional offline mode of "queuing—registration—payment—report collection" to the new mode of "online transaction—offline diagnosis and treatment."

The overall architecture of the mobile Internet hospital cloud platform is divided into three parts: the user access layer, the external network business service layer, and the internal network data interaction layer. In the user access layer, users enter the system using mobile terminals such as smartphones via WeChat or Alipay service windows. In the external network business service layer, data interaction security between the internal and external networks is ensured through security authentication and protection provided by devices such as firewalls, intrusion prevention systems, and network gateways. The internal network data interaction layer is mainly responsible for facilitating the interaction between external networks and internal hospital systems such as HIS (Hospital Information System), LIS (Laboratory Information System), and PACS (Picture Archiving and Communication

System) through business interface service middleware. As shown in Fig. 9.5, the entire system includes functional modules covering hospital information, intelligent guidance, and appointment registration for pre-hospital, in-hospital, and post-hospital processes.

By using the mobile Internet hospital cloud platform, the treatment process has been optimized. In the traditional treatment mode, patients were unfamiliar with the routes to various departments in the hospital and had to run back and forth for medical consultations and payments, which also involved long waiting times. This not only caused inconvenience for patients but also reduced the operational efficiency of the hospital. Through the mobile Internet hospital cloud platform, first-time patients can access the mobile hospital via WeChat or Alipay service windows, perform operations such as registration, payment, and application processes online, thus significantly reducing the service pressure at hospital windows. This resolves the "three long and one short" issue—long registration, waiting, and payment times, and short consultation times—effectively alleviating doctor–patient conflicts, significantly improving efficiency, and saving valuable work time. At the same time, the mobile Internet hospital cloud platform also establishes a bridge for doctor–patient communication. In the traditional treatment mode, interaction between patients and doctors only occurred within the hospital. However, with the mobile Internet cloud platform, patients can communicate with doctors throughout the entire process, from pre-hospital appointments to in-hospital consultations and post-hospital feedback, thus establishing a comprehensive bridge for doctor-patient communication.

9.4.2 Multi-Center Intelligent Medical Information Platform

After more than a decade of rapid informatics, a large amount of clinical medical data has been accumulated in various medical and research institutions. However, these clinical medical data generally face issues such as complex data types, weak integration and analysis techniques, significant heterogeneity between institutions, incomplete data-sharing strategies, and a lack of collaborative analysis methods under privacy protection. These issues severely hinder the development of large-scale, multi-center, high-quality clinical data research. There is an urgent need for concentrated efforts to break through core technologies related to the deep utilization of multi-center clinical data. This would involve constructing a cross-institutional, multi-center medical big data platform to break the barriers of single-center, centralized data analysis, thereby effectively enhancing the accuracy and effectiveness of decision support models in real clinical applications.

9.4.2.1 Observational Health Data Sciences and Informatics (OHDSI)

The Observational Health Data Sciences and Informatics (OHDSI) platform, led by institutions such as Columbia University, provides solutions for medical big data analysis focused on drug research. OHDSI conducts high-throughput observational studies using consistent and standardized methods. Its data network includes over

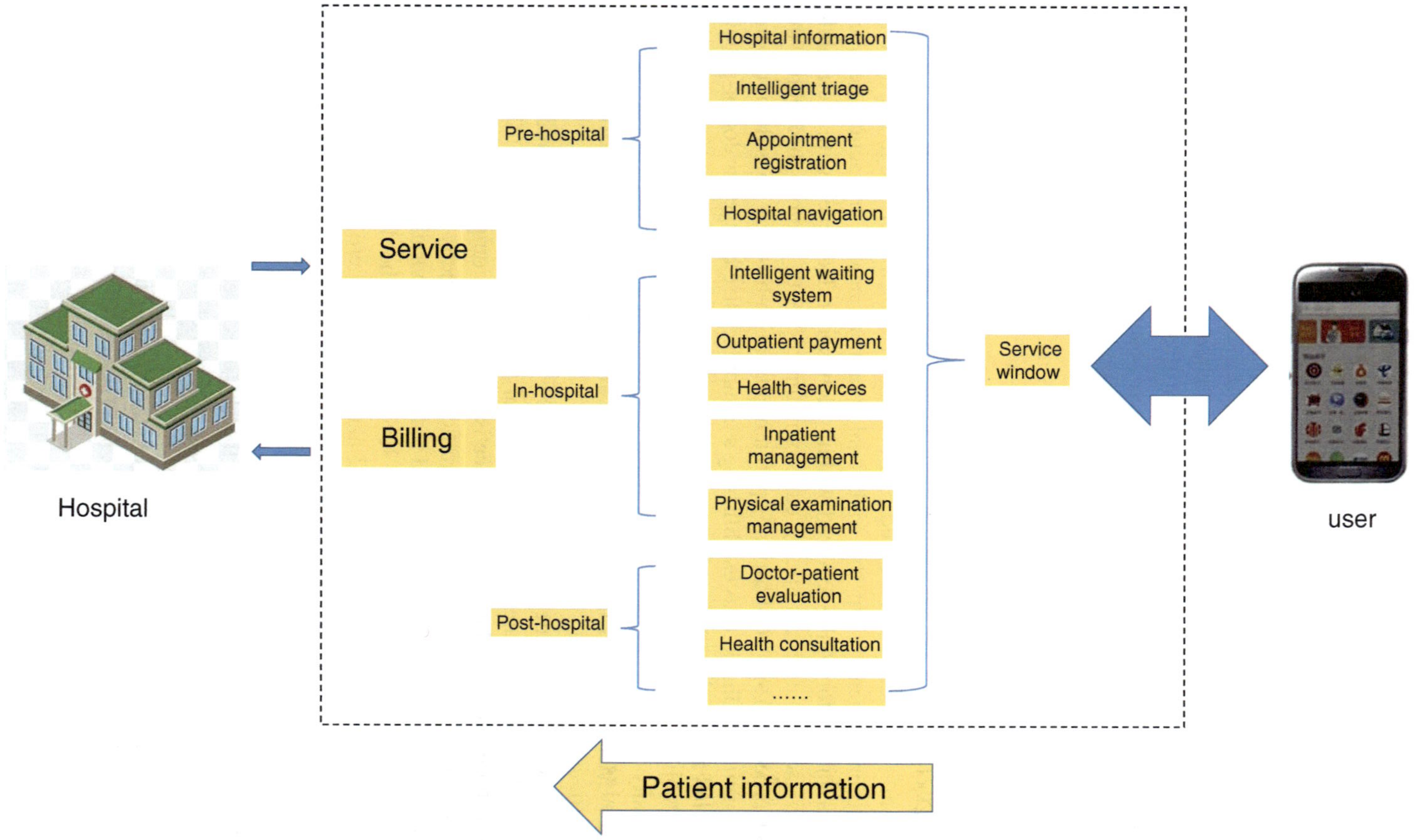

Fig. 9.5 Functional module diagram of the mobile Internet hospital cloud platform system at the 454th Hospital of the People's Liberation Army

100 medical databases from more than 20 countries. By using a common data model (CDM) and standardized terminology sets, OHDSI integrates medical records of a billion patients through a distributed network. Each data partner in the network maintains full control over their patient-level data, which allows for the creation of precise research cohorts that can significantly reduce biases caused by insufficient data or imprecise research cohorts in traditional studies, leading to more scientific and objective research conclusions [1, 2].

A brief introduction to the CDM designed by OHDSI follows. It includes 16 clinical event tables, 10 vocabulary tables of standardized terminology sets, 2 metadata tables, 4 health system data tables, 2 health economics data tables, 3 standardized derived tables, and 2 outcome model tables. This "person-centered" model links all clinical event tables to the patient table. Additionally, the CDM covers 30 specific domains, including disease conditions, medical costs, and drugs. In the OHDSI CDM, content is represented by concepts, using the same concept as the sole standard. Each event record is fully standardized, and the concept table contains detailed information about each concept. The standardized terminology closely related to the concepts includes detailed information on concepts, concept relationships, and other related concepts. Together, these form the foundation for OHDSI's interoperability with researchers, ensuring that researchers can obtain reproducible and comparable results [3].

9.4.2.2 Zhijiang Laboratory Multi-Center Intelligent Medical Information Platform

To further break the barriers of medical information data, achieve multi-center clinical data sharing and deep utilization, in 2020, the "Multi-Center Intelligent Medical Information Platform" developed by the Network Health Big Data Center of Zhijiang Laboratory officially became the first major project to enter the Zhijiang Laboratory Digital Health Achievement Transformation Base. This is the country's most complete multi-center clinical data collaborative utilization platform that supports cross-national research.

The "Multi-Center Intelligent Medical Information Platform" is based on independently developed semi-automatic Chinese clinical data cleansing, transformation, and mapping tools. It has recorded real clinical records of over 20.10 million patients from multiple large tertiary hospitals in Zhejiang Province. The platform offers more than 70 efficient data processing and intelligent analysis tools, including clinical cohort construction and intelligent medical imaging labeling. Notably, it features ultra-large-scale complete electronic medical record knowledge graph technology, covering 18 clinical terminology sets, 4.79 million terms, over 35 million medical relationships, and 96 million medical literature knowledge entries. This technology can break knowledge barriers and fully mine the vast dormant data within various medical institutions. Additionally, it employs high-performance homomorphic encryption technology for multi-center clinical data security and privacy protection, with a security level 248 times higher than existing solutions, effectively solving the practical challenges of clinical data ciphertext mining.

9.5 Summary

With the continuous improvement of medical informatics and automation, the growth of medical big data in China is explosive, and the demand for its application is also increasing. To make good use of this valuable foundational resource, on the one hand, it is necessary to have a clear understanding of the characteristics of big data, promoting the development of big data storage, processing, analysis, and visualization technologies. On the other hand, it is essential to establish medical big data platforms to manage, analyze, and apply medical big data, thereby creating a good ecosystem for medical big data platforms and introducing relevant national and industry standards for these platforms. Currently, the country is gradually introducing related policies to promote the governance and utilization of medical big data and the construction and implementation of medical big data platforms.

References

1. Hripcsak G, Ryan PB, Duke JD, et al. Characterizing treatment pathways at scale using the OHDSI network. Proc Natl Acad Sci U S A. 2016;113(27):7329–36.
2. Hripcsak G, Duke JD, Shah NH, et al. Observational health data sciences and informatics (OHDSI): opportunities for observational researchers. Stud Inform Control. 2015;216:574–8.
3. Xin Z, Li W, Miao S, et al. Analysis of treatment pathways for three chronic diseases using OMOP CDM. J Med Syst. 2018;42(12):260.

Internet Hospitals

10

Contents

10.1 Overview of Internet Hospitals ... 276
10.1.1 Introduction to Internet Hospitals ... 276
10.1.2 Development History of Internet Hospitals ... 276
10.1.3 Current Status of Internet Hospitals Domestically and Internationally ... 277
10.2 Internet Hospital Technology System ... 279
10.2.1 Internet Hospital Technology Framework ... 279
10.2.2 Internet Hospital System Framework ... 280
10.2.3 Main Functions and Implementation of Internet Hospitals ... 281
10.2.4 Interconnection with In-Hospital Systems ... 281
10.2.5 Security Construction of Internet Hospitals ... 282
10.3 Internet Hospital Service Model ... 283
10.3.1 Online Consultation ... 283
10.3.2 Online Prescription ... 284
10.3.3 Hierarchical Medical System ... 284
10.4 Issues in the Development of Internet Hospitals ... 285
10.4.1 Potential Security Risks ... 285
10.4.2 Operational Difficulties ... 286
10.4.3 Talent Scarcity ... 287
10.4.4 Relevant Laws and Policies ... 287
10.5 Case Studies ... 289
10.5.1 Implementation of Physical Community Internet Hospitals ... 289
10.5.2 Innovative Internet Hospital Combining Tertiary Hospitals and Internet Enterprises ... 291
10.5.3 Role of Internet Hospitals During the COVID-19 Pandemic ... 291
10.6 Summary ... 293

In recent years, the field of medical services has seen the emergence of new forms, with Internet hospitals standing out as a prominent example. Based on physical hospitals, Internet hospitals leverage Internet information technology to deeply integrate medical and health services. This integration allows patients to use their

J. Li et al., *Healthcare Information Systems*, Innovative Medical Devices,
https://doi.org/10.1007/978-981-97-9551-2_10

mobile phones or other mobile devices to access and experience a full range of services, including intelligent medical guidance, appointment registration, online consultations, medication delivery, appointment scheduling for tests and examinations, viewing electronic medical reports, making payments, and providing feedback on their medical experiences. These services play a positive role in promoting hierarchical diagnosis and treatment and improving patient experiences, showcasing enormous development potential.

10.1 Overview of Internet Hospitals

10.1.1 Introduction to Internet Hospitals

An Internet hospital is a new type of outpatient medical service that provides healthcare through Internet technology. With its potential to deliver comprehensive outpatient services, the Internet hospital has become a popular trend in China in recent years. Through websites or smartphone application platforms provided by Internet hospitals, patients can consult doctors from top hospitals in major cities directly from their homes or local clinics. By overcoming time and geographical barriers, Internet hospitals help alleviate the issue of "difficult access to medical care" to a certain extent.

Internet hospitals are categorized into two types based on their organizing entities:

The first type is the physical Internet hospital dominated by hospitals. Most of these Internet hospitals are dominated by tertiary hospitals with strong capabilities, and special departments are set up by the hospitals to be responsible for the operation of Internet hospitals, which mainly provide the staff of the medical institutions with appointment registration, triage, rediagnosis of some common chronic diseases, online appointment for examination and inspection, online follow-up, remote consultation and two-way referral services.

The second type is the Internet medical platform based on entity medical institutions led by Internet enterprises, which has good technical ability, operation management ability and innovative development thinking, and cooperates with entity hospitals and invites medical staff of entity hospitals to provide online medical services for patients.

10.1.2 Development History of Internet Hospitals

With the development of information technology, computers and IT (information technology) began to be applied in hospitals, gradually enabling the digitization of medical information storage and laying a solid foundation for the formation of Internet hospitals. Since their inception, Internet hospitals have evolved from a simple information display model to a diversified business model. Initially, they could only offer basic functions such as appointment registration, online payments, report queries, and text consultations. Over time, they developed to provide online appointment consultations, offline examinations and treatments, prescription transfers, health management follow-ups, and full-process coverage before, during, and after consultations.

On the one hand, as a supplement to traditional medical services, Internet hospitals have helped meet the growing health needs of the public and significantly improve medical efficiency. On the other hand, issues such as ethical risks and information leakage during the operation of Internet hospitals raise doubts about their future prospects. Therefore, in addition to technical support and guarantees, it is necessary to fully leverage government policy guidance, strengthen the construction of legal and regulatory systems, emphasize the integration of various social resources, and enhance the management of hospital medical applications for Internet hospitals to become more widely adopted and developed. Although Internet hospitals currently cannot completely replace offline hospitals, they have become an indispensable part of hierarchical diagnosis and treatment. As public living standards improve and attention to health increases, Internet hospitals will eventually become normalized.

10.1.3 Current Status of Internet Hospitals Domestically and Internationally

Internet hospitals are an inevitable product of "Internet + Healthcare," aligning with China's policy of vigorously promoting hierarchical diagnosis and treatment, as well as the current market ecosystem. The policy development of Chinese Internet hospitals can be divided into two phases: the first phase (2005–2017) and the second phase (from 2018 onward). Overall, the first phase emphasized the construction of information infrastructure, the integration of medical resources, and the design of development models. The second phase focuses on the systematic development of service and payment models, prioritizing the conversion of resources into effective services.

In 2005, the State Food and Drug Administration first allowed the online sale of over-the-counter drugs, promoting the exploration of innovative Internet pharmaceutical services. In 2014, the National Health and Family Planning Commission (now the National Health Commission) allowed remote medical service providers to create medical services. In 2015, the State Council incorporated the "Internet + Healthcare" model into the national medical and health service system, promoting health informatization services and smart medical services to benefit all people. Additionally, the State Council issued guidelines on building a hierarchical medical service system, utilizing information technology and big data to reform the existing hospital-centered model. In December 2015, the first Internet hospital in China, Wuzhen Internet Hospital, was established, marking the transition of the "Internet + Healthcare" model from concept to physical construction. In 2017, the State Council promoted the construction of medical institution alliances, implementing hierarchical medical service models, and strengthening the support and training of primary medical institutions by higher medical institutions through digital technology. The construction of population health information systems was listed as a key project by the State Council and the National Health and Family Planning Commission. Furthermore, the National Health and Family Planning Commission allowed doctors to practice at multiple sites and officially permitted doctors to work for Internet-based medical institutions.

In 2018, the development of Internet hospitals achieved milestone progress. The National Health Commission and the State Administration of Traditional Chinese Medicine issued policies such as the "Administrative Measures for Internet Diagnosis and Treatment (Trial)," "Regulations for the Management of Telemedicine Services (Trial)," and "Administrative Measures for Internet Hospitals (Trial)." These policies clarified the access, practice, and supervision rules of Internet hospitals. In 2019, the National People's Congress promulgated the "Drug Administration Law of the People's Republic of China," explicitly supporting the development of "Internet + Healthcare" hospitals and allowing the online sale of prescription drugs at the legislative level. The National Healthcare Security Administration has issued a policy guideline on "Internet plus health" medical service pricing and medical insurance payment, aiming to support insurance coverage in Internet hospitals.

According to the National Health Commission, as of February 2021, China had over 1100 Internet hospitals, with 7700 secondary and higher hospitals providing online services. The online appointment diagnosis rate of tertiary hospitals had exceeded 50%, and over 90% of tertiary public hospitals had achieved information sharing within the hospital. Nationwide, 30 provinces had established Internet medical service supervision platforms. Although China's new healthcare reform has made substantial progress in providing equitable access to healthcare and improving financial risk protection mechanisms over the past decade, there are still significant disparities compared to developed countries in terms of healthcare quality, non-communicable disease control, healthcare expenditure control, public satisfaction, and medical resource allocation. At present, China's Internet hospitals still have many limitations and problems to be solved, such as uneven construction level, low efficiency of data sharing, low public recognition, shortage of professional talents, insufficient profitability, and imperfect corresponding regulatory policies.

In countries with advanced Internet levels, the application and development of Internet hospitals started earlier and are more widespread. For example, Athena Health, a data-driven healthcare system founded in the United States in 1997, collaborates with various healthcare organizations to open networks to care facilities, providers, and other partners through improved clinical records and patient engagement services, seeking and eliminating barriers to achieving smarter healthcare experiences. WellDoc, founded in 2005, primarily uses information technology to assist in chronic disease management, making it easier for individuals to manage chronic diseases and improve their quality of life. The company is globally leading in AI-driven guidance for managing multiple chronic diseases and comorbidities. For instance, its diabetes management platform BlueStar uses a smartphone app to remind patients to take medication, track diet, sleep, and exercise, provide personalized health guidance, store patient records, and upload data to the cloud to timely alert doctors and nurses for relevant actions.

The UK has a mature Internet hospital system, with the National Health Service (NHS), established in 1948, being the most representative. It has grown to be the world's largest public healthcare system, funded by the government, and available to everyone living in the UK without requiring full payment. Albasoft focuses on providing cost-effective solutions for Scotland's healthcare sector, integrating with existing clinical databases and providing detailed patient record analysis to ensure basic healthcare services. eSCro, a custom-developed medical practice software by Albasoft, guides general practitioners in obtaining the necessary information for each medical payment, covering all details of individual treatment processes, and is fully integrated into Scotland's healthcare system. Additionally, there are Internet service systems aimed at individuals or specific diseases, such as Cellnovo, the world's first mobile diabetes management system comprising an insulin patch pump, activity monitor, and automatically connected wireless smartphone. This system provides optimal insulin injection management while ensuring extensive freedom of movement for diabetes patients. Acutus Medical is a top-tier atrial fibrillation ablation mapping system that integrates ultrasound and proprietary mapping platforms, providing unprecedented precision in the electrocardiogram of complex arrhythmias and guiding ablation treatment in real time.

Denmark also has a mature and convenient central healthcare data network system, such as Sundhed.dk and MedCom. Sundhed.dk, launched in 2003 by the Danish Ministry of Health and local authorities, is Denmark's official public health service portal. It offers an online platform for users to find information about diseases, treatments, and healthcare services, including doctor visits, health journals, laboratory results, and organ donation consent. Today, the platform has become a supplier of nationwide IT-related health solutions, with the vision of helping Danish citizens take control of their health. MedCom, launched in 2005, is an electronic national laboratory test order solution, fully implemented in all 2100 general practitioner clinics and 1000 private specialist clinics within 3 years. It includes 42 biochemistry laboratories, 14 microbiology laboratories, and 16 histopathology and cytology laboratories. Today, over 6,000,000 laboratory test orders (100%) are processed electronically each year.

10.2 Internet Hospital Technology System

10.2.1 Internet Hospital Technology Framework

The construction of an Internet hospital technology framework can be divided into five parts: user entrance, business service layer, access control layer, in-hospital business, and provincial regulatory platform. The user entrance refers to the multiple ways users can access the Internet hospital, primarily designed using Hypertext Markup Language version 5 (HTML5) and Bootstrap technology. This allows the program to be accessed via different types of terminals after compilation, with an adaptive interface to maintain esthetics across devices. The business service layer showcases the specific services provided by the Internet hospital, such as appointment booking, online consultations, and electronic prescriptions. Function implementation adopts a front-end and back-end separation model, decoupling development for concurrent development and improved project efficiency. The front-end needs to support cross-platform operation for better compatibility and efficiency, while the backend generally uses Java, managed by the Spring framework for unified lifecycle management. The access control layer uses a 3-layer architecture, which enhances system design concepts of high cohesion and low coupling, thereby improving scalability and security. In-hospital systems must interact with the Internet hospital, including appointment and payment information from outpatient systems, test results from laboratory and medical imaging systems, and patient records from electronic medical record systems. This data exchange is managed by the access control layer to ensure both in-hospital system security and compliance with national standards. Additionally, Internet hospitals need to be supervised by regulatory platforms, such as using unified video channels, electronic health card services, and unified payment services, requiring all diagnostic records and electronic medical bills to be uploaded to the regulatory platform.

10.2.2 Internet Hospital System Framework

Based on the content included in the Internet hospital model, its system framework is generally divided into three parts: online systems, offline entities, and cloud databases.

The online system is the most crucial component of the Internet hospital, including subsystems for appointment booking, online diagnosis, electronic medical records, and online settlement and evaluation. The appointment booking subsystem needs to provide not only simple registration and appointment functions but also necessary self-diagnosis features to help patients diagnose their conditions based on symptoms, reducing misregistration issues. The online diagnosis system currently supports checks for common, chronic, and recurrent diseases. The electronic medical record subsystem records all patient consultations and corresponding prescriptions on the platform and can integrate with local hospital electronic medical record systems under appropriate conditions. The online settlement and evaluation subsystem offers payment functions for registration, consultation, and some medications.

Offline entities compensate for the shortcomings of the online system and include medical institutions (physical hospitals, medical testing agencies, public health departments), patients, networked pharmacies, and insurance agencies. Many diseases, especially those with complex symptoms, may lead to misdiagnosis if judged solely by the patient or online diagnosis. Therefore, direct diagnosis and treatment are necessary, supported by the online appointment system.

The cloud database is crucial for the normal operation of the Internet hospital, including detailed historical medical records accessible only to the patient and anonymized public case databases. The cloud database, based on Internet technology, allows each person to have a separate sub-information repository. When patients need to diagnose conditions again, necessary information can be extracted from their sub-information repository for reference, aiding in diagnosis and treatment.

According to the timing of the medical process, the system architecture of an Internet hospital can be divided into pre-diagnosis, diagnosis, and post-diagnosis stages. Pre-diagnosis includes online consultation before visiting the hospital, collecting relevant professional health information, deciding whether to visit based on their condition, and choosing suitable medical institutions based on service evaluations and costs, then registering through the appointment booking subsystem, which includes triage. During diagnosis, hospitals or medical testing institutions enter examination reports, imaging data, medical process records, and treatment plans into the electronic medical record system. Patients can view their process records and electronic prescriptions online, with medication delivered by third-party logistics companies or collected from nearby networked pharmacies, and insurance reimbursement involving uploading electronic prescriptions to insurance agencies. Post-diagnosis involves recording mutual evaluations between patients, doctors, pharmacies, and hospitals, providing service evaluation references for other patients and feedback for medical institutions to improve services.

10.2.3 Main Functions and Implementation of Internet Hospitals

Current Internet hospitals mainly include three parts: online medical platforms and communities, online medical services, and mobile medical services. These functions are primarily implemented through Internet medical workstations, patient application platforms, doctor–patient interaction frameworks, and unified payment and reconciliation platforms.

Internet medical workstations provide a unified management backend, supporting real-time communication among doctors, pharmacists, and nursing staff, with capabilities for instant messaging via text, audio, and video, facilitating medical record discussion and collaboration while preserving patient privacy with access logs for auditing. The patient application platform, typically based on mobile devices, supports individual accounts, enabling patients to access online services of self-diagnosis and treatment information queries. The doctor–patient interaction framework supports various communication forms, including text, video, questionnaires, and online consultation logs. The unified payment and reconciliation platform integrates business applications with payment services, managing orders, payments, queries, and operation logs.

10.2.4 Interconnection with In-Hospital Systems

Data integration is crucial to realizing core medical services online. It is necessary to analyze the data structure of existing main information systems and external data to build a heterogeneous data integration system. Internet hospitals need to establish a unique patient master index for each patient seen in the hospital, online revisits, and online consultations, enabling master data management based on various standard dictionaries. An electronic medical record standard dataset and clinical data center should be established, storing all diagnostic data centrally in an intranet database. With the patient master index, all current and past diagnostic information can be integrated into a single user interface, providing a complete and unified patient view, enabling data integration and sharing across intranet and Internet systems. Therefore, Internet hospitals need to interface with HIS, LIS, PIS, PACS, and other systems. These local information systems vary, using different suppliers' hardware, database management systems, and utility software.

HIS is a set of applications used to manage healthcare data, acting as a centralized database that collects and stores all information related to patients, doctors, and staff, optimizing information flow to support patient care and hospital management tasks. Healthcare professionals can access patient health information anytime for quick diagnoses. HIS also includes systems for handling data related to hospital operations management or healthcare policy decisions, essential for Internet hospital functions like appointment booking and online consultations.

LIS and PIS are necessary for the automation, modernization, and standardization of laboratory management, enabling users to share samples and results across laboratories, integrating results and tracking samples in multiple laboratory environments. Internet hospital integration with LIS and PIS allows doctors to query test results based on patient information to assess disease progression.

PACS has rapidly developed with advances in digital imaging, computer, and network technology, aimed at solving medical image acquisition, display, storage, transmission, and management. PACS's basic functions include connecting different imaging devices, storing and managing images, and calling and post-processing images. PACS contains patients' medical image information, crucial for doctors to diagnose and treat patients.

All data exchanges and application service interactions in the medical network are conducted through the hospital integration platform. Through standard interface specifications, the hospital data integration platform supports data interoperability between different heterogeneous systems, quickly deploying applications and enabling collaborative communication between medical subsystems. Building the hospital data integration platform avoids data isolation caused by single-point access to multiple different systems, allowing the hospital to manage business uniformly based on the platform, enhancing information sharing and efficiency, and adapting to the increasing demand for Internet applications.

10.2.5 Security Construction of Internet Hospitals

The development of informatization and the application of information technology also face security issues. Medical information records hold a special status, requiring strict privacy protection and secure storage and processing. Therefore, the security construction of Internet hospitals is crucial. The security issues of Internet hospitals mainly include: access to Internet applications may lead to malicious attacks from large data and traffic, threatening hospital systems; there may be malicious theft of medical data leading to patient privacy leakage; the hospital cannot visualize the entire data access process; diversified Internet access leads to inconsistent and irregular connection methods; traditional medical architecture cannot support Internet access needs, facing expansion and performance improvement issues.

Medical information security and privacy protection are global concerns. Due to poor regulation and technical vulnerabilities, hospital information and patient privacy leakages occur, causing significant economic loss and social impact. Internet hospital network construction generally needs to meet the following points: integrating third-party cloud protection mechanisms, shielding malicious Internet attacks through traffic traction, DDOS cleaning, attack interception, and traffic reinjection; managing external application requests and access processes, solving unified identity authentication, access authorization, data encryption and decryption, and data transmission security to prevent malicious data theft; addressing overreliance on vendors for hospital system interface development, defining technical standards for open services to ensure flexible and convenient platform expansion and easy integration with hospital systems, guaranteeing normal operation of business and operation platforms; ensuring no single point of failure affects the entire system, preventing data loss in case of failure; providing flexible access capabilities for the business security open platform, supporting system capacity expansion without changing software architecture.

The overall security architecture of Internet hospitals generally includes modules such as terminal users, cloud protection, internal monitoring, service security open platform, and hospital business systems. Terminal users can access convenient online services like registration, consultation, queuing, payment, and medication collection via App, WeChat, browsers, etc.; the platform shields malicious attack traffic from the Internet through cloud protection, re-injecting cleaned and intercepted traffic into the Internet healthcare service security open platform to protect the platform from malicious attacks; internal monitoring detects vulnerabilities in time, further ensuring platform security; the service security open platform acts as the only entry point for Internet business and hospital system interaction, reducing hospital exposure to the Internet; in hospital business systems, data is transmitted through gateways and the business security open platform, ensuring the security and reliability of data transmission.

10.3 Internet Hospital Service Model

10.3.1 Online Consultation

The disparity in medical resource distribution often leaves patients in rural and remote areas without access to high-quality medical services. In physical hospitals, the time doctors can spend with each patient is limited, with an average communication time of less than 3 min in large outpatient departments. This is especially insufficient for patients with chronic diseases like diabetes, who require more comprehensive disease education and information. Online consultations allow healthcare professionals to provide health consultations and follow-up services via Internet communication technologies such as text, audio, and video. This breaks the constraints of time and geography, enabling early screening of potential patients and reducing the risk of cross-infection.

Studies have shown that compared to traditional medical services, online consultations in Internet hospitals increase the time doctors spend with each patient, improve the accessibility of high-quality medical services, and alleviate the issue of "difficult access to healthcare" to some extent. This promotes a more rational distribution of healthcare resources and improves the balance between supply and demand in China's healthcare system.

In practice, online consultations cannot completely replace offline visits; patients still need to go to hospitals when necessary. However, online consultations can become a crucial part of hierarchical medical systems. As the public's living standards and awareness of health improve, online consultations meet a real demand and hold the potential for more innovation. They are anticipated to become a normalized service, extending the benefits of modern medical technology to more people.

10.3.2 Online Prescription

An online prescription is an electronic medical document issued by a registered physician as a credential for patient medication. It is reviewed, dispensed, and verified by a pharmacist with the necessary professional qualifications. Unlike traditional paper prescriptions, online prescriptions follow a standardized input format to integrate with hospital or pharmacy databases. Unlike current hospital electronic medical records, patients can access their online prescriptions. Online prescriptions must adhere to regulations such as the "Prescription Management Measures." Physicians should have access to the patient's medical records and may only issue online prescriptions for common or chronic diseases diagnosed in a physical medical institution. All prescriptions must have an electronic signature from the physician and be validated by a pharmacist to become effective. After issuing an electronic prescription, patients can choose online drug purchases or delivery services. The prices of medications prescribed online should be consistent with those in physical hospitals or partner pharmacies. Currently, the online pharmacy service model relies heavily on manual operations, which are cumbersome, inefficient, and risky.

10.3.3 Hierarchical Medical System

China's large population and uneven medical resource distribution lead to a lack of trust in primary healthcare institutions. People tend to go to large hospitals even for minor illnesses, exacerbating the problem of "difficult access to healthcare." Community health service centers, which play a crucial role in health management, suffer from simple services, lack of diversity in service forms, and insufficient capability of medical personnel. Traditional medical models show that patients requiring referral often avoid it due to complicated referral procedures, lack of information sharing, repeated tests, and delays in treatment, leading to wasted medical resources and overburdened large hospitals.

Since 2015, the Chinese government has implemented a "hierarchical diagnosis and treatment" policy, which classifies diseases by severity, mode of onset and difficulty of treatment to optimize medical resources. The development of Internet information technology has brought hope to solve this problem. Establishing a two-way referral model within the medical union under the Internet hospital model allows for efficient referrals and better resource allocation. On the one hand, community health service centers or small grass roots hospitals can initiate applications for referral with the help of the Internet hospital platform; On the other hand, secondary and tertiary hospitals can also send patient referral information to community health service centers or grass roots small hospitals through the Internet hospital platform, and the doctors of the two Internet hospitals will evaluate the referral application after receiving it, and choose to accept or refuse to accept the referred patients according to the knowledge base. The information in the referral request includes patient electronic medical records, laboratory and imaging reports, electronic prescriptions, the department to be referred, etc. The two-way referral mode under the Internet hospital model can not only facilitate patients to seek medical treatment, but also rapidly strengthen the sharing of physician resources, hospital bed resources, hospital hardware and software resources in the medical consortium, so as to improve the overall medical service ability of regional medical institutions, strengthen the coordinated and efficient development of institutions in the medical consortium, and alleviate the problem of "difficulty in seeing a doctor" of residents.

10.4 Issues in the Development of Internet Hospitals

At present, affected by many factors such as the scarcity of network doctors and the small coverage of medical insurance, the development of Internet hospitals is far from mature, and there are many problems: the standard system of Internet medical market has not been fully established, the industry norms have not been fully formed, the entry threshold of Internet hospitals is low, there is a lack of practice norms, and the supervision and management mechanism is loose. The service innovation of Internet hospital still needs to be further promoted with the support of corresponding policy intervention.

10.4.1 Potential Security Risks

Internet hospitals involve two main stakeholders: hospitals and enterprises. Hospitals serve as the foundation for Internet hospital construction, extending their services online to provide remote follow-up care. Enterprises provide the technical support to maintain platform operations, and when they lead Internet hospital initiatives, their focus is often on increasing revenue and profitability. Without strict government regulation, these enterprises could cause major medical accidents and severe social repercussions. Unlike traditional healthcare regulation, the Internet hospital model involves spatially separated patients, doctors, platforms, and regulatory bodies, complicating risk management. Traditional mechanisms for patient supervision, medical personnel credentialing, service scope and quality control, and administrative oversight are less effective in this context.

Additionally, the lack of face-to-face communication during online consultations poses significant challenges. Doctors cannot directly observe patients, raising concerns about the accuracy and truthfulness of the information provided. Patients, in turn, may struggle to verify doctors' identities and qualifications, potentially eroding trust and leading to withheld information. This increases the risk of misdiagnosis and delayed treatment. The indirect communication via text or images also exacerbates information asymmetry, potentially escalating doctor-patient conflicts.

Privacy breaches are the most serious security concern for Internet hospitals. Unauthorized access or cyberattacks could threaten hospital information systems and lead to the malicious theft of medical data. Internet hospital infrastructure must prioritize security measures and develop appropriate response strategies.

Additionally, Internet medical services face inherent limitations, as they are merely an extension of traditional medical services and must adhere to medical ethics reviews.

10.4.2 Operational Difficulties

The operation of an Internet hospital has very large hidden costs. In addition to the platform construction and maintenance of Internet hospitals, personnel management and business coordination during each operation generate additional expenses.. Not only that, the working hours of doctors in the online consultation mode of Internet hospitals are several times higher than that of offline consultation, and the human cost is greatly increased. In addition, the Internet operation also has the problem of whether the pricing is reasonable, and the service price and medical insurance payment are not clear. In the process of online diagnosis and treatment, it is not clear whether the diagnosis and treatment service fee between the upper and lower medical institutions is charged according to the standard of third-level A hospital or the standard of grass roots medical and health institutions. If the unit price of online diagnosis and treatment is too high, many patients may think that the value of online services is not as good as offline services; On the contrary, if the unit price is too low, doctors and hospitals and cooperative technology suppliers will lose enthusiasm, but will limit the long-term large-scale development of Internet hospitals. In addition, the Internet hospital must also solve the problem of medical security payment system. At this stage, there is still a big gap between whether Internet medical projects are self-funded projects or included in basic medical insurance in different regions, so it is very important to formulate standardized medical insurance standards and reasonable medical insurance reimbursement ratio. In addition, Internet hospitals break through geographical restrictions, and cross-provincial medical treatment nationwide may become the norm in the future. If medical insurance payments are limited to the province, it will in turn curb the development of Internet hospitals.

10.4.3 Talent Scarcity

In 2014, the National Health and Family Planning Commission (now the National Health Commission) issued a notice allowing eligible doctors to practice at multiple locations. The 2018 "Internet Diagnosis and Treatment Management Measures (Trial)" further allowed physicians with over three years of practice in physical medical institutions to register for Internet hospital practice. However, most doctors are already burdened with substantial offline responsibilities, leaving little time and energy for online consultations. Older experts, unfamiliar with Internet technologies, find it challenging to participate in Internet hospital services. Hospital administrators' varying levels of understanding and recognition of Internet hospital value and trends further complicate matters. Additionally, there is a disconnect in the training and utilization of health information technology professionals, with notable skill gaps in data analysis and operational management.

In response, the development of medical talent under the "Internet+ healthcare" initiative has seen some progress. Higher education institutions are establishing medical information management programs, and various regions are incorporating Internet medical talent training into their development measures, aiming to create talent hubs and integrate resources.

10.4.4 Relevant Laws and Policies

The implementation of Internet hospital is related to people's life safety and health, and must be run on a standardized track, while the actual and effective supervision and management depends on the relevant laws and policies of the state. The implementation of Internet hospitals is crucial for people's safety and health and must adhere to standardized practices. Effective supervision and management rely on relevant state laws and policies.

In 2015, the State Council issued the "Guiding Opinions on Actively Promoting the 'Internet Plus' Action Plan," proposing to "popularize new models of online medical and health services, develop Internet-based medical and health services, support third-party organizations in building medical information sharing service platforms for medical imaging, health records, test reports, electronic medical records, etc., and gradually establish a standard system for cross-hospital medical data sharing and exchange." At the same time, it emphasized the need to "construct and perfect a system for monitoring, evaluating, supervising, managing, standardizing, and certifying network security, as well as enhancing innovation capabilities.

Pay attention to the security risks brought about by integration, improve the security management and technical measures for network data sharing and utilization, explore the establishment of a data security flow certification system based on administrative reviews and third-party evaluations, improve the management system for cross-border data flow, and ensure data security."

In 2016, the General Office of the State Council issued the "Guiding Opinions on Promoting the Construction of a Graded Diagnosis and Treatment System" and the "Guiding Opinions on Promoting and Regulating the Development of Big Data Applications in Health and Medicine," proposing to accelerate the informatization of medical and health services. It aimed to improve the capabilities of primary medical services, perfect the service network, operational mechanisms, and incentive mechanisms, guide high-quality medical resources to the grassroots level, and gradually establish a graded diagnosis and treatment system that suits the national conditions. At the same time, it emphasized the need to strengthen the construction of legal regulations and standards, the establishment of a trusted network system, and the enhancement of health and medical data security, as well as the cultivation of a talent team in health and medical informatization.

In 2018, the General Office of the State Council issued the "Opinions on Promoting the Development of 'Internet Plus Medical Health,'" proposing to allow medical institutions to provide Internet-based medical services for the follow-up treatment of some common diseases and chronic diseases, thus clarifying the development direction for Internet hospitals. In the same year, the National Health Commission and the Administration of Traditional Chinese Medicine formulated the "Interim Measures for the Management of Internet Hospitals," the "Interim Measures for the Management of Internet Diagnosis and Treatment," and the "Regulations for the Management of Telemedicine Services (Trial)." These documents clarified that the national health administrative departments and the competent authorities for traditional Chinese medicine are responsible for the supervision and management of Internet medical activities nationwide. Local health administrative departments at all levels (including the competent authorities for traditional Chinese medicine) are responsible for the supervision and management of Internet medical activities within their jurisdictions. They emphasized the access principles and practice rules for Internet hospitals and Internet medical activities, and defined the legal liability relationships for Internet hospitals. Article 27 of Chapter 4 in the "Interim Measures for the Management of Internet Hospitals" states that "Internet hospitals should establish processes for preventing and handling adverse events in Internet medical services, implement measures to protect personal privacy information, and strengthen content review management of the Internet hospital information platform." Article 30 points out that "provincial health administrative departments and the registration authorities of Internet hospitals, through the provincial Internet medical service supervision platform, jointly implement supervision over Internet hospitals, focusing on the supervision of personnel, prescriptions, medical practices, patient privacy protection, and information security. Internet hospitals should be incorporated into the local medical quality control system, and related services should be included in the performance assessment and medical institution evaluation by administrative departments, implementing integrated online and offline supervision to ensure medical quality and safety."

In 2019, the National Medical Products Administration issued the "Drug Administration Law of the People's Republic of China," further specifying the action direction and implementation path for "Internet Plus Medical Health Plus Drug Distribution." In the same year, the General Office of the State Council issued the "Key Tasks for Deepening the Reform of the Medical and Health Care System in 2019," which required the National Healthcare Security Administration to formulate charging and healthcare policies for Internet medical services by September 2019. Subsequently, the central government issued the "Guiding Opinions on Perfecting the Pricing and Healthcare Payment Policies for 'Internet Plus' Medical Services," which clarified the five basic principles that "Internet Plus" medical service pricing projects should meet, providing guidance on the pricing of Internet services and healthcare policies. The specific prices, healthcare reimbursement scope, and proportions need to be formulated by each province and city based on their own situations.

In 2020, under the impact of the COVID-19 pandemic, Internet hospitals faced new opportunities and challenges. The General Office of the National Health Commission issued the "Notice on Further Promoting the Development and Standardized Management of Internet Medical Services," which clarified that all regions should further promote the integration of Internet technology and medical services, play the positive role of Internet medical services, emphasizing that all regions should adhere to the bottom line of medical quality and patient safety. No experiments or explorations should break existing laws and regulations, and continuous efforts should be made to standardize the access and practice management of Internet diagnosis and treatment and Internet hospitals, and to strengthen supervision.

Internet medical regulation is a complex system engineering that requires quality supervision from the medical industry on one hand and the assurance of Internet information security on the other. This requires cooperation from government departments, medical institutions, Internet companies, and patients. It is necessary to improve Internet medical-related laws, innovate regulatory systems using informatization, clarify the rights and responsibilities of all parties involved, and ensure medical quality and safety.

10.5 Case Studies

10.5.1 Implementation of Physical Community Internet Hospitals

In 2020, the General Office of the National Health Commission issued the "Notice on Further Improving the Appointment and Consultation System and Strengthening the Construction of Smart Hospitals," which required the acceleration of the establishment and improvement of the appointment and consultation system, the creation of a comprehensive smart hospital system, and strongly promote the development of

Internet diagnosis and treatment, as well as Internet hospitals.. Primary medical and health institutions, especially community hospitals, can become the best pilot projects for Internet hospitals. Using Internet hospital communication technology, online remote consultations and two-way referrals can be conducted, providing community residents with better medical resources and a more convenient medical experience, which helps promote the construction of a graded diagnosis and treatment system.

The Pengpu New Village Street Community Health Service Center in Jing'an District, Shanghai, is the first physical community Internet hospital in China, officially launching on April 26, 2020. The construction of this community Internet hospital adopted a self-built model, in accordance with the unified planning of the District Health Commission. The platform uses a unified software platform, "Healthy Jing'an," for both residents and doctors, avoiding the need for investment in external network security protection. All data generated by the Internet hospital business is stored on the district-level platform, mitigating legal risks that may arise from third-party cooperation. The community Internet hospital implements a full-process closed loop management system, covering all medical and health service functions of the community health service center through online, offline, and online+offline models. This includes pre-consultation triage, online consultations with patients during consultations, doctors providing online diagnosis and treatment and prescribing medications, home delivery of pharmaceuticals, and post-consultation online follow-up surveys and chronic disease daily management. The entire business process design incorporates various steps to ensure medical safety, such as pre-prescription review, physician certification, and pharmacist certification, to ensure compliance with the requirements of the Internet hospital management methods.

The physical Internet hospital has broken through the spatial limitations between doctors and patients, bringing great convenience to the residents of Pengpu New Village Street. In 2020, the outpatient volume of the community Internet hospital reached 860,000 visits, with a daily high exceeding 5000 visits, making it the hospital with the largest outpatient volume among the medical institutions affiliated with Jing'an District. Besides providing residents with high-quality medical services without leaving their homes, the community Internet hospital also continuously improves its functions to meet the growing demands of the residents. In 2020, services such as nucleic acid testing appointments and electronic billing were implemented on the "Healthy Jing'an" WeChat public account. The first batch of medical institutions offering nucleic acid testing services included five large and small hospitals within Jing'an District, allowing citizens to make appointments for tests based on the testing times offered by each hospital. The electronic billing service is the first regional medical electronic billing service platform in Shanghai and quickly covered all 26 public medical institutions in the region. With the full coverage of medical electronic billing, an effective closed loop will be formed between medical electronic billing and medical payment, streamlining the payment and billing process into "one-stop service" for patients seeking treatment in Jing'an District.

However, the physical community Internet hospital still faces challenges such as the difficulty of changing medical habits quickly, the need for further improvements in user experience, and the limitations of online diagnosis and treatment. Nevertheless, with the continuous maturation of related technologies, community Internet hospitals are certain to become one of the fundamental models in the medical field, providing practical solutions for the medical needs of the general public.

10.5.2 Innovative Internet Hospital Combining Tertiary Hospitals and Internet Enterprises

Zhejiang University School of Medicine's First Affiliated Hospital (Zhejiang First Hospital), founded in 1947, is a large, comprehensive tertiary hospital integrating medical care, education, and research. It serves as the medical, teaching, and research center of Zhejiang Province, encompassing six campuses with nearly 5000 open beds, spanning a total area of 521 acres. It serves as the medical, teaching, and research center of Zhejiang Province, with six campuses and nearly 5000 open beds across a total area of 521 acres. Zhuojian Technology, a high-tech enterprise in the Internet industry, has provided diverse Internet solutions for large and medium-sized hospitals and the healthcare ecosystem since its establishment in 2011.

The "Zhejiang First Internet Hospital," established on February 16, 2016, was the first online campus of a public tertiary hospital in China. Supported by Zhuojian Technology, it utilizes Zhejiang First Hospital's high-quality medical resources to create a seamless integration of online consultation appointments, offline examinations, and drug delivery, creating a closed-loop medical service system. This model optimizes resource allocation, improves medical efficiency, and fosters positive doctor-patient interactions.

Initially, the "Zhejiang First Internet Hospital" provided a relatively simple patient care process, covering common steps: patients could book online consultations with specific departments, consult with doctors remotely, receive electronic prescriptions, and choose home delivery of medications or pick them up at physical locations.

At its inception, the hospital offered 12 departments, including general outpatient, diabetes, and cardiovascular specialties, with 12 specialist doctors available for consultation. On its first day, 1045 patients registered online, with 108 successfully connecting with doctors for consultations, resulting in eight electronic prescriptions being issued.

10.5.3 Role of Internet Hospitals During the COVID-19 Pandemic

During the COVID-19 pandemic, how to fully leverage the role of grassroots and community general practitioners in epidemic prevention and control, and how to guide residents to seek medical treatment in an orderly manner and reduce unnecessary cross-infections have become key focuses. In February 2020, the National

Health Commission successively issued the "Notice on Strengthening Informatization Support for the Prevention and Control of the COVID-19 Pandemic," the "Notice on Doing a Good Job in Providing Internet Medical Consultation Services during Epidemic Prevention and Control," and the "Notice on Further Implementing Scientific Prevention and Precision Control Measures, and District-Based Classification Requirements to Manage Medical Services during the Pandemic." These notices aimed to actively promote remote medical services and standardize Internet-based medical consultation services, including but not limited to online health assessments, health guidance, health education, consultation guidance, follow-up visits for chronic diseases, and psychological counseling.

The role of Internet hospitals during the COVID-19 pandemic mainly manifested in two aspects. On the one hand, since the main transmission routes of COVID-19 are respiratory droplets and close contact, patients visiting physical Internet hospitals could increase the risk of cross-infection. However, through Internet hospitals, patients could receive quality medical services without leaving their homes, greatly reducing direct contact between patients and healthcare providers, effectively cutting off the virus transmission route, and improving the safety of medical visits. This was facilitated by functions such as fever clinic consultations and nucleic acid testing appointments, which smoothly carried out pre-hospital screening for fever patients. On the other hand, due to the impact of the pandemic, patients' willingness to seek medical treatment decreased significantly. At this time, Internet hospitals played a huge positive role, promoting a change in patients' medical habits, with contactless medical treatment becoming a new trend in medical development .

During the pandemic, hospital-led physical Internet hospitals, such as Wuhan University People's Hospital, West China Second University Hospital, and Shenzhen Nanshan Hospital, quickly launched online consultation services, adding AI-guided consultations and online consultation functions specific to COVID-19. Meanwhile, Internet medical platforms led by Internet companies provided online voluntary consultations, greatly reducing the pressure on physical hospitals and cooperating with pharmacies nationwide to ensure the online supply of medications for chronic disease patients.

In addition, some Internet hospitals also established platforms specifically for the COVID-19 pandemic. For example, the Guangdong Second Provincial General Hospital, in collaboration with an Internet hospital, launched a COVID-19 online service platform. This platform provided online medical services to the public and non-professional medical staff, with key functions including automatic screening for COVID-19, monitoring of related symptoms, online consultations, psychological counseling, and a COVID-19 knowledge center. By the end of June 2020, a total of 96,642 people had used the automatic screening system 161,884 times and the symptom monitoring system 7,795,194 times. The number of daily general online consultations increased from 30 before the pandemic to 122 during the pandemic, and then decreased to 73 after the pandemic. During the pandemic, psychological counseling services were provided to 636 individuals.

The establishment of Internet hospitals broke down the spatial distance between patients and hospitals/doctors. On the one hand, it expanded the channels for patients to consult and purchase medications, reducing the time and cost of visiting a doctor, allowing patients to enjoy quality medical resources without leaving their homes. On the other hand, traditional physical medical services are limited by time and space, especially during the COVID-19 pandemic, leading to unmet daily medication or treatment needs for some chronic disease patients. In desperation, they chose to delay treatment, missing treatment opportunities and damaging their health. The launch of Internet hospitals broke through these limitations, providing a certain degree of protection for the health of some patients. Moreover, Internet hospitals effectively integrated resources accumulated in physical hospitals, improving the efficiency of medical resource allocation, and consequently enhancing the economic benefits of hospitals.

In summary, Internet hospitals not only effectively supported pandemic prevention and control but also strongly promoted lean hospital operation management. During the COVID-19 pandemic, the emergence of Internet hospitals greatly improved the efficiency of medical services and resource utilization, enhancing the overall resilience of hospitals and ensuring their healthy and sustainable development. In the future, when facing similar public health emergencies, Internet hospitals will provide a new model for protecting people's health.

10.6 Summary

Internet hospital is a new type of Internet medical service model, which develops rapidly based on the practical requirements. Compared with the traditional hospital model, it has great advantages in improving the patient's medical experience, improving the intelligent management level of hospitals, and promoting hierarchical diagnosis and treatment. However, the current Internet hospital is still in the stage of development and exploration, and there are still some problems such as the limited scope of patients and departments, the large risk of medical data security, and the imperfect policy and regulatory system, which has great room for improvement. However, with the modernization and informatization of hospitals, the gradual collapse of "information island", the improvement of information interconnection between medical institutions at all levels, the further optimization of diagnosis and treatment processes and the improvement of relevant laws and regulations, and the protection of medical service quality and medical information security, Internet hospitals will become an inevitable trend in the future development of the medical industry.

Proactive Health Systems

11

Contents

11.1 Overview of Proactive Health Technology 296
11.1.1 Concept of Proactive Health 296
11.1.2 Overview of Proactive Health Systems 298
11.1.2.1 Contract Management Services 298
11.1.2.2 Population Management Services 298
11.1.2.3 Health Data Monitoring 299
11.1.2.4 Drug Traceability Systems 299
11.1.2.5 Chronic Disease Diagnosis and Treatment Systems 299
11.1.2.6 Rehabilitation Management Systems 299
11.1.3 The Development History of Proactive Health 300
11.2 Key Technologies for Proactive Health 301
11.2.1 Proactive Health Monitoring Technology 301
11.2.1.1 Precision 302
11.2.1.2 Convenience 302
11.2.1.3 Enrichment 303
11.2.1.4 Integration 303
11.2.1.5 Wearability 303
11.2.2 Health Status Identification and Risk Warning Technology 303
11.2.2.1 Primary Prevention of Diseases 304
11.2.2.2 Secondary Prevention of Diseases 304
11.2.2.3 Tertiary Prevention of Diseases 305
11.2.3 Proactive Health Intervention and Management Techniques 305
11.2.3.1 Contract Management Intervention Model 306
11.2.3.2 Self-Management Intervention Model 306
11.2.3.3 Family Management Intervention Model 306
11.2.3.4 Community Intervention Model 306
11.3 Case Analysis 307
11.3.1 Intelligent Health Management Systems 307
11.3.1.1 Apple Health 307
11.3.1.2 Miao Health 307
11.3.2 Digital Health Family Service Systems 308
11.3.2.1 Geometry Technology Smart Toilet 308
11.3.2.2 AliHealth Family Doctor 309
11.4 Summary 310

J. Li et al., *Healthcare Information Systems*, Innovative Medical Devices,
https://doi.org/10.1007/978-981-97-9551-2_11

The concept of proactive health was introduced in China in 2015, but the underlying principles of proactive health have been popular for a long time. Proactive health emphasizes the identification and assessment of an individual's health status through long-term, continuous health monitoring and tracking. It utilizes various medical approaches to intervene in health behaviors, primarily to improve the individual's health. With the development of big data and artificial intelligence, the typical applications of proactive health systems have evolved into AI-based health management systems. These systems use health monitoring to gather large amounts of data, employ data-driven health assessment methods such as risk prediction models, and are supported by artificial intelligence to provide health management and intervention services. Current systems, such as family doctor health management systems and intelligent health management systems, all reflect the principles of proactive health.

11.1 Overview of Proactive Health Technology

11.1.1 Concept of Proactive Health

The "Dictionary of Science and Technology" defines "medicine" as "a system of scientific knowledge and practical activities aimed at protecting and enhancing human health, preventing, and treating diseases." The "Dictionary of Natural Science Disciplines" defines it as "medicine, in a narrow sense, can be considered synonymous with medical science; in a broad sense, it should be understood as a comprehensive term for medical science and healthcare services." The "Encyclopedia Britannica" defines medicine as "the practice of maintaining health, preventing, diagnosing, and treating diseases." Narrowly defined, medicine emphasizes the treatment of diseases and the restoration of effective bodily functions, while broadly defined, it also includes Chinese health preservation practices and the derived Western nutrition science. Therefore, proactive health is also included in the broad definition of medicine.

Proactive health is a medical model that enhances bodily functions or reverses chronic diseases by actively applying controllable stimuli to the human body, increasing its micro-level complexity, and promoting diverse adaptation. It emphasizes long-term continuous dynamic tracking of an individual's behavior system throughout their life cycle, identifying and assessing individual states, evolutionary directions, and degrees. By choosing lifestyle elements and fully utilizing subjective initiative, it aims to improve health behaviors. Various medical means are comprehensively used for controllable proactive interventions in human behavior, prompting self-organizing adaptive changes in the body to enhance functions, eliminate diseases, and maintain a healthy state. Therefore, proactive health can be considered a medical model that actively places the human body in a controllable, non-equilibrium state to stimulate self-organizing capabilities and achieve disease elimination and health promotion.

Modern medicine, supported by precise analytical tools, attempts to maintain various bodily indicators within normal ranges through treatments like drugs and surgery. In contrast, proactive health explores another path, attempting to distance the body from a non-equilibrium state through behavioral interventions, thereby stimulating self-organizing behavior and achieving overall functional enhancement for disease prevention and treatment. Proactive health views the human body as a complex system with strong self-repair and evolutionary abilities, establishing a new medical model based on new scientific paradigms and big data technology. The difference between proactive health and modern disease medicine lies in proactive health's emphasis on overall health promotion and disease prevention, while disease medicine focuses on localized treatment and disease prognosis. Future national health assurance and the "Healthy China Initiative" require balancing both medical models, emphasizing proactive disease prevention and effective disease treatment. Essentially, the proactive health medical model is a new smart medical model. The development of the Internet of Things, new materials, intelligent sensors, wearable devices, big data technology, and artificial intelligence provides the material basis for collecting and processing continuous dynamic big data of the human body. Disease medicine refers to providing appropriate treatment methods based on the patient's condition. As a single medical model for treating specific diseases, disease medicine no longer suits the current trends of chronic disease development. Proactive health is a new medical model based on continuous dynamic real-time monitoring and comprehensive analysis. It represents a new exploration of shifting from primarily passive treatment to self-initiated proactive health interventions.

In fact, the concept of "proactive health" exists in other countries with similar proposals. For example, the American College of Sports Medicine proposed the concept of "Exercise is Medicine (EIM)" in September 2007, the Japanese government launched and implemented the "National Health Promotion Movement," and Singapore proposed the concept of "Healthy Citizens." Comparatively, proactive health is not only a Chinese proposal but also a more systematic Chinese approach. It is a future plan proposed by China for the health medical model in the big data era, resonating with new explorations initiated simultaneously by Western developed countries. China has inherent advantages in health data resources, market scale, and user demand, making it more likely to break through the constraints of European and American competitors in this field. Smart wearables, big data, and artificial intelligence provide technical support for proactive health by collecting multidimensional, real-time human health signals to achieve comprehensive, all-weather continuous monitoring and analysis. This shifts the center of disease prevention and treatment from hospitals to communities and even households, thereby enhancing national health awareness and literacy and promoting the advancement of health technology. Additionally, the development of health products, health service models, and the health industry can provide more resources and market space for national economic development, fostering the growth of the health industry and social economy.

11.1.2 Overview of Proactive Health Systems

A proactive health system integrates online health management with offline health monitoring. It can be either a commercial profit-oriented system or a nonprofit service-oriented system. Online management allows for a comprehensive examination of a user's health status during medical visits, aiding doctors in diagnosis. Offline daily check-ups combined with physical examinations can promptly screen for major diseases, enabling early detection and treatment.

A complete and professional proactive health system is composed of three teams: the core team, the support team, and the auxiliary team. The core team must at least include family doctors, physician assistants, and health managers. The support team includes pharmacists, public health physicians, nutritionists, psychological counselors, laboratory technicians, specialists, exercise rehabilitation therapists, and traditional Chinese medicine physicians. The auxiliary team mainly includes social workers (such as health volunteers and social care groups), pharmaceutical service providers (such as logistics delivery and pharmaceutical companies), and medical service providers (such as appointment scheduling, referral services, long-term care providers, nursing homes, home care services, and clinics).

Although the level of informatics is deepening, the role of humans remains irreplaceable. Each role should perform its duties and responsibilities. Due to the different human resource structures in various regions, the structure of the core team may vary. However, a new core team needs to work collaboratively within the scope of health management. This means that, compared to traditional basic medical and public health services, the core team is more involved in tasks such as communication with patients and external resources, identifying patient-centered needs, activating and engaging patients, quality tracking of contracted populations, and batch interventions. These tasks require teamwork to be accomplished.

A proactive health system must at least include the following functions.

11.1.2.1 Contract Management Services

The contract management function supports family doctors in providing continuous health assessment and management services to patients. It allows for personalized configuration of health assessments and management services according to individual needs, maintaining unique service content. Using health cards, ID cards, or social security cards for identity verification, it establishes complete and continuous health monitoring records for patients, offering a range of services such as health assessments and the formulation of individualized health plans.

11.1.2.2 Population Management Services

Population management targets both contracted and non-contracted populations. Specific functions include viewing the health risk status of all populations, screening target intervention groups, and mandating health interventions to achieve comprehensive health management. Health interventions may include organizing regular check-ups for high-risk groups. For contracted populations, it allows viewing specific health monitoring data and providing individualized health management services, enabling proactive management by creating a plan for each contracted individual.

11.1.2.3 Health Data Monitoring

By collecting, analyzing, and managing data from electronic medical records systems, medical insurance systems, and population health data, the system automatically handles population data for common chronic diseases and disease quality indicator data. It offers data visualization and analysis tools to provide reference for health management decisions concerning regional chronic disease populations and for monitoring the effectiveness of governmental healthcare expenditures and budget retention.

11.1.2.4 Drug Traceability Systems

By establishing a unique code for each item, the system can track each box of medicine from coding on the production line through various distribution stages, including distributors and pharmacies. Each batch of medicine's warehousing, out-warehouse, and inspection processes is recorded via scanning, ensuring full traceability of drug circulation. This guarantees the quality and safety of medications for patients and ensures strict adherence to medical prescriptions.

11.1.2.5 Chronic Disease Diagnosis and Treatment Systems

Leveraging more accurate risk prediction models derived from medical big data analysis, the system can conduct risk assessments, screen high-risk patients, manage controllable risk factors, and achieve personalized risk interventions. It integrates optimal treatment pathways mined from complex medical knowledge bases (including clinical guidelines, medical literature, and expert knowledge) with best clinical practices identified through data analysis, achieving cognitive decision support to provide standardized and personalized treatment for patients. Chronic disease management, particularly for common conditions like hypertension and diabetes, is crucial. Patients need to adhere to dietary habits, lifestyle routines, and medication instructions, promoting a balanced diet, smoking cessation, alcohol limitation, appropriate exercise, regular routines, stress reduction, self-monitoring, and continuous management and supervision.

11.1.2.6 Rehabilitation Management Systems

Comprehensive supervision of family doctor teams' work is essential to support the performance evaluation and performance-based compensation management of these teams. By promoting the implementation of services through an objective, reasonable, and effective performance indicator system, we can guide family doctor teams toward effective and compensated contractual services. This ensures that high performance is rewarded appropriately, protects the rights of contracted patients, and better supports the healthy development of the contractual service model. This is a necessary component of a commercialized proactive health management system.

The construction of a proactive health system is a long-term and continuous process. On the one hand, it requires dynamic adjustments based on the changing health needs of the local population and the actual situation of health service system construction to meet evolving needs. On the other hand, building a proactive health system is a systematic transformation of the healthcare service system itself. It is a process of establishing new institutions in the health field, which needs to be carried out step by step, with top-level design and phased advancement.

11.1.3 The Development History of Proactive Health

With the changing spectrum of human diseases, lifestyle-related diseases have become one of the leading causes of death. The reductionist approach of modern antagonistic medical models faces significant challenges. Although modern science and technology have greatly advanced the development of modern medicine and improved the precision of human body measurements, they have been less effective in addressing lifestyle diseases. Analysis of data from the National Bureau of Statistics between 2008 and 2017 reveals that China's total health expenditure has been increasing rapidly each year. It is projected that by 2035, total health expenditure will exceed 22 trillion yuan. Currently, the number of healthcare workers has surpassed 11 million. However, the number of people suffering from diseases continues to rise.

In 2015, the Ministry of Science and Technology organized an expert group to draft the "13th Five-Year Plan for Digital Healthcare and Health Promotion," which proactively focused on health-centric technological planning for the population and health of China. Experts like Li Xiangchen from the General Administration of Sport proposed proactive interventions as an important means to combat the outbreak of chronic diseases, specifically highlighting exercise as a key intervention method. This proposal received strong endorsement from the expert group and was actively promoted to include exercise in health promotion plans. The subsequent series of reports garnered attention from then Vice Premier Liu Yandong, who summarized the opinions in the reports under the term "proactive health." This concept received national support and was included as a special focus in key research and development plans. Thus, "proactive health" became an original concept proposed by China for the global health initiative.

On February 14, 2017, the General Office of the State Council issued the "Medium- to Long-Term Plan for the Prevention and Treatment of Chronic Diseases in China (2017–2025)," which outlined the work needed for chronic disease prevention and treatment in the coming years. The goal was to reduce the disease burden, increase the expected healthy lifespan for residents, and strive for comprehensive and life cycle health protection for the people. By 2025, the risk factors for chronic diseases are expected to be effectively controlled, achieving health management for the entire population across their lifespan.

On May 16, 2017, the Ministry of Science and Technology, in collaboration with the National Health and Family Planning Commission, the General Administration of Sport, the China Food and Drug Administration, the State Administration of Traditional Chinese Medicine, and the Logistics Support Department of the Central Military Commission, issued the notice on the "13th Five-Year Plan for Health and

Medical Science and Technology Innovation." This plan prioritized people's health as a strategic development priority, aimed to build a comprehensive national health and medical science and technology innovation system, enhance China's health and medical science and technology innovation capabilities, and significantly strengthen the role of scientific and technological innovation in improving public health and promoting the health industry. Proactive health was officially included in the special plan.

On June 25, 2019, the State Council issued the "Opinions on Implementing the Healthy China Initiative", which clearly stated the need to accelerate the shift from a disease-centered approach to a people-centered health approach, implementing the Healthy China Initiative. At the national level, a Healthy China Action Promotion Committee was established to coordinate the organization, implementation, monitoring, and evaluation of related work. The "Healthy China Action (2019–2030)" was formulated and issued, emphasizing the integration of prevention and early disease prevention into various policies and measures. This marked the inclusion of proactive health as an important component of China's future health protection system.

With the development of the economy and society, especially the accelerated aging of China's population and changes in the disease spectrum, the demand for health among Chinese citizens has increased rapidly. People not only hope for "easy access to good medical care" but also pay more attention to disease prevention, the improvement of individual functions, good health status, and the extension of healthy life expectancy. Thus, beyond advancing disease prevention research, there is a need to focus on proactive and preventive health strategies. This involves constructing a new theoretical system for health promotion that organically integrates and complements the current disease treatment-centered medical system, actively exploring new models for the sustainable development of the national health protection system.

Moreover, it is necessary to strengthen the systematic layout of health promotion technology research and build a technical product support system for behavioral intervention, proactive disease health management, and services centered on community and family, with continuous service both inside and outside hospitals. This will enhance health protection capabilities and autonomy, reduce excessive reliance on disease treatment, improve the overall health quality of the population, and promote the development of health promotion technology.

11.2 Key Technologies for Proactive Health

11.2.1 Proactive Health Monitoring Technology

In the 1970s, the International Health Systems Company, Inc. first introduced sensors into the field of medical diagnostics and monitoring, marking the debut of the concept of exercise and health monitoring in the medical domain. Thanks to advancements in sensor technology, today's health monitoring technologies exhibit superior sensitivity, accuracy, and stability. Additionally, there has been a proliferation of various methods for collecting biological signals to fulfill different types of monitoring functions.

The development of health detection technologies relies on the progression of sensor technology. Biomedical sensors are classified into electrophysiological, biochemical detection, cardiopulmonary monitoring, and motion monitoring categories. Traditionally, electrophysiological signal collection has involved direct contact between electrodes and the skin. However, innovations now include capacitive electrodes, flexible dry surface electrodes, and new material-based electrodes such as carbon nanotube or micro-wire array electrodes, which can collect electrocardiogram (ECG) signals through clothing.

Innovations in cardiopulmonary monitoring sensors are a research focus for many scientists. The European Union's fifth Framework Program for Information Technology (FP5) included a health initiative aimed at achieving real-time monitoring of vital signs like ECG and respiration. This led to the development of wearable fabric sensors that ensure user comfort without causing any discomfort.

Recently, wearable sensors for monitoring biochemical parameters have also emerged. Under the EU's sixth Framework Program for Information Technology (FP6) and its special BIOTEX initiative, a fabric-based wearable biosensor was developed to monitor the pH and Na + content in sweat. Motion detection sensors are typically utilized in rehabilitation and routine health care. Some wearable devices employ accelerometers and gyroscopes to monitor movements, gait, and posture.

Proactive health monitoring devices can be categorized based on their usage into wearable, mobile, portable, implantable, remote health monitoring devices, and terminals. Proactive health monitoring technologies need to facilitate the easy collection of residents' physical parameter data. Therefore, miniaturized, integrated, and wireless health monitoring devices suitable for home or community use are ideal. In recent years, common household health monitoring devices include smart wristbands or watches, body fat scales, thermometers, glucometers, ECG monitors, and portable electronic blood pressure monitors, with smart wristbands and watches being the most popular digital health monitoring products. Additionally, regular hospital check-ups also constitute a method of health monitoring.

With ongoing technological advancements, it is anticipated that proactive health monitoring devices will exhibit the following trends in the future.

11.2.1.1 Precision

The barriers to medical testing technology are lowering, and the accuracy of portable devices such as electronic blood pressure monitors, glucometers, and thermometers will gradually meet medical-grade requirements.

11.2.1.2 Convenience

Product operation will become more convenient, with the operation methods tending toward traditional devices, requiring low learning costs and being accessible for the elderly without obstacles.

11.2.1.3 Enrichment

More medical tests can be completed at home, such as routine urine tests and complete blood counts.

11.2.1.4 Integration

Current devices are mostly for single-item testing, requiring users to use various devices separately to test multiple indicators. In the future, devices will integrate multiple sensors to simultaneously test various physiological indicators.

11.2.1.5 Wearability

Future product designs will tend toward convenience, ensuring that long-term wear is comfortable and easy. Data will be automatically detected, recorded, and uploaded to the cloud while users wear the products.

The large amount of data generated during health monitoring will provide services for health status identification and risk warning. This data can be categorized into resident health information (such as physical indicators, vital signs, behavior, exercise, diet, sleep, mental, psychological, and social aspects) and body parameter data (such as blood pressure, blood glucose, electrocardiogram, blood oxygen, body fat percentage, respiratory signals, and scene recognition related to chronic disease management). Throughout this process, user privacy protection and data security are of utmost importance. Currently, the application of sensor networks in health monitoring devices is gradually becoming more intelligent and wireless, so special attention must be paid to issues such as data privacy, data integrity, data timeliness, and data security.

11.2.2 Health Status Identification and Risk Warning Technology

Health status identification and disease risk warning technology involves the comprehensive analysis of human health conditions using physiological indicators obtained from examinations and tests. These physiological indicators come from different medical devices, and their data structures are not uniform. Therefore, it is necessary to have technologies for the integration, fusion, storage, cleaning, and analysis of multidimensional, dynamic, heterogeneous, and multilevel personal health monitoring information. This allows for the integration and cleaning of health information from multiple different devices, converting it into uniformly structured data for subsequent analysis. Additionally, open data interface access technology, unstructured personal health data privacy protection mechanisms, and health data service security control mechanisms and access technologies are required to ensure the secure access and storage of user data.

Automatic health status identification and disease risk warning require risk prediction based on a large amount of health monitoring data. Classification techniques in the field of information technology can predict unknown categories based on a large amount of known labeled data, which aligns with the requirements of health status identification and automatic disease risk warning technology. Health monitoring data have characteristics such as diversity, temporality, inconsistency, redundancy, heterogeneity, and privacy. To address these characteristics, classification methods suitable for medical data, such as support vector machines and decision trees, can be chosen.

Clinical prediction models, also known as clinical prediction rules or risk scores, refer to the use of multifactor models to estimate the probability of having a certain disease or the probability of a certain outcome occurring in the future. Clinical prediction models include diagnostic models and prognostic models. Diagnostic models focus on estimating the probability of currently having a certain disease based on the clinical symptoms and characteristics of the study subjects and are mostly used in cross-sectional studies. Prognostic models focus on estimating the probability of disease recurrence, death, disability, and the occurrence of complications within a certain period in the future based on the current disease state and are mostly used in cohort studies.

Diagnostic and prognostic models also share similarities, such as outcomes being mostly binary classifications, though in some cases they may involve continuous indicators such as blood pressure, blood lipids, blood glucose, pain scores, and quality of life scores. The effect indicators studied are the absolute risk of the outcome occurring, that is, the probability of occurrence, rather than relative risk effect indicators such as risk ratio (RR), odds ratio (OR), or hazard ratio (HR). From a technical perspective, both models face challenges in the selection of predictive factors, modeling strategies, and the evaluation of model performance.

The use of clinical prediction models can span the entire course of a disease, including prevention, treatment, and prognosis stages. They can aid in health status identification and disease risk warning, playing a crucial role especially in the tertiary prevention system of diseases.

11.2.2.1 Primary Prevention of Diseases

Clinical risk prediction models can provide patients and doctors with a quantified risk value (probability) of developing a certain disease in the future based on current health status. This offers a more intuitive data foundation for health education and behavioral interventions and also involves proactive health interventions as discussed in Section 11.2.3. For example, the Framingham Risk Score, based on heart disease research, clearly indicates that lowering blood lipids and blood pressure can reduce the probability of coronary heart disease.

11.2.2.2 Secondary Prevention of Diseases

Clinical prediction models, especially diagnostic models, often utilize non-invasive, low-cost, and easily collectible indicators, such as physiological data obtained from health monitoring. These models provide highly sensitive and specific diagnostic solutions to achieve the disease prevention concept of "early detection, early diagnosis, and early treatment," which holds significant importance in health economics.

11.2.2.3 Tertiary Prevention of Diseases

Prognostic models can provide a quantified estimate of the probabilities of disease recurrence, death, disability, and complications. This guides the formulation of rehabilitation plans and targeted treatments, preventing complications or disease recurrence, promoting the recovery of related functions, improving patient quality of life, and reducing disease mortality.

11.2.3 Proactive Health Intervention and Management Techniques

Health management refers to the entire process of monitoring, evaluating, and intervening in the health of individuals or groups. It is a forward-looking health assurance service. Health management is generally based on modern biomedical and digital information management technologies, focusing on the health of individuals or groups. By conducting health risk assessments of health risk factors, it provides targeted interventions and guidance.

The concept of health management was first proposed in the United States in the late 1950s. It emerged in the context of medical insurance institutions conducting systematic health management for their insurance clients (including patients or high-risk groups) or medical service clients. The goal was to significantly reduce the probability of disease occurrence or progression through effective control, thereby lowering actual medical expenses and reducing medical insurance compensation losses. In China, the "Healthy China 2030" Planning Outline, implemented in 2016, is guided by the construction of "big health." It elevates the improvement of national health management to a national strategic level, proposing that public health should shift from passive medical treatment to proactive prevention, continuously enhancing the public's awareness of self-health management. This provides new opportunities for the development of health intervention and management.

Health management focuses on controlling health risk factors and is based on the previously mentioned health status identification and disease risk warning. After evaluating the health status and disease risk of individuals or groups, it formulates personalized health management plans and intervention measures. Health management advocates maintaining health balance through health preservation methods and means such as diet, exercise, and psychological adjustment to achieve the purpose of disease prevention, embodying the characteristics of primary, secondary, and tertiary prevention.

Precise health management requires proactive health interventions for users. Types of proactive health interventions include disease prevention knowledge, nutritional intervention plans, exercise intervention plans, psychological intervention plans, and various solutions covering common diseases and sub-health conditions. The service targets can be divided into sub-health populations, rehabilitation populations, and others, with different management categories for different groups. For sub-health populations, timely and effective management and intervention are needed, such as encouraging early to bed and early to rise, exercise, and stress relief to alleviate sub-health conditions, and urging regular check-ups to prevent and control potential diseases. For rehabilitation populations, it is necessary to guide them to follow medical advice strictly and minimize or eliminate the influence of adverse factors such as mental, psychological, and bad habits.

Proactive health intervention models are divided into four categories.

11.2.3.1 Contract Management Intervention Model

The contract management intervention model refers to fixing the responsibilities and obligations between health managers and those being managed in the form of a contract (health agreement).

11.2.3.2 Self-Management Intervention Model

Self-management intervention provides knowledge and skills through course teaching, enabling the managed individuals to autonomously carry out interventions under effective guidance.

11.2.3.3 Family Management Intervention Model

The family management intervention model involves educating the patient's family members or combining regular home visits by health managers to conduct intervention training. This method aims to improve the compliance of the managed individuals and enhance their quality of life.

11.2.3.4 Community Intervention Model

Community intervention refers to a series of planned and organized activities conducted within a residential community to create a health-promoting environment. It aims to change people's behaviors and lifestyles and reduce risk factors, thereby promoting health and improving the quality of life of the community members.

In the field of computer software, there are currently two main types of software applied to health management. The first type focuses on health risk assessment, converting health data into health reports and related health guidance through risk assessment models. Relevant domestic products include the digital precision health management platform "Miao Health," which tracks health data from multiple aspects such as exercise, diet, sleep, and stress. It provides users with multidimensional, customized health behavior intervention plans, reasonably plans daily health tasks, and offers functions such as health record management, personal comprehensive health index scoring, abnormal indicator interpretation, and disease risk prediction. The second type primarily provides health management services through interventions, such as exercise health apps like Keep and Gudong, diet health apps like Mint Health, sleep health apps like Pillow and AutoSleep, mental health apps like BigHealth, and comprehensive apps like Xiaomi Health and Apple Health.

11.3 Case Analysis

11.3.1 Intelligent Health Management Systems

With the rapid development of the economy, people's demand for health is continuously increasing. The public's health management philosophy has gradually shifted from "treating illness" to "preventing illness," thereby making health management, a subdivision of the broader healthcare field, increasingly significant.

The progress in medical technology is advancing rapidly. Data intelligence technologies such as deep learning, machine learning, and data mining integrate and refine previously difficult-to-utilize data, including disease status, medical history, and various physiological signs, playing a significant role. An intelligent health management system can conduct long-term, continuous, dynamic monitoring of individual data, assess the health status and its evolving risks, and achieve proactive lifestyle-based interventions and health management. By fully utilizing artificial intelligence technology, intelligent health management systems can provide patients with more scientific and effective health guidance, offer interventions for a healthier lifestyle, and significantly mobilize patients' enthusiasm and initiative. This helps patients better improve their personal health, truly achieve disease prevention, monitor body indicators, protect health, enhance the quality of life, and reduce medical expenses.

11.3.1.1 Apple Health

Apple Inc. integrates data from the Apple ecosystem, including iPhone, Apple Watch, and commonly used third-party applications, allowing users to view a wide range of information in one place. Users can not only check their long-term health trends but also delve into the daily details of various health indicators.

The Apple Watch, as a data collection terminal, can capture a wealth of user health information. In terms of exercise, it can collect user workout data, calculate calories, and provide motivation as needed, helping users better record their exercise information. For body metrics, it can monitor heart rate and blood oxygen levels. Real-time heart rate and blood oxygen monitoring can provide users with more detailed health data records and offer warnings when indicators are abnormal. Additionally, it can record users' sleep data, enabling them to better understand their sleep conditions.

Apart from the Apple Watch, the iPhone is also equipped with an accelerometer, gyroscope, and GPS, which can track physical training, steps, and various types of daily activities.

Furthermore, to obtain more data, the Health app can integrate data from numerous third-party apps, forming a more complete ecosystem.

11.3.1.2 Miao Health

Miao Health is a digital precision health management platform that provides users with a comprehensive, one-stop health service solution. Miao Health collects and aggregates users' health information through smart wearable devices, offering personalized health solutions and health risk assessments. For users with potential health risks, it provides access to third-party services.

In terms of health management, Miao Health is based on professional medical models. It performs disease risk assessments and matches them with insurance underwriting rules to deliver underwriting conclusions and future risk analyses. By strengthening daily health management, it enhances risk control for insured populations, achieving an effective integration of health management and insurance.

For mobile health and fitness, Miao Health offers customized health tools for smart hardware users, providing professional medical health interpretations. It continuously monitors users' health behaviors across multiple dimensions and intelligently pushes relevant information.

11.3.2 Digital Health Family Service Systems

The concept of digital health (eHealth) first appeared in 2000. It refers to a range of medical information systems that, through the application of the Internet and other related technologies in the healthcare industry, improve the efficiency, effectiveness, and quality of medical services delivered to patients. The advent of eHealth has provided new solutions for recording health information, personal involvement in disease diagnosis and treatment, and health management.

The healthcare and Internet industries are gradually exploring the development potential of the digital health field. In recent years, China has seen a growing aging population and has entered an aging society. The common family structure today is the "421 model," which includes 4 elderly people, 2 adults, and 1 child in a household. Adults work outside, while the elderly take care of the children. Both the elderly and the children are susceptible to illnesses. Therefore, real-time monitoring of the health conditions of the elderly and children is very important.

In summary, it is very necessary to establish a digital health family service system that monitors and measures the health of patients with chronic diseases, the elderly, and infants.

11.3.2.1 Geometry Technology Smart Toilet

Geometry Technology is a home health management service platform that utilizes big data technology through the Internet to provide users with services such as home health monitoring, real-time health indicator monitoring, assistance in chronic disease control and treatment, and health management through health data analysis.

The first product from Geometry Technology—the fully automatic intelligent health monitoring toilet—is now on the market. This toilet features a detection device and biochip developed by Geometry Technology at its core, compatible with three major detection technologies, covering a wide range of indicators. Most smart toilets on the market have functions such as buttocks cleaning, seat heating, warm air drying, automatic deodorizing, and silent seating. However, the highlight of this smart toilet is its health monitoring function.

Urine, as one of the most important metabolic products of the human body, can reflect changes in health status from multiple perspectives. In addition to providing alerts, warnings, and early screening for kidney disease, urinary system diseases, diabetes, and the three highs (hypertension, hyperglycemia, hyperlipidemia), continuous urine monitoring can also be applied in various daily life and work scenarios. Since urine contains a wealth of detectable substances and indicators, it helps to obtain in-depth health information about the human body. Additionally, as toilets are now essential household items, Geometry Technology developed this smart toilet as an entry point. This system breaks through traditional urine testing indicators and is compatible with mainstream detection methods—dry chemistry, electrochemistry, and immunoaffinity. Its unique structural design allows the toilet to collect urine from people of different genders and ages.

This health function can be used by more than five family members. Using fingerprints for identification, it automatically recognizes individual users. Each user will have their own daily health data. The toilet is also compatible with various chips and can automatically match and switch users, thus forming an entry point for family health monitoring.

The toilet can obtain continuous health data from individuals through its fully automatic urine detection function. This data is analyzed by a backend artificial intelligence system and medical team, and through an app, it provides users with dynamic health assessments and action suggestions, enabling users to understand their physical condition in a timely manner.

11.3.2.2 AliHealth Family Doctor

AliHealth targets the elderly, launching the "Parental Care Plan" to provide intelligent chronic disease management services for families and parents. The aim is to establish real-time interactive chronic disease management among parents, children, and doctors through smart hardware, Internet, and data technology. This plan helps children better understand their parents' health conditions, avoiding situations where parents hide their illnesses, avoid treatment, or seek inappropriate medical advice. The "Parental Care Plan," leveraging Ali's Internet, technology, and platform advantages, creates the AliHealth service platform. It forms regular health analysis reports based on blood glucose test results, providing scientific advice for blood glucose monitoring and management for the elderly and their families. For instance, if the service platform does not detect the elderly's blood glucose data or if there are anomalies in the uploaded blood glucose data, it will promptly remind the elderly and their children to conduct blood glucose tests through various methods such as app notifications, SMS, and phone calls. If an adjustment to the blood glucose management plan is needed, the corresponding contracted family doctor will provide telephone consultation services based on the prompts. Additionally, the platform will offer comprehensive care and supervision services through smart devices, automatically recording patient data and presenting it in intuitive charts.

11.4 Summary

Although the concept of proactive health has been proposed, there is still a significant gap between its maturity in both basic theoretical aspects and methodological tools compared to current disease medicine. Proactive health is not a simple accumulation of other medical experiences, methods, and technologies but requires the construction of a complete theoretical system distinct from passive medicine.

Proactive health is based on long-term human data to identify and intervene in the overall functional status of individuals, requiring higher precision, lower power consumption, and real-time online intelligent health devices. With the development of Internet technology, the precision and quantity of data obtained by various monitoring devices are increasing. Meanwhile, with the advancement of artificial intelligence technology, AI will be able to replace medical workers in performing a large amount of mechanical and repetitive work. Building a complete and mature proactive health system in the future will require the joint efforts of the medical, Internet, and other industries.

Intelligent Systems for Medical and Elderly Care Combination

12

Contents

12.1 Overview of Integrated Medical and Care Intelligent Systems ... 312
12.1.1 Concept of Integrated Medical and Care ... 312
12.1.2 Concept of Integrated Medical and Care Intelligent Systems ... 313
12.1.3 Current Status of Integrated Medical and Care Intelligent Systems ... 314
12.1.4 Development History of Integrated Medical and Care Intelligent Systems ... 315
12.2 Main Functions and Applications of Integrated Medical and Care Intelligent Systems ... 316
12.2.1 Telemedicine ... 316
12.2.2 Health Risk Assessment and Health Plan Development ... 317
12.2.3 Assisted Chronic Disease Management ... 318
12.2.4 Health Education ... 318
12.2.5 Dietary and Medication Guidance ... 319
12.2.6 Community Care ... 319
12.3 Key Technologies of Integrated Medical and Nursing Care Intelligent Systems ... 320
12.3.1 Comprehensive Assessment and Chronic Disease Risk Assessment for the Elderly ... 320
12.3.2 Aging-Friendly Human–Computer Interaction Technology ... 323
12.4 Case Studies ... 325
12.4.1 Case Study: Zhejiang Elderly Care Hospital ... 325
12.4.2 Elderly Health Intervention and Management Technology ... 326
12.4.2.1 Remote Monitoring ... 326
12.4.2.2 Enhanced Contrast for Clear Information Viewing ... 327
12.4.3 Smart Health and Care System Integrating Medical Treatment and Elderly Care ... 327
12.5 Summary ... 329
References ... 329

J. Li et al., *Healthcare Information Systems*, Innovative Medical Devices,
https://doi.org/10.1007/978-981-97-9551-2_12

Integrated medical and care is the latest concept proposed in the twenty-first century, which represents the newest direction of development in China's elderly care service industry. The integrated medical and care intelligent system can effectively assist in the implementation of integrated medical and care policies and promote the sustainable development of China's elderly care service industry. This chapter is divided into four parts. Firstly, it introduces the concepts and development history of integrated medical and care and integrated medical and care intelligent systems. Secondly, it presents the main unit modules of the integrated medical and care intelligent system, including remote consultation, health education, community care, and other functions. Next, it introduces the key technologies of the integrated medical and care intelligent system, including adaptive human–computer interaction technology, elderly health assessment technology, etc. Finally, it analyzes the Zhejiang Elderly Care Hospital as an example of the integrated medical and care system.

12.1 Overview of Integrated Medical and Care Intelligent Systems

12.1.1 Concept of Integrated Medical and Care

Integrated medical and care refers to the integration of medical resources with elderly care resources, combining professional medical technology examinations and advanced equipment with rehabilitation training, daily learning, daily diet, and professional elderly care. "Medical" refers to services such as early identification of major diseases, necessary examinations, treatments, rehabilitation training, including disease prognosis, evaluation observation, examinations, functional rehabilitation, diagnosis and treatment care, early intervention for major diseases, and end-of-life care. "Care" includes physiological and psychological care, medication and safety, daily dietary care, functional training, daily learning, daily activities, critical life signs analysis, physical condition analysis, regular weight and nutrition monitoring, and other services.

The concept of integrated medical and care is based on the consideration of China's current situation. Currently, there is one elderly person among every six people in the country, and by 2040, it is estimated that there will be one elderly person among every three people. On the one hand, the elderly have a higher prevalence of diseases than the general population, especially a higher proportion of chronic disease patients, leading to a stronger dependence on medical services. On the other hand, many elderly people live alone without care, and the treatment level in community clinics is low. Large hospitals cannot provide detailed life care for the elderly, and minor illnesses and long-term bedridden conditions of the elderly will further strain resources in large hospitals. However, most elderly care institutions only provide simple life care services without much medical services, and there is also a severe shortage of beds in nursing homes. The concept of integrated medical and care has emerged, leading to a new model of elderly care integrating medical and care services.

With the strong promotion of the government, integrated medical and care has become one of the key directions of recent policies. Various integrated medical and care projects have been developed, mainly differentiated by positioning into three types: medical-oriented, care-oriented, and balanced integration of medical and care. Medical-oriented projects mainly establish rehabilitation departments, geriatrics departments, and other affiliated nursing institutions within large hospitals, providing professional care services for dementia, disability, and semi-disabled elderly people. Care-oriented projects mainly provide daily medical treatment and emergency services for elderly people with certain self-care abilities through nursing apartments or community secondary and below hospitals. Balanced integration projects usually combine a continuous care apartment or community with a tertiary specialty hospital featuring elderly diseases and disease rehabilitation. The functions of "medical" and "care" can complement each other, and they also have a good referral mechanism.

12.1.2 Concept of Integrated Medical and Care Intelligent Systems

An intelligent system is a computer system capable of exhibiting human-like intelligent behaviors. Intelligence encompasses a broad range of functions, generally referring to the higher-level activities of the human brain. Such systems can automatically acquire and apply knowledge, think and reason, solve problems, and even learn autonomously.

The integrated medical and care intelligent system applies intelligent systems to medical and elderly care, mainly relying on basic medical methods, using modern information technology as a platform, applying intelligent Internet of Things technology, artificial intelligence technology, and related advanced equipment, utilizing integrated module design concepts, integrating intelligent monitoring, intelligent medical and care rooms, intelligent diagnosis, and intelligent care modules into a whole, thus forming a model system that changes the traditional medical and care work philosophy. The integrated medical and care intelligent system includes multiple modules such as medical and nursing workstations, pharmacy management, physical examination management, medical management, cost management, logistics management, residential management, etc. Through this system platform, the elderly can use smart devices such as wireless health monitoring devices and elderly phones for information interaction with medical and nursing staff, family members, and service centers.

12.1.3 Current Status of Integrated Medical and Care Intelligent Systems

The popularization of modern Internet and smart electronic products has provided crucial media and support for integrated medical and care intelligent systems. Technologies commonly used in the Internet and smart electronic products, such as RFID, sensor, network communication, big data processing, have been applied to various medical products. With the rapid promotion of mobile communication programs, people can also perform medical behaviors such as registration, follow-up visits, prescribing, and doctor–patient communication through mini-programs. The concepts and applications of cloud computing, cloud management, and big data have provided technical support for elderly chronic disease patients to enjoy comfortable home care services. Additionally, new functions are continuously being added to the integrated medical and care intelligent system, driving vigorous development in this field.

Under the active promotion of national and local policies, Mudanjiang City in Heilongjiang Province has successfully developed the "360 Integrated Medical and Care Intelligent System" with integrated medical and care as the theme. The system "mainly includes indoor and emergency two parts, adding sensors in both parts to monitor the elderly's body temperature, weight, and corresponding clinical physiological changes in real-time. Firstly, by predicting the comfort of the crowd, the indoor intelligent hardware devices can be automatically adjusted, and information analysis and transmission can be carried out on the intranet and platform network in different times, places, and environments. Secondly, an intelligent management platform can be deployed, and perception layer information can be analyzed to provide big data retrieval and analysis functions to relevant departments. It can also exchange information and data with franchisees and cooperative medical institutions. Finally, the intelligent information system can provide convenience for the elderly and their families in operating related functions and accessing data."

With the assistance of this system, the elderly and their families can quickly understand relevant medical and care information through the platform and can also select suitable family doctors through recommendation mechanisms and doctor evaluation. Doctors can access their patients' health records in the 360 Integrated Medical and Care Intelligent System, conduct accurate health assessments based on patients' physical data, provide the most suitable medical services for patients, and improve the follow-up work of medical services. For government departments, the 360 Integrated Medical and Care Intelligent System has rich data. With the data analysis function of this platform, government departments can complete data reports of various departments in a short period and conduct comprehensive and detailed analysis of these reports, thereby providing certain data support for government personnel in formulating relevant regulations and policies.

12.1.4 Development History of Integrated Medical and Care Intelligent Systems

The development of integrated medical and care intelligent systems has been driven by the continuous promotion of national integrated medical and care policies. Discussing the development history of these systems requires examining China's integrated medical and care policies.

The inception of integrated medical and care policies began in 2011. In December 2011, the State Council issued the "Social Pension Service System Construction Plan (2011–2015)," proposing that "the construction of the social pension service system should be based on home-based care, community-based support, and institutional support, focusing on the actual needs of the elderly, prioritizing the service needs of difficult elderly people such as lonely, high-aged, living alone, and disabled with low income, and taking into account the requirements of improving and enhancing pension service conditions for all elderly people." Although this policy did not explicitly propose the concept of integrated medical and care, the rehabilitation care needs of the elderly had already attracted national attention, and contemplation on how to better care for the elderly had begun. However, the concept of integrated medical and care had not yet been proposed, so integrated medical and care intelligent systems had not yet emerged.

In September 2013, the State Council issued the "Opinions on Accelerating the Development of the Elderly Care Service Industry," officially listing "actively promoting the integration of medical and healthcare with elderly care services" as one of the six main tasks to accelerate the development of the elderly care service industry. It specifically stated, "Explore new models of cooperation between medical institutions and elderly care institutions. Medical institutions and community health service institutions should establish health records for the elderly, establish contractual service relationships between community hospitals and the elderly for family medical care, and provide services such as home visits, health examinations, and health consultations. Accelerate the pilot of remote medical services for elderly care institutions. Medical institutions should provide priority and preferential services for the elderly seeking medical treatment." This policy marked the beginning of China's integrated medical and care policy and was a milestone in the country's elderly care service industry. However, it only proposed cooperation between medical institutions and elderly care institutions without elucidating the concept of integrated medical and care as a new proprietary term.

In March 2015, the State Council issued the "Outline of the National Medical and Health Service System Plan (2015–2020)," which formally defined the concept of integrated medical and care and elaborated on the importance of cooperation between medical institutions and elderly care institutions in a subsection. In November 2015, the State Council forwarded the "Guiding Opinions on Promoting the Integration of Medical and Health Care with Elderly Care Services" jointly issued by the Ministry of Civil Affairs and eight other departments, requiring comprehensive deployment to further promote the integration of medical and health care with elderly care services. It also specified the five key tasks that need to be completed for this integration. This document clarified many concepts of integrated medical and care and marked another important milestone in the development of integrated medical and care. Since then, the concept of integrated medical and care has been frequently mentioned, but at this time, it was just the emergence of the concept of integrated medical and care, and subsequent development focused on policy improvements and promotion, without involving integrated medical and care intelligent systems.

Since 2016, related policies of integrated medical and care have gradually shifted from macro design to specific implementation approaches. Documents such as the "Work Points of the National Health and Family Planning Commission for 2016," "Key Tasks Division Plan for Integrated Medical and Care," "13th Five-Year Plan for Health and Hygiene," and "Healthy China Action (2019–2030)" have implemented the lofty goal of integrated medical and care into practical action. Integrated medical and care has gradually become well-known, incorporating work such as nutrition, medical association construction, and chronic disease prevention and control into its services. The content of relevant documents has become more accurate, and the procedures have become more detailed. At this time, integrated medical and care intelligent systems aimed at integrated medical and care began to flourish.

Driven by policies over the years, the development goals of integrated medical and care intelligent systems have continuously evolved. With the popularization of modern Internet and smart electronic products in recent years, these systems have added more functions and optimized various aspects, gradually becoming comprehensive information management systems that integrate health records, appointment management, family doctor management, medication management, nursing management, cost management, personnel management, warehouse management, elderly banking, reception management, change records, statistical queries, health management, intelligent calls, and basic management.

12.2 Main Functions and Applications of Integrated Medical and Care Intelligent Systems

12.2.1 Telemedicine

The key to telemedicine lies in two aspects: "remote" and "consultation." "Remote" currently refers to modern communication tools such as network information platforms, which are characterized by their speed and accuracy and can serve as a medium for communication even over long distances. "Consultation" is a working method for hospital doctors, mainly including the analysis of patient medical records, diagnosis of conditions, and then determining a treatment plan based on the diagnosed condition. Telemedicine refers to the use of modern communication tools to enable remote communication between doctors and patients, a method that can break through geographical limitations and is a convenient new way of consulting.

Telemedicine offers numerous advantages. For instance, it can greatly reduce patients' travel time and economic costs in appropriate settings and for home healthcare. It allows for the effective management and allocation of emergency medical services resources in remote areas by transmitting images to key medical centers. It enables doctors to overcome geographical limitations, share patient records and diagnostic images, and thereby promote further clinical research. It also provides better medical education to healthcare personnel in remote areas.

With the help of an integrated medical and healthcare intelligent system, doctors can access a patient's basic information in the database and, using their professional knowledge and guidance from the medical support system, provide remote rehabilitation guidance to patients from two aspects: medical interventions such as surgery and medication and daily care measures including diet and activity.

12.2.2 Health Risk Assessment and Health Plan Development

Health risk assessment is primarily used to describe and evaluate the likelihood of an individual developing a specific disease or dying from it in the future. The purpose of this assessment is to estimate the probability of health-related events occurring within a specific time frame for a patient, and it is not intended to provide a definitive diagnosis. In simple terms, health risk assessment is a quantitative method of evaluating an individual's health status and the risk of future disease or death. It mainly includes assessing health status, future risk of disease or death, and providing a quantitative evaluation.

Health programs are health management service plans developed by the healthcare industry for individuals and social groups to improve the quality of medical visits, prevent and reduce the incidence of diseases, delay the progression of conditions, increase the effectiveness of treatments, control medical costs, and reduce the medical expenses of relevant institutions and individuals. These plans are executable and have a significant impact, featuring both standardization and personalization. By implementing health plans, it is possible to achieve timely intervention in conditions, reduce medical expenses, effectively prevent diseases, enhance health awareness, promote health recovery, and improve the quality of life.

Through health risk assessment and the development of health programs, individuals can gain a comprehensive understanding of health risk factors and be encouraged and assisted to modify unhealthy behaviors. It also allows for the development of personalized health intervention measures and the evaluation of their effectiveness.

In the intelligent medical and elderly care system, the health risk assessment module generally uses computational models such as the Holf model and regression models to assess the current health risks and predict the probability of developing a chronic disease within a certain period in the future. Based on this, doctors can establish stage management goals, measures, and plans for patients to prevent the onset or further development of diseases. This includes dietary guidance plans, exercise guidance plans, medication plans, etc.

12.2.3 Assisted Chronic Disease Management

Chronic diseases are characterized by insidious onset, non-contagiousness, long duration, and complex etiology and can cause significant damage to vital organs such as the brain, kidneys, and heart over time. They can easily affect patients' labor capacity and quality of life, and medical expenses are expensive, which can increase the economic burden on society and families.

Chronic disease management is a medical behavior and process, mainly involving continuous monitoring, regular testing, assessment, and comprehensive intervention management of chronic diseases and their risk factors. Specific processes include evaluation of the effectiveness of chronic disease management, comprehensive management of chronic disease populations, early warning and comprehensive intervention, prediction of chronic disease risks, and early screening for chronic diseases.

For managers of chronic disease management, it involves managing and intervening in various aspects such as diet, mental health, and behavioral habits for chronic disease patients and high-risk groups, as well as promoting correct concepts, skills, and knowledge of chronic disease management. However, in most cases, chronic diseases are caused by improper lifestyles, and patients cannot rely solely on doctors with limited management capabilities; they must also self-manage and develop a sense of "I am responsible for my health." In most cases, doctors primarily provide education and guidance.

With the assistance of the integration of medical and nursing care intelligent system, doctors can search for the basic information of the patient and all recorded examination information in the database, clarify the object of chronic disease management, and further, under the guidance of medical auxiliary systems, utilize their professional knowledge to effectively manage patients with targeted measures, mainly focusing on biomedical monitoring, medication, and supervising patients' compliance with medical instructions, etc.

12.2.4 Health Education

Health education is a planned, organized, and systematic social educational activity aimed at encouraging individuals to adopt behaviors and lifestyles beneficial to health, reducing or eliminating factors affecting health, preventing diseases, promoting physical health, and improving personal quality of life. Health education can help people develop good hygiene habits, prevent abnormal deaths, diseases, and disabilities, enhance people's educational concepts, understand, support, and advocate national health policies, and collectively build a healthy social environment.

The integration of medical and nursing care intelligent system can select populations based on specific labels such as region, age, and occupation and provide corresponding graphic and textual reports. When healthcare personnel conduct health education for specific populations, they can adopt different methods based on the population labels provided by the system.

12.2.5 Dietary and Medication Guidance

Dietary guidance refers to the formulation of dietary guidance recommendations based on the knowledge of nutrition and health sciences, combined with the patient's own situation, which meets the nutritional health status and basic needs of Chinese residents.

Medication guidance involves doctors using their pharmaceutical knowledge to explain to patients the importance of adequate, timely, and course-based drug use for disease treatment. They also explain possible adverse reactions during medication and corresponding coping measures, scientifically guiding patients on the correct and reasonable use of drugs.

With the assistance of the integration of medical and nursing care intelligent system, doctors can find the basic information of patients and all recorded examination information in the database and further standardize the dietary and medication of patients under the guidance of medical auxiliary systems.

12.2.6 Community Care

Community care combines knowledge and skills from public health and nursing, emphasizing both disease prevention and care. It relies on organized social forces, is community-based, and serves individuals, families, and populations to promote and maintain health. The core of community care is to enhance health, focusing on disease prevention, targeting the entire community, including both the sick and healthy populations.

In the field of community care, most elderly people are equipped with a smart terminal device, which can connect various sensors to read the elderly's physical data, such as heart rate, respiration, blood pressure, etc. The relevant data is then transmitted to a remote server via a serial port or wireless connection. Healthcare personnel can remotely view and analyze the data, and family members can also view the elderly's health data and corresponding health analysis reports through mobile apps and other mobile applications.

With the assistance of the integration of medical and nursing care intelligent system and social forces collaborating with hospitals, basic information and examination records of all individuals in the community can be found in the database, further providing services to the population within the community.

12.3 Key Technologies of Integrated Medical and Nursing Care Intelligent Systems

12.3.1 Comprehensive Assessment and Chronic Disease Risk Assessment for the Elderly

The integrated medical and nursing care intelligent system assesses the physical health and predicts risks for the elderly population through comprehensive assessment and chronic disease risk assessment technologies.

Comprehensive geriatric assessment (CGA) is a multidimensional, interdisciplinary diagnostic process used to determine the clinical condition, pathological risks, residual skills, short-term and long-term prognosis, and personalized treatment and care plans for elderly individuals with functional impairment and frailty. The effectiveness of CGA depends on the executing unit of CGA and the individual physical condition of elderly and frail patients. Over the decades, CGA and nursing quality have been significant challenges. From the perspective of improving nursing quality and reducing hospitalization events, most elderly subjects can benefit from CGA.

Comprehensive geriatric assessment is one of the cornerstones of modern geriatric care. It was first used in the late 1930s in the UK to conduct comprehensive assessments of elderly individuals who were vulnerable medically, socially, functionally, or psychologically. In 1988, CGA was defined as a multidisciplinary diagnostic process that identifies, describes, and interprets various problems in elderly individuals and develops a coordinated care plan. Furthermore, it involves the examination and assessment of elderly individuals' problems by community health workers and the diagnostic evaluation and management of these problems by an experienced multidisciplinary team trained in geriatric medicine. Research is exploring the clinical utility of CGA programs in emergency departments, geriatric orthopedics departments, and patients with cancer and cognitive impairments [1]. Long-term care (LTC) refers to a variety of services that help meet the medical and non-medical needs of patients with chronic diseases or disabilities.

CGA is sometimes referred to as geriatric assessment and management. Although specific criteria for assessment in comprehensive geriatric assessment programs have not yet been agreed upon, the main components of CGA include functional status, activity capacity, gait speed, cognitive ability, emotional status, economic status, nutritional status, comorbidities and polypharmacy, scales for geriatric syndromes (delirium, urinary incontinence, visual or hearing impairment), scales for specific diseases (gait dysfunction, Parkinson's disease, and Alzheimer's disease), nursing goals, and advanced care plans. CGA uses geriatric assessment tools and tests to compile a list of health problems and then develops personalized geriatric intervention plans based on it. Most CGAs use an interdisciplinary team approach to assess patients, interpret results, and gather expertise to achieve common goals. Typically, CGA relies on a core team, including a physician (usually a geriatrician), a nurse, and a social worker. An extended team composed of physical and occupational therapists, nutritionists, pharmacists, psychiatrists, psychologists, dentists, audiologists, podiatrists, and ophthalmologists may also participate in the baseline assessment or serve as consultants.

The US government introduced the resident assessment instrument (RAI) for comprehensive geriatric assessment, requiring regular admission treatment after entering nursing homes. interRAI is a non-profit collaboration network of researchers and clinicians from more than 30 countries dedicated to improving care for disabled or complex patients by developing, evaluating, and implementing comprehensive assessment tools. Each interRAI tool is developed for specific populations, and the interRAI network forms a comprehensive health information system, sharing a common language to ensure consistency in clinical concepts across various tools. Each interRAI tool consists of projects, outcome measures, assessment protocols, case mix algorithms, and quality indicators. These tools undergo rigorous testing to determine their reliability and effectiveness. interRAI tools can detect residents' needs and potential risks, providing information for personalized care plans and monitoring.

Additionally, many tools exist for comprehensive assessment of the elderly, such as the Older Multidimensional Functional Assessment Questionnaire (OMFAQ) and the EASY-Care Standard. OMFAQ, an early comprehensive assessment questionnaire, is commonly used in China to investigate the health issues of elderly individuals in the community and to analyze influencing factors. However, OMFAQ requires a lot of questions and consumes a longer time, a challenge that is addressed by the EASY-Care Standard. Comprehensive assessment tools for specific elderly populations include the Geriatric Assessment in Hematology (GAH) for evaluating elderly patients with certain hematologic malignancies and the Long Term Care Comprehensive Geriatric Assessment (LTCCGA) for assessing elderly individuals in need of long-term care, helping healthcare professionals identify their care needs and make care decisions. Moreover, there are other tools such as the Abbreviated Comprehensive Geriatric Assessment (aCGA), the Vulnerable Elders Survey 13 (VES13), the Geriatric 8 (G8), and the Korean Cancer Study Group Geriatric Score 7 (KG7).

Addressing the lack of geriatrics and evidence-based medicine experts, the United States has developed rapid screening tools based on genetic algorithms to enhance the ability of nursing home physicians to identify and treat geriatric syndromes. Japan has developed the Kihon Index to address this issue, France has developed the Gerontopole screening tool, and the United States has also developed rapid geriatric assessment (RGA) as part of health insurance health checks. Currently, RGA has been successfully applied to over 1500 elderly individuals, demonstrating that simple exercise programs and nutritional interventions can improve muscle wasting and cognitive decline.

A recent study explored the ability of nursing home residents to perform self-comprehensive geriatric assessments using two different mobile devices: a 6-inch tablet and a 3.7-inch smartphone [2]. Both devices were optimized, with 92.9% of participants able to complete the assessment using the 6-inch tablet and 20% able to use the 3.7-inch mobile smartphone. This exploratory study suggests that nursing home residents can use mobile devices for self-assessment of their health status.

Chronic non-communicable diseases, commonly known as chronic diseases, involve multiple systems such as the cardiovascular system, endocrine system, digestive system, respiratory system, etc. The most typical examples include atherosclerosis, diabetes, hypertension, intervertebral disc herniation, osteoporosis, etc., characterized by insidious onset and long course. Chronic disease risk assessment technology first collects a set of health risk factors (including biomedical indicators, psychological health indicators, and social life indicators) and then constructs a chronic disease risk assessment model based on these indicators, which is used to study the quantitative dependence and regularity between chronic disease risk factors and incidence and mortality rates. The following sections will discuss the technologies, methods, and content of chronic disease risk assessment from three aspects: risk factor screening, risk assessment model construction, and model quality assessment.

1. Chronic Disease Risk Factor Screening: The assessment of chronic disease risk factors first requires the selection of risk factors. Since the occurrence and development of chronic diseases are closely related to biological inheritance, lifestyle habits, social psychology, and other factors, the selection of risk factors should be comprehensively considered. Most of the risk factors for chronic diseases are obtained based on cohort studies because cohort studies can incorporate disease onset time factors into chronic disease risk factor research.
2. Construction of Risk Assessment Models: Chronic disease risk assessment models are generally divided into two categories: statistical model-based risk assessment and artificial intelligence-based risk assessment. In risk assessment based on statistical models, the most common analysis methods for the impact of risk factors on disease occurrence are multivariate linear regression and multivariate logistic regression. After determining potential risk factors and disease status, the regression coefficients in the statistical model reflect the strength of the association between risk factors and disease status, and the strength of the impact of current risk factor status on individual chronic disease risk is also determined with the determination of regression coefficients. For example, evaluation models for individual cardiovascular disease risk, such as the "Framingham Risk Score" [3], and breast cancer risk assessment models, such as the "Breast Cancer Risk Assessment Tool (Gail model)" [4]. Risk assessment based on artificial intelligence methods generally uses artificial intelligence methods such as neural networks or support vector machines, constructs models based on prior knowledge, and substitutes risk factor variables into predictive models to predict the impact of current risk factor status on individual health.
3. Quality Assessment of Risk Assessment Models: Common quality assessment methods include scale assessment, global model fitness assessment, and ROC curves.

Future chronic disease risk assessment should follow the principles of evidence-based medicine, fully utilize the advantages of public health big data, focus on the joint effects of multiple risk factors, and also consider the ethical issues involved in predicting the risk of chronic disease incidence.

12.3.2 Aging-Friendly Human–Computer Interaction Technology

When faced with new technological products and services, elderly individuals often encounter numerous difficulties in their usage due to personal characteristics and inadequate consideration of aging-related design during product development. With the development of the smart aging industry, more and more companies are conducting user research targeting elderly users, and various smart health and aging products centered around elderly users are being developed and promoted. Aging-friendly human–computer interaction (HCI) technology is widely applied in smart health and aging products. This technology starts from the perspective of elderly users, fully considering their physiological and psychological characteristics, and systematically explores innovative research ideas and design methods for aging-friendly human–computer interaction to meet the diverse and complex usage scenarios of elderly users.

Human–computer interaction refers to the interaction between users and product service systems, including image interaction, natural interaction (voice interaction and touch gestures), and adaptive interaction based on affective computing and context-awareness technologies, all of which are applied in smart health and aging products. This requires accurate acquisition of user needs through extensive experiments and research on the behavior habits of elderly users, which can be explored from the following aspects:

1. Aging-Friendly Image Interaction:
   Image interaction is an important part of aging-friendly design. Images can clearly express content, nature, direction, principles, and images, mainly composed of text, graphics, symbols, signs, forms, etc. The design of images in aging products should be concise, easy to recognize, and should attract the attention of elderly users to key information, taking into account characteristics such as visual decline and weak visual perception among the elderly population.
2. Enhanced Contrast for Clear Information Viewing:
   In aging-friendly design, attention should be paid to whether the contrast between information and background in the interface is sufficient for elderly people to clearly identify, which involves adjustments to color gamut. For example, in color selection, it is necessary to ensure that the color gamut span between information and its background in the interface is at least 5 to make it clear for elderly people to see the information.
3. Conveying Consensus for Understanding Content:
   After ensuring that elderly people can see the information in the interface clearly, the design also needs to have clearer semantic information for them to understand. The key lies in whether these pieces of information can "convey consensus." To achieve "conveying consensus" in design, it is necessary to

express it mainly in pure text or graphics and text, avoiding the sole appearance of graphic symbols. In addition to adding text to icons, adjustments can also be made to the design of icons themselves, incorporating factors such as era and group environment, making the graphic representation in line with the commonly used and inherent content in the elderly generation and daily life, allowing elderly people to easily understand the meaning conveyed by the graphics.

4. Cognitive Association for Finding Clickable Areas:

   In aging-friendly interfaces, more cognitive anchors that can be associated with life experiences need to be introduced to help elderly people find clickable areas on the interface smoothly. For example, areas that can be clicked in the interface can be emphasized by projection or highlights to help elderly people associate them with their cognitive understanding of physical buttons in life. Additionally, weaken content that may interfere with cognitive clicking to ensure that the visual focus remains on clickable areas.

5. Behavioral Guidance for Completing Clicks:

   In aging-friendly design, subconscious cues can also be used as invisible guides in the interface to help elderly people complete target behaviors smoothly. For example, behavior actions and results can be included in the text of buttons, and behavioral buttons can be added to some non-specific clickable areas, leveraging the subconscious's invisible guiding role to help elderly people complete target behaviors smoothly.

6. Aging-Friendly Voice Interaction:

   "Speaking" and "listening" are one of the most natural ways of communication in the human–computer interaction process, with intelligent voice technology as its embodiment, which has been widely applied on various intelligent terminals. Daily human–computer interactions can be simply divided into two processes: one is issuing commands to the system, and the other is the system feedback to us. From the perspective of "issuing commands to the system," voice commands involve "saying" the tasks that we want the system to complete and then having the computer system understand and execute them. For elderly people, compared to learning to operate complex interaction logic on small screens with intelligent terminal apps, voice commands allow them to more directly and simply "express their needs" to easily obtain corresponding services. From the perspective of "system feedback to us," voice technology can also provide elderly people with a more natural way of receiving information. By using speech synthesis technology, information that needs to be read on smart terminals can be output to the elderly population with declining vision through voice broadcasting, allowing them to "listen" instead of "see." "Voiceprint recognition" is a technology that recognizes the identity of speakers through speech. Voiceprint recognition works on the principle that differences in vocal organs and structures cause significant differences in the voiceprint diagrams of any two people. Indonesia is the first country to apply voiceprint recognition on a large scale in a national social security institution, allowing retired elderly people to remotely complete identity authentication and survival verification through their voices when receiving pensions without leaving their homes.

7. Multidimensional Synchronous Interaction:

   Elderly users often have difficulty in timely and correctly recognizing and providing feedback during image interactions due to problems such as visual decline and reduced reaction speed. Against this background, natural interaction has been widely used in smart health and aging products, such as real-time collection of physiological data generated by elderly users during interactions through wearable physiological measurement devices. However, physiological signals are easily affected by external environmental factors. Therefore, when designing human–computer interaction methods for smart health and aging products targeting elderly users, single-dimensional interaction methods are often not objective and accurate enough. Multidimensional synchronous interaction refers to the simultaneous recording of multiple parameter data during the same period based on the analysis of the usability of smart health and aging products, using techniques such as electroencephalography (EEG) measurement, measurements of electrocardiogram (ECG), galvanic skin response (GSR), and eye movements, combined with analysis of elderly people's action events and facial expression behaviors. Relevant calculation parameters are designed according to different interaction goals to verify multiple dimensions of data synergistically. This method can explore the implicit needs of elderly users, thus obtaining more objective and accurate conclusions.

12.4 Case Studies

12.4.1 Case Study: Zhejiang Elderly Care Hospital

Zhejiang Elderly Care Hospital (located in Gongshu District, Hangzhou, affiliated with the Traditional Chinese Medicine Hospital and Gongchenqiao Community Health Service Center) was established in 1995. It was the first Grade B tertiary (3B) Chinese medicine geriatric hospital in Zhejiang Province integrating medical treatment, traditional Chinese medicine rehabilitation, and nursing. The hospital adopts the concept of "medical care for the elderly" and has overcome the traditional separation between medical treatment and elderly care. It integrates medical treatment, nursing, rehabilitation, basic elderly care facilities, living assistance services, and accessible activities to provide various specialized medical services for the elderly. The hospital is equipped with professional disease rehabilitation trainers and psychological counselors. It provides 24-hour care for elderly patients with conditions such as stroke, Alzheimer's disease, advanced-stage cancer, bedridden elderly, and those who have lost the ability to live independently. Leveraging the advantages of traditional Chinese medicine, the hospital conducts projects such as Chinese herbal medicine, acupuncture, and physical rehabilitation training, forming a distinctive feature in Chinese medicine rehabilitation.

Within its service range, the hospital has established a "self-testing + home diagnosis + intelligent diagnosis and treatment" integrated smart medical room. Equipped with health integration machines, rehabilitation training, and other medical equipment, elderly individuals can independently complete over 20 tests including height, weight, blood pressure, electrocardiogram, fat content, and blood oxygen level using the health integration machines. After completing the examination, they can access their electronic health records anytime through a smartphone. Additionally, healthcare providers can integrate cloud platforms with big data to monitor dynamic changes in various test data of elderly individuals. By using cloud-based medical models for index analysis and result evaluation, potential health risks can be identified in a timely manner. For elderly individuals with mobility limitations, the smart medical room is equipped with portable smart examination boxes, allowing healthcare providers to conduct testing and medical services directly at their homes.

12.4.2 Elderly Health Intervention and Management Technology

With the development of emerging information technologies such as telemedicine, the Internet of Things (IoT), and cloud computing, traditional health management has become more closely integrated with modern technology, emphasizing the broad implications of "intelligence." The development of elderly health intervention and management will help address the significant health demands brought about by China's accelerated aging population under the reality of insufficient medical resources, improve the high economic burden of medical care services, and promote autonomous elderly care, contributing to achieving healthy aging and aging in place. With the popularization of smart products, the acceptance of smart products by the elderly has gradually increased, providing more possibilities for the extensive application of health intervention and management technology in the field of elderly health services.

Smart health management is mainly applied in the field of elderly health management for remote monitoring, health information interconnection, chronic disease management, psychological assessment, lifestyle improvement, and health education. Chronic disease management, psychological assessment, lifestyle improvement, and health education have been described in detail in Sects. 12.2 and 12.3. The following will focus on the application of smart health management in remote monitoring and health information interconnection.

12.4.2.1 Remote Monitoring

In recent years, the development of wearable devices has fully utilized the characteristics of wireless sensors to collect real-time, continuous, and complete health information. These devices including smart bracelets, rings, necklaces, earrings, belt buckles, smart vests, T-shirts, shoes, etc. are used to monitor parameters such as blood pressure, heart rate, pulse, body temperature, blood oxygen saturation, skin conductivity, and gait. In addition to ordinary physiological and environmental monitoring, some monitoring devices can also identify food types, estimate food intake and nutrition, record daily and weekly activities, including exercise and sedentary time, accurately locate geographical positions, and monitor and alert for falls, which are especially suitable for elderly individuals with Alzheimer's disease and risk of falls. These monitoring devices can transmit monitoring data to remote servers or software clients through Bluetooth, Wi-Fi, Zigbee, and GPRS wireless transmission networks, enabling healthcare providers to provide feedback and suggestions to users in a timely manner.

12.4.2.2 Enhanced Contrast for Clear Information Viewing

Personal health records (PHRs) are considered crucial tools for improving individual health behaviors and outcomes, facilitating users to dynamically understand their health status. Users can transmit, manage, and maintain their own and their family's health records through websites, software, mobile applications, or monitoring devices and can decide whether to open the record information to third parties. In addition to the elderly themselves, caregivers can fully utilize network platforms to authorize healthcare providers they trust to jointly manage the health of the elderly.

12.4.3 Smart Health and Care System Integrating Medical Treatment and Elderly Care

With the support and guidance of national policies, many companies have developed their own integration of medical and elderly care with smart health systems. These systems have been put into operation in collaboration with multiple hospitals and elderly care institutions, effectively alleviating the pressure on medical work in our country to a certain extent. The integration of medical and elderly care with smart health systems connects elderly friendly smart terminals and intelligent health detection devices to create a management system that integrates medical treatment, rehabilitation, care, and nursing. It helps elderly care institutions transition from simple living care to actively providing integrated health and elderly care services such as hospitalization treatment, rehabilitation care, stable period living care, and end-of-life care, addressing the health and elderly care needs of the elderly. Through cloud platforms, institution mobile apps, WeChat public accounts, etc., data interoperability is achieved, operations are streamlined, duplicate data recording is avoided, and the efficiency of institutional staff is improved. At the same time, real-time statistics on institutional operations are collected, linked to civil affairs systems, and widely applied in institutions such as medical and elderly care integration, elderly care institutions, nursing homes, care centers, and home-based care.

The integration of medical and elderly care with smart health systems consists of smart health interconnection products as the "front end" of service and a smart elderly digital platform as the "back end," forming an intelligent product service system. Through the integration of medical and elderly care with smart health systems, health records are established, and effective connections are made between hospitals, elderly care service institutions, and care teams. By precisely analyzing rehabilitation service needs, services such as medical rehabilitation for disabled and demented elderly individuals, early non-pharmacological interventions for Alzheimer's disease, home visits, and family support are provided.

Smart health interconnection products are designed with elderly users as the central elements of product composition. They use various sensors, processors, and software to achieve interoperability between users and their environments. Meanwhile, by installing various types of smart interconnection products in the homes of elderly users, continuous 24-hour uninterrupted services are provided, such as smart home products, wearable health management devices, portable health monitoring devices, self-service health monitoring devices, smart elderly care monitoring devices, and specially equipped elderly care service robots, offering nursing, companionship, rehabilitation, and other services.

The smart elderly digital platform, based on artificial intelligence, knowledge graphs, and other technologies, provides services for elderly users and related users based on their needs for living care, chronic disease management, home health care, etc. Its functions cover health record management, vital signs monitoring and early warning, care guidance and assistance implementation, indoor environment regulation and control, indoor accident warning and intervention, etc.

The health record management function provides intelligent health record storage, retrieval, and other services, providing a basis for elderly care service institutions to understand the physical health status of elderly care service recipients and formulate care plans. The vital signs monitoring and early warning function monitors the vital sign data of elderly care service recipients in real time through wearable devices and promptly alerts doctors to take emergency measures in case of abnormal situations. The care guidance and assistance implementation function formulate targeted care plans and remind and guide elderly care service recipients to engage in care activities and routines through wearable devices such as text displays and vibrations. The indoor environment regulation and control function adjusts the environmental temperature, humidity, etc., based on the health record information and vital sign data of service recipients, through the linkage with smart home interconnection products. The indoor accident warning and intervention function monitors and controls facilities and equipment with potential safety hazards, issues alerts in case of abnormal operation, and reminds elderly care service recipients to handle them in a timely manner through the Internet of Things.

The integration of medical and elderly care with smart health systems enhances the level of service management through informationization and other means, effectively improves the efficiency of care staff, provides personalized guidance for the elderly population, reduces institutional operating costs, enhances patient stickiness, promotes the interconnection between government supervision, institutions, home-based, and community-based elderly care services, realizes intelligent and diversified development, empowers the elderly care industry, achieves the goal of disease prevention and control, reduces the burden on society and families, enhances the self-care ability of the elderly, effectively reduces national medical insurance expenditures, and improves the utilization rate of limited elderly care resources.

12.5 Summary

The integrated medical and elderly care intelligent system applies smart systems to the fields of healthcare and elderly care. It primarily relies on basic medical methods and uses modern information technology as a platform, leveraging intelligent IoT technology, artificial intelligence, and advanced equipment. It also incorporates an integrated module design concept to structure modules such as intelligent monitoring, intelligent medical and elderly care rooms, intelligent consultations, and intelligent nursing. This creates a model that transforms traditional concepts of healthcare and elderly care model.

The integrated medical and elderly care intelligent system is a platform that integrates various modules to address the practical issues in implementing the policies of combining medical and elderly care. From the current national policies on integrated medical and elderly care, it is evident that there are still many challenges. These include the low level of community healthcare services, a shortage of personnel with high professional technical skills, unfamiliarity of some nursing staff with the procedures required for their services, an unreasonable allocation of medical resources, and a simplistic approach to care among some nursing staff. These are urgent issues that need to be resolved during the implementation of the integrated medical and elderly care policies and are also the direction for the optimization of the integrated medical and elderly care intelligent system. In addition, innovations in medical informatics technology will also bring about significant changes to the integrated medical and elderly care intelligent system, allowing it to play a greater role and further promote the development of the elderly care industry.

References

1. Ngandu T, Lehtisalo J, Solomon A, et al. A 2 year multidomain intervention of diet, exercise, cognitive training, and vascular risk monitoring versus control to prevent cognitive decline in at risk elderly people (FINGER): a randomised controlled trial. Lancet. 2015;385(9984):22552263.
2. Panza F, Solfrizzi V, Lozupone M, et al. An old challenge with new promises: a systematic review on comprehensive geriatric assessment in long term care facilities. Rejuvenation Res. 2018;21(1):314.
3. Reddy R, Mahendra J, Gurumurthy P, et al. Identification of predictable biomarkers in conjunction to Framingham risk score to predict the risk for cardiovascular disease (CVD) in non cardiac subjects. J Clin Diagn Res. 2015;9(2):2327.
4. Vargas AC, Silva LD, Lakhani SR. The contribution of breast cancer pathology to statistical models to predict mutation risk in BRCA carriers. Fam Cancer. 2010;9(4):545553.

GPSR Compliance

The European Union's (EU) General Product Safety Regulation (GPSR) is a set of rules that requires consumer products to be safe and our obligations to ensure this.

If you have any concerns about our products, you can contact us on ProductSafety@springernature.com

In case Publisher is established outside the EU, the EU authorized representative is:

Springer Nature Customer Service Center GmbH
Europaplatz 3
69115 Heidelberg, Germany

Batch number: 10732044

Printed by Printforce, the Netherlands